Antimicrobial Resistance

NIPA® GENX ELECTRONIC RESOURCES & SOLUTIONS P. LTD.
New Delhi-110 034

About the Editors

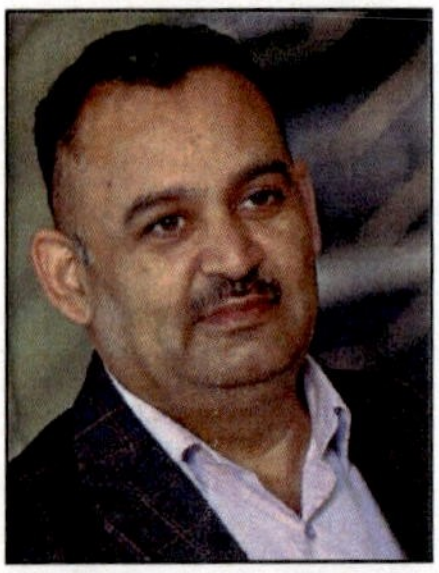

Prof (Dr) Amit Kumar, Professor & Head, Division of Animal Biotechnology, College of Biotechnology at Sardar Vallabhbhai Patel University of Agriculture & Technology Meerut, India is a Veterinary Microbiologist working in the field of Antimicrobial Resistance (AMR) and vaccinology for more than 20 years. His major contributions include the reporting of various MRSA, VRSA and ESBL producing bacterial pathogens of different bacterial species of animals and human origin. It includes the molecular detection of auto inducer genes in AMR super bugs like Staphylococcus, Klebsiella, *E. coli* and Pseudomonas, which can be targeted for the inhibition of expression of autoinducer genes to avoid resistance transmission. These led to publication of the first report of multi drug resistant (MDR) bacterial species with phylogenic linkage to similar microbes reported in other countries. His current focus is on the development of alternate therapy by exploiting quorum sensing mechanism of drug resistant bacteria to mitigate anti microbial resistance. He has delivered more than 25 invited lectures on AMR on various forum including national and international workshop, seminar, symposium. He has in his credit more than 100 research papers, 50 book chapters and compiled 10 books as an editor.

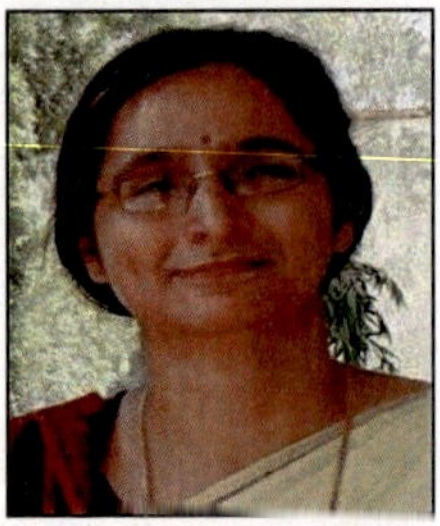

Dr Anu Rahal, Principal Scientist, Division of Animal Health, ICAR-CIRG, Mathura is a veterinary pharmacologist with specialization in pharmacokinetics. She has an experience of almost 25 years and in recent past engaged in field of green pharmaceuticals and drug development based on indigenous knowledge based system through advanced validation methods. She is engaged in the selection of phytoconstitutents, their molecular mechanisms involved in host microbial interaction, its survival and reproduction. The recently developed anti brucellosis polyherbal formulation might be a major break though in this field and formulation is in the process of commercialization. Similarly, development of poly herbal formulation for the prevention and cure of bovine anaplasmosis is another significant contribution. She has nearly 65 reviews, research papers, short communications published in various journals of international and national reputes. She has edited 5 books and contributed 23 book chapters.

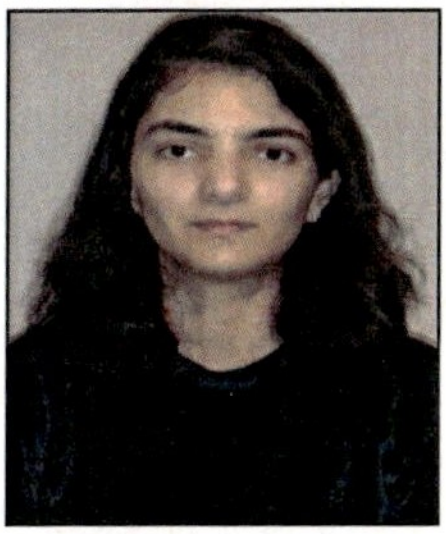

Dr Yanshi a veterinary graduate with specialization in public health is currently working as a Scientist in the Public Health Government Agency of the United Kingdom on epidemiology of various zoonotic pathogens. She graduated with a Bachelor of Veterinary Science and Animal Husbandry from Govind Ballabh Pant University of Agriculture and Technology, Pantnagar, post graduated in Public Health from School of Medicine, University of Nottingham, UK. She has also worked at Royal Veterinary College, London in the One Health Poultry Hub. In her career, she has participated in 14 training courses, 13 workshops, 10 conferences, 5 symposiums and seminars with remarkable publications in different languages. Her main focus is on the epidemiological studies involving zoonotic pathogens particularly multi drug resistant bacteria involved in human diseases.

Antimicrobial Resistance
Scenario, Impact and Future Perspectives

Amit Kumar
Professor & Head
Division of Animal Biotechnology
College of Biotechnology
Sardar Vallabhbhai Patel University of Agriculture & Technology
Meerut, Uttar Pradesh, India

Anu Rahal
Principal Scientist
Division of Animal Health
ICAR-CIRG
Mathura, Uttar Padesh, India

Yanshi
Scientist
Public Health Government Agency
United Kingdom

NIPA® GENX ELECTRONIC RESOURCES & SOLUTIONS P. LTD.
New Delhi-110 034

NIPA® GENX ELECTRONIC RESOURCES & SOLUTIONS P. LTD.

101,103, Vikas Surya Plaza, CU Block
L.S.C.Market, Pitam Pura, New Delhi-110 034
Ph : +91 11 4386 0225, 9717133558, 9540816132
E-mail: newindiapublishingagency@gmail.com
Website: www. niparesources.com

Print ISBN: 978-93-5887-804-2

ebook ISBN: 978-93-58873-87-0

NIPA® also publishes books in a variety of electronic formats. Some content that appears in print may not be available in electronic books, and vice versa

Composed and Designed by NIPA®.

Preface

The role of antibiotics is increasingly being challenged by the emergence of resistant bacteria. The majority of available antibiotics including third generation antibiotics are appearing ineffective in the treatment of bacterial infections. The condition is graver for the treatment of patients suffering from chronic infections and asking for support of intensive care units. This is because of bacteria resistance to commonly used antimicrobials. Bacterial resistance is not new for the scientific community. The studies conducted in recent past had clearly indicated the presence of resistance genes in the bacterial population never exposed to antimicrobial. The bacteria came earlier than the concept of antibacterials and for their survival smartly developed strategies to overcome the exposure of any adverse conditions including presence of antimicrobial in their environment. The addition of newer antimicrobial or antibiotics exposed this microbial population and very smartly, they adapt it either by adopting phenotypic measures like production of biofilms that inhibit the penetration of any undesired molecules particularly large size molecules as happened with vancomycin. Further, expression or acquisition of certain genes responsible to alteration in any enzymic pathway leading to alteration or inhibition of entry through influx pump, enhancing expulsion through efflux pump, alteration of target sites of antimicrobial drugs are some examples of genetic resistance as happens against penicillin and quinolones group of antibiotics. More smartly, these microbes have mechanism to transfer and acquire such genes to nearby bacterial population through quorum sensing. Thus, to deal with such a smart and versatile enemy, it is imperative to perform continuous monitoring, exploration of mechanisms of resistance development and transfer with detection of new and more effective target sites in these pathogens with lesser chances of resistance development.

The current scenario of AMR is very alarming and almost none of the available antibiotic is completely safe. The recent report of colistin resistance in newly born kids in Nigeria is showing the picture of upcoming challenges to humanity. It is the reason that AMR is expected to cause about 50 million deaths per year by 2050 and it is expected to push about 28 million people, mostly residing in developing countries, into poverty by 2050. Recognizing the impact of AMR on society, World Health Organisation (WHO) came up with a global action involving multi-sectoral action needed to combat AMR in 2015. It was accepted by Food and Agriculture Organisation (FAO) in 2016 leading to United Nations

General Assembly (UNGA) passing a resolution for the countries across the world to commit to address AMR in a concerted way. In recent G-20 summit held in New Delhi in 2023, Leaders' Declaration committed to address AMR as part of One Health.

Considering all these factors a project was proposed to address all these issues related to emergence of AMR and Multi drug resistant bacteria with compilation of information to understand AMR development, acquisition and transfer mechanism. It included amalgam of experienced as well as budding experts to get the update of recent development with new approaches possibly applicable in addressing AMR. The compilation of their expertise manuscript have evolved in the shape of a book entitled "Antimicrobial Resistance: Scenario, Impact and Future Perspectives". It will be available to all the stakeholders related to AMR with new insights of AMR mechanism and approaches to overcome it. In recent past while working on AMR, these microbes always surprised us. The chapters involving those surprises will spark curiosity among readers and will also motivate readers to explore further to have better prevention as well as containment of AMR for safe and secured future of humanity through availability of safe food with better and effective therapeutics.

Editors

Contents

1

Antimicrobial Resistance A Global Challenge: Need for One Health Approach

Vamshi Krishna Sriram[1], J Shiva Jyothi[2] and Ambily R[3]

[1 & 2]College of Veterinary Science, Warangal, P.V.Narsimha Rao Telangana Veterinary University, Hyderabad, Telangana, India
[3]College of Veterinary and Animal Sciences, Mannuthy, Thrissur, Kerala Veterinary and Animal Sciences University, Kerala, India

Abstract

Antimicrobial resistance (AMR) stands as a critical global health challenge, threatening the efficacy of currently available antimicrobial agents thus compromising the health care in human and veterinary perspective and complicating the treatment of infectious diseases. The rapid emergence and spread of multidrug resistant pathogens necessitate a multifaceted approach that transcends disciplinary boundaries. This chapter examines origin and spread of AMR, drivers of AMR, explores its global implications in human and veterinary medicine, and emphasizes the indispensable role of the One Health approach in addressing this global concern. By integrating perspectives from human health, animal health, and environmental science, One Health strategies offer comprehensive solutions to combat antimicrobial resistance effectively in the near future thus safeguarding the currently available antimicrobials.

Introduction to Antibiotic Discovery

Antibiotics are the drugs that are used to treat illnesses caused by bacteria in humans and animals. These act by killing or inhibiting the growth and multiplication of bacteria. Antibiotics were considered as "magic bullets" that selectively kills microbes responsible for disease causation, but at the same time would not affect the host (Zaman *et al.*, 2017).

Louis Pasteur in 1877, first discovered the properties of antibacterial compounds with the inhibition of anthrax by saprophytic bacteria. In 1928, Alexander Fleming observed that the growth of *Staphylococcus aureus* in petri dishes was inhibited by substances produced by the fungus *Penicillium chrysogenum*, which led to the discovery of the first antibiotic, penicillin (Aminov, 2017). Selman Waksman, discovered multiple antibiotics from filamentous actinomycetes living in the soil and defined an antibiotic as "a compound made by a microbe to destroy other microbes". Following the discovery of Penicillin, various antimicrobial compounds such as sulphonamides, aminoglycosides, tetracyclines, lipopeptides, oxazolidinones, glycopeptides, streptogramins, and quinolones were discovered in the "Golden era" of antibiotics during the period from the 1940s to the 1960s and most of the antibiotics still in current use were discovered during that period (Salam *et al.*, 2023). Millions of metric tons of newer classes of antibiotics have been produced in last 60 years since its inception.

Classification of Antibiotics

There are several ways of classifying antibiotics and are presented in the Table 1.

Table 1: Classification of antibiotics

A.	**Mechanism of action**	**Examples**
	Cell wall synthesis inhibitors	Penicillins and Cephalosporins
	Protein synthesis inhibitors	Tetracyclines, Aminoglycosides Macrolides
	DNA and RNA synthesis inhibitors	Quinolones, Ancyamycins
	Inhibitors of various metabolic pathways	Sulphonamides and Trimethoprim
B	**Chemical Nature**	
	Beta-lactams	Penicillins
	Macrolides	Erythromycin Azithromycin
	Tetracyclines	Chlortetracycline Oxytetracycline
	Quinolones	Ciprofloxacin Enrofloxacin
	Aminoglycosides	Gentamicin Streptomycin
	Sulphonamides	Sulphadiazine Sulphadimidine
	Glycopeptides	Vancomycin
	Oxazolidinones	Linezolid

C	Spectrum of action	
	Narrow spectrum	Pencillin G Bacitracin
	Broad spectrum	Third and Fourth Generation Cephalosporins
D	**Mode of action**	
	Bacteriostatic	Tetracyclines Sulphonamides Macrolides
	Bactericidal	Aminoglycosides Penicillins Cephalosporins Quinolones

(*Source*: Ebimieowei Etebu and Ibemologi Arikekpar.,2016; Inbaraj et al., 2019)

Antimicrobial Resistance (AMR)

Antimicrobial resistance was reported to occur when a bacteria which is previously sensitive to a particular antibiotic drug becomes resistant to the inhibitory action of that antibiotic. Since the discovery of antibiotics, there has been a gradual decline in antibiotic discovery with concomitant evolution of drug resistant pathogens. Resistance of bacteria to antibiotics have been recognized almost since the dawn of the antibiotic era (Zaman *et al.*, 2017).

Origin and Spread of Antibiotic Resistance

Bacteria are naturally resistant to certain classes of antibiotics. This resistance was documented even before the beginning of the usage of the antibiotics in fighting the infection. In 1945 itself, Sir Alexander Fleming foresaw the dangers of inappropriate usage of penicillin and the emergence of resistance. The imprudent usage of broad spectrum antibiotics in hospital settings as a solution for nosocomial infections increases resistance (Lowy, 2003). Antibiotics generally eliminates the majority of bacteria in a colony. However, there may exist a different colony of bacteria that are genetically mutated which can lead to resistance (Alanis AJ, 2005). Antibiotics induce selective pressure and the genes responsible for resistance development act in association with selective pressure (Zaman *et al.*, 2017). The resistant bacteria can directly transfer the genetic material to other bacteria by plasmids, which signifies that natural selection is not the only mechanism by which resistance evolves. The antibiotic resistance in bacteria transfer through vertical and horizontal gene transfer mechanisms. Through vertical gene transfer the genetic information, including any mutations will be passed, from one generation to the next within a family. Whereas antibiotic-resistance genes are rapidly disseminated across several bacterial species by Horizontal gene transfer (HGT). Native bacteria in the environment serve as a reservoir for ARGs, which can then be passed on to pathogens through HGT (D'Costa *et al.*, 2006). HGT can occur through transformation, transduction, and conjugation, as well as other mechanisms (Vikelsand *et al.*, 2019). The resistant bacteria subsequently remain untouched gaining more strength against the antibiotics (Zaman *et al.*, 2017). Bacteria may collect multiple resistance traits over a period of time and can become resistant to multiple classes of antibiotics and develop multidrug resistance (MDR) referred to as a super bug (Avorn *et al.*, 2001).

For example, within six years of the production of the aminoglycosides, aminoglycoside-resistant strains of *Staphylococcus aureus* were isolated (Gootz TD, 1990). Resistance to methicillin, the first of the semisynthetic penicillinase-resistant penicillin to target strains of penicillinase-producing *Staphylococcus aureus* was reported soon after its introduction in 1961 (Jevons, 1961). Similarly, resistance to fluoroquinolones, which were introduced to treat Gram-negative bacterial diseases in the 1980s, was emerged by chromosomal mutations in the DNA gyrase and ParC genes of the bacteria (Lowy, 2003). The clinical isolates of vancomycin-resistant *Staphylococcus aureus* (VRSA) were found in 2002, after 44 years of introduction of Vancomycin to the market (Appelbaum P, 2006)

Mechanisms of Antibiotic Resistance

Several bacterial species evolved different strategies to survive in the presence.

Table 2: Strategies of antibiotic resistance

Resistance strategy	**Example**
Altered permeability of the cell wall or cell membrane decreasing the drugs penetration into the microbial cell	Penicillins B-lactams Tetracyclines Aminoglycosides Streptogramins
Activation or expression of efflux pumps	Tetracyclines Macrolides Aminoglycosides Penicillins Fluoroquinolones Sulphonamides
Target alteration	Glycopeptides Tetracyclines Aminoglycosides Macrolides Fluoroquinolones

Resistance strategy	Example
Drug inactivation or enzyme modification	B-lactams Tetracyclines Aminoglycosides Streptogramins

(*Source*: Irfan *et al.*, 2022)

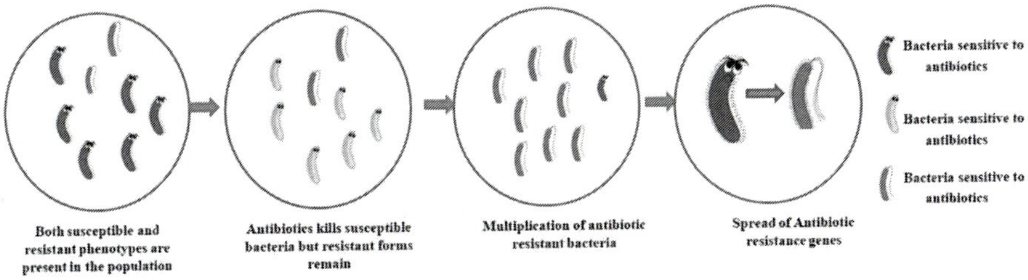

Fig. 1: How antibiotic resistance emerges and spreads among bacterial populations

Drivers of AMR

Antimicrobial resistance is a complicated and multifaceted issue that is influenced by a variety of factors as follows

- The biggest driver of AMR is excessive or unrestricted use of antimicrobials in humans and animals by exerting selective pressure.
- Using sub therapeutic doses or for improper duration of time in animals and human medicine.
- Overuse of broad-spectrum antibiotics which can cause selective pressure on commensal bacteria and expose them to secondary infections.
- Antibiotic overuse in agriculture, farm animals, aquaculture systems as growth promoters and for prophylaxis.
- Taking antibiotics for the incorrect duration or using antibiotics when they are not needed, such as for viral infections, can both contribute to the development of multidrug-resistance (MDR) in an organism.
- Poor hygienic measures and protocols in hospital environments to help.
- Keep the spaces clean, which lead to an increase in AMR in bacteria
- Contamination of water systems during floods with resultant spread of resistant bacteria in sewage.
- International travel and trade, which can result in the spread of resistant bacteria and resistance genes.

- Lack of rapid and accurate diagnostics to aid in the proper use of antibiotics.
- Lack of awareness on the adverse consequences of excessive and unnecessary antibiotic usage and lack of awareness on AMR policies and monitoring systems.

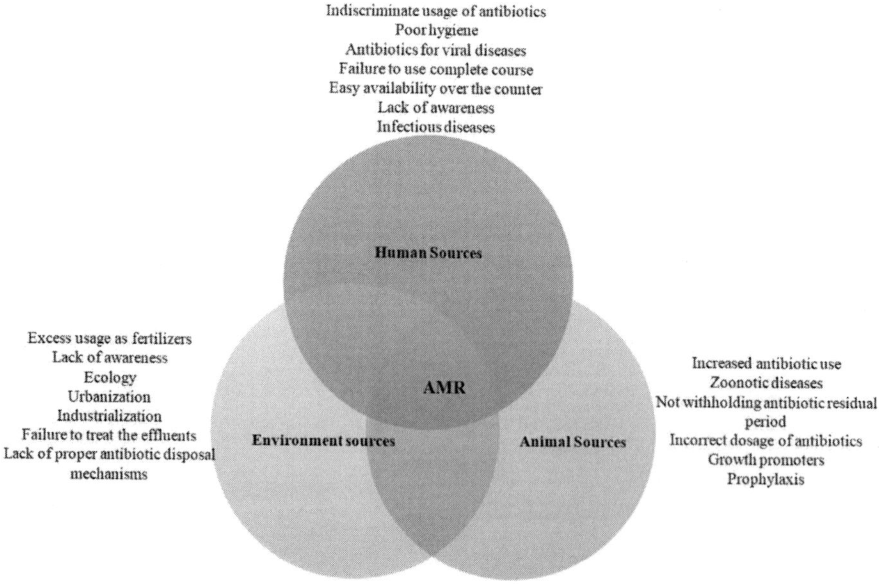

Fig. 2: The drivers of Antimicrobial resistance

Antimicrobial use in Humans, Animals and Plants

- Although antimicrobials were being used since decades, the resistance development differs with antibiotics. Vancomycin, the antibiotic in which the resistance developed slowly were highly valued for their continued ability to treat infections that could not be treated with other commonly used antimicrobials. Today, the increasing vancomycin resistance is a concern such as vancomycin-resistant enterococci (VRE), resulting in high mortality particularly in hospitals (Collignon and McEwen, 2019).
- Antimicrobials are being widely used in farm animals, food animals, pets, aquaculture systems, and bees. Antimicrobials are used for therapeutic, prophylactic, and for growth promotion in animal production. Worldwide, the volume of antimicrobials used in animals is estimated to be much greater than for humans.

- Most classes of antimicrobials used in humans including broad-spectrum beta-lactams and quinolones are often prescribed for animals (Jans *et al.*, 2018). Antimicrobials such as tetracycline, triazoles, and streptomycin which are intended for use in both humans and animals are being used therapeutically in plants. AMR can be easily transferred between and within different ecosystems and populations; resistant zoonotic bacteria can be found in the soil; and from there, they can infect plants, vegetables, and fruits. It has been documented that the use of antimicrobials in agriculture induces antibiotic-resistant fungi transmitted from the environment to humans (FAO, 2018).
- Some classes of antimicrobials such as carbapenems are extensively intended for human use only and others such as flavophospholipol and ionophores for animal use only (FAO, 2016).
- The doses of antimicrobials are often higher in aquaculture than those prescribed for livestock. Residues of antimicrobials thus may remain in fish products and can remain in aquatic environments for a long time through excreta. These residues spread rapidly in water bodies, exerting selective pressure (Velazquez-Meza *et al.*, 2022).

Consequences of Excessive Antimicrobial Use

In recent years global consumption of antibiotics climbed by 65 % from 2.11 billion defined daily doses (DDDs) at 2000 to 34.8 billion defined daily doses (DDDs) at 2015, primarily in low-income countries (Klein *et al.*, 2018). India's antibiotic usage increased from 3.2 billion to 6.5 billion DDD doses.

Antimicrobial resistance is among the critical global public health crises nowadays. The WHO reports that AMR is dangerously high worldwide and morbidity and mortality are increasing (Larsson and Flach, 2022). It is expected to reduce global gross domestic product (GDP) by 1.1–3.8% by 2050. These include a $60–$100 trillion loss in economic productivity, increased treatment costs and inability to achieve universal health coverage and the Sustainable Development Goals (SDGs).

The following are the risks that have been associated with the overuse of antibiotics

1. Increased emergence of antimicrobial resistance among pathogens causing human, animal and plant diseases
2. The overuse of antibiotics can lead to the emergence of more severe diseases.

3. Inappropriate use of antibiotics can lead to prolonged illness increasing the hospital duration days.
4. Overuse of antibiotics can create an opportunity for opportunistic infections or the overgrowth of drug-resistant bacteria, leading to further complications.
5. Antibiotic resistance can increase mortality rates.
6. Overuse of antibiotics contributes to increased healthcare costs adding to the financial burden on healthcare systems and individuals.
7. Inappropriate use of antibiotics increases the likelihood of experiencing adverse effects, some of which can be severe or even life-threatening.
8. Lack of effective antibiotics leads to ineffective treatment of infections, leading to re-attendance for hospitals thus prolonging the illness.
9. Some of the examples of multidrug resistant bacteria include *E.coli, Staphylococcus aureus, Klebsiella pneumoniae, Acinetobacter baumannii, Pseudomonas aeruginosa*, and *Enterobacter*. The term "ESKAPE" is often used as acronym for these six highly drug-resistant bacteria.
10. More recently, carbapenem-resistant Enterobacteriales (CRE), carbapenem resistant *Klebsiella pneumoniae* (CRKP), methicillin-resistant *Staphylococcus aureus* (MRSA), ESBL-producing Enterobacteriales, vancomycin-resistant *Enterococcus* (VRE), multidrug resistant *Pseudomonas aeruginosa*, and multidrug-resistant *Acinetobacter* are among the top most encountered superbugs worldwide.

Methods of Detecting AMR

Method	**Advantages**	**Disadvantages**	**Examples**
Culture based (Kirby-Bauer Disk diffusion / Minimum Inhibitory Concentration testing)	Gold standard Routinely used Inexpensive Relatively precise convenient	Not suitable for non culturable bacteria Errors in Repeatability	Commercial platforms include VITEK® system MicroScan-Walkaway system, The Biolog Microbial Identification
Molecular techniques for detecting Antibiotic Resistance Genes (ARGs) (PCR / qPCR / Epic PCR)	Suitable for even non culturable microbes Relatively rapid Sensitive than culture method	Relatively expensive Require reference laboratories	GeneXpert® AMPLICOR® (ROCH)

Method	Advantages	Disadvantages	Examples
Metagenomics and Whole genome sequencing technologies	Can identify ARGs in diverse ecological samples Highly sensitive	Expensive Require reference laboratories and expertise to analyze the data	Illumina PacBio® HiFi technology
Mass Spectrometry (MALDi-ToD MS)	Rapid, very accurate, and can process larger volumes than regular molecular techniques	Requires an isolated bacterium and access to a specialized database, and the initial setup investment is costly	MALDI Biotyper® (Bruker) and VITEK® MS (bioMérieux).

(*Source*: Irfan *et al.*, 2022)

Strategies to Combat Antimicrobial Resistance

Antimicrobial resistance is a serious concern affecting not humans but also animals, plants, and the environment. Neither only government establishments nor independent organizations in any country can tackle the problem of emerging AMR, without a synchronized effort. An orchestrated coordination and collaboration within and between multiple sectors is the need of the hour to contain and combat AMR across the globe. Healthcare industries including pharmacy, agriculture, finance, trade, education, and nongovernment organizations at national and international levels should work hand by hand to mitigate the grave effects of AMR. Multisectoral collaboration can be both horizontal and vertical. Horizontal collaboration is across sectors and departments within the country, i.e., multi stakeholder forums, and vertical collaboration involves different levels within a country, a region, and internationally.

In April 2014, the World Health Organization (WHO) recognized AMR as a "significant universal challenge." WHO launched the Global Antimicrobial Resistance and Use Surveillance System (GLASS) in 2015 to fill knowledge gaps and inform strategies at all levels. The World Health Assembly, the governing body of all WHO member nations, announced the Global Action Plan on Antimicrobial Resistance (WHO, 2015), encouraging member countries to adopt comparable national action plans by May 2017. The US Food and Drug Administration officially announced measures to evaluate AMR outbreaks (Huang *et al.*, 2019). World AMR Awareness Week (WAAW), an official campaign initiated by WHO since 2015, and celebrated from 18 to 24 November every year to raise awareness, understanding and best practices in the public to prevent AMR. WHO along with the Food and Agriculture Organization of the United Nations (FAO), the UN Environment Programme (UNEP) and the World Organisation for Animal Health (WOAH) formed as

Quadripartite Joint Secretariat on Antimicrobial Resistance as one Health approach to drive multi-stakeholder engagement in AMR. This Quadripartite has supported establishment of the Global Leaders Group on AMR in November 2020.

As of November 2023, 178 countries had developed AMR national action plans aligned with the GAP. To ensure sustained progress, countries need to establish a functioning multisectoral AMR governance mechanism, prioritize activities, develop a costed operational plan, mobilize resources (both domestic and external), and effectively implement their plan. Monitoring mechanisms are needed to track progress, identify challenges and report periodically. To globally track the progress in AMR national action plan implementation, countries have committed to completing the multisectoral annual Tracking AMR Country Self-Assessment Survey (TrACSS) that was launched in 2016 with results published at https://www.amrcountryprogress.org/.

One Health Approach to Combat AMR

One health is an approach for the improvement of public health through the promotion and collaboration of multidisciplinary areas as it takes in the contributions from different scientific discipline. The World Health Organisation (WHO) highlighted the one health approach as a guide for the global action plan and framework on AMR as it is one among the top three major public health threats and has been ranked third as the leading cause of death after cardiovascular diseases (WHO 2015, 2017). The categories of people involved in this approach are the pharmacists, physicians and patients along with other health care and epidemiology professionals. As far as the animal Healthcare health representatives are concerned, veterinarians and agricultural workers are included, while ecologists and wildlife experts are represented as environmental experts (CDC, 2023).

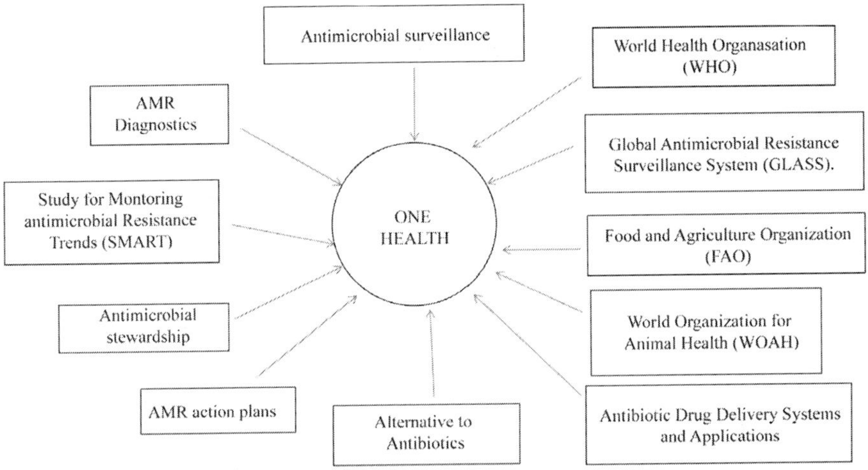

Fig. 3: One Health approach to mitigate the development of Antimicrobial resistance in bacteria

The important strategies for addressing AMR from the One Health approach include:

1. Organizing public awareness campaigns there by educating people about the harm caused by the indiscriminate use of antibiotics which in turn decreases the inappropriate prescriptions.
2. Improving the living standards by improving the personal and environmental hygiene to prevent the diseases or infections can significantly reduce the demand for antimicrobial usage.
3. Unnecessary usage of antibiotics for prophylaxis, growth promoters and in animals and agriculture should be considered dangerous, as it has been documented that animal excretes a significant percentage (75%–90%) of antimicrobials without being metabolized and dispersed into the environment.
4. Establishment of data and surveillance on AMR about the current cases can predict the future threats.
5. Development of rapid and accurate diagnostics will allow administration of correct antimicrobials and prevent unnecessary prescription of antibiotics.
6. Efforts to identify potential alternatives for antibiotics from natural resources and vaccines directed against antibiotic-resistant bacteria have to be made as an alternative strategy. According to recent findings

on compounds derived from plants, such polyphenolics, alkaloids, and other plant extracts, plants are being considered as untapped sources of potential antimicrobials. However, the antimicrobial potential of several phytochemical compounds including polyphenolics, alkaloids, and flavonoids has yet to be investigated (Islam *et al.*, 2021, Al-Amin *et al* ., 2022, Foyzun *et al.*, 2022, Mustafa *et al.*, 2022) Moreover, the big challenge is to transfer and translate some of these precious discoveries out of laboratories into hospital practices.

7. With advances in biotechnology, genetic engineering, and synthetic chemistry, opportunities for research on innovative alternative therapies have to be widened, thereby bringing an optimistic approach in tackling to the emergent AMR problem.
8. Increase in the investments in research and development and the need for skilled personnel to address AMR. Training of skilled professionals such as microbiologists, pharmacists, infectious disease specialists, nurses, infection control specialists, veterinarians, and epidemiologists and working in coordination with an effort to reduce the indiscriminate usage of antibiotics.
9. Incentives to promote investment in new drugs and in the improvement of existing drugs.
10. Building a global coalition for real action against AMR involves the coordination between medical, veterinary and plant health specialists using One Health approach is important to effect change.

Conclusion

Antimicrobial resistance represents a formidable global challenge that demands collective action and interdisciplinary collaboration. The One Health approach recognizing the interconnectedness of human, animal, and environmental health provides a blueprint for addressing the multifaceted dimensions of AMR. By embracing the principles of One Health and implementing coordinated interventions, and antimicrobial stewardship programs the stakeholders can mitigate the spread of antimicrobial resistance, thus pave the way to preserve the efficacy of antimicrobial agents, and uphold the human, animal and environmental health and well-being.

References

Al-Amin MY, Lahiry A, Ferdous R, Hasan MK, Kader MA, Alam AK, Saud ZA, Sadik MG. 2022. Stephania japonica Ameliorates Scopolamine-Induced Memory Impairment in Mice through Inhibition of Acetylcholinesterase and Oxidative Stress. Adv. Pharmacol. Pharm. Sci. 8305271.

Alanis AJ., 2005. Resistance to antibiotics: Are we in the post-antibiotic era? . Arch Med Res., 36:697–705. 10.1016/j.arcmed.2005.06.009

Aminov, R., 2017. History of antimicrobial drug discovery: major classes and health impact. In: Biochem. Pharmacol., Antibiotics - Meeting the Challenges of 21st Century Health Care: Part I 133, pp. 4–19. https://doi.org/10.1016/j. bcp.2016.10.001

Appelbaum P., 2006. The emergence of vancomycin-intermediate and vancomycin-resistant Staphylococcus aureus. Clin Microbiol Infect., 12:16–23. 10.1111/j.1469-0691.2006.01344.x

Avorn J, Barrett JF, Davey PG, *et al.*,2001. Antibiotic resistance: Synthesis of recommendations by expert policy groups. WHO/CDS/CSR/DRS/2001.10 .

CDC. One Health Basics. Available online: https://www.cdc.gov/onehealth/basics/index.html (accessed on 22 February 2024).

Collignon PJ and McEwen SA., 2019. One Health—Its importance in helping to better control antimicrobial resistance. Trop Med Infect Dis., 4(1): 22.

D'Costa VM, McGrann KM, Hughes DW, Wright GD., 2006. Sampling the Antibiotic Resistome. Science, 311, 374–377.

Ebimieowei Etebu and Ibemologi Arikekpar., 2016. Antibiotics: Classification and mechanisms of action with emphasis on molecular perspectives. Int. J. Appl. Microbiol. Biotechnol. Res. 90-101.

Food and Agriculture Organization (FAO). 2016. Drivers, dynamics and epidemiology of antimicrobial resistance in animal or production. Available at: http://www.fao.org/3/ai6209e.pdf.

Food and Agriculture Organization (FAO). 2018. Antimicrobial resistance and foods of plant origin summary report of an FAO meeting of experts FAO antimicrobial resistance working group. Available at: www.fao.org/ antimicrobial-resistance

Foyzun T, Mahmud AA, Ahammed MS, Manik MIN, Hasan MK, Islam KMM, Lopa SS, Al-Amin MY, Biswas K, Afrin MR. 2022.Polyphenolics with Strong Antioxidant Activity from Acacia nilotica Ameliorate Some Biochemical Signs of Arsenic-Induced Neurotoxicity and Oxidative Stress in Mice. Molecules 2022, 27, 1037.

Gootz TD., 1990. Discovery and development of new antimicrobial agents . Clin Microbiol Rev., 3:13–31. 10.1128/CMR.3.1.13 15.

Huang QM, Horn MA, Ruan SG. 2019. Modeling the Effect of Antibiotic Exposure on the Transmission of Methicillin-Resistant Staphylococcus Aureus in Hospitals with Environmental Contamination. Math. Biosci. Eng. MBE, 16, 3641–3673.

Irfan M., Almotiri A., AlZeyadi ZA., 2022. Antimicrobial Resistance and Its Drivers—A Review. Antibiotics, 11, 1362. https://doi.org/10.3390/ antibiotics11101362

Islam MA, Zaman S, Biswas K, Al-Amin MY, Hasan MK, Alam A, Tanaka T, Sadik G. 2021. Evaluation of cholinesterase inhibitory and antioxidant activity of Wedelia chinensis and isolation of apigenin as an active compound. BMC Complement. Med. Ther. 2021, 21, 204.

Jans C, Sarno E, Collineau L, Meile L, Stärk KDC and Stephan R., 2018. Consumer exposure to antimicrobial-resistant bacteria from food at Swiss retail level. Front Microbiol., 6(9): 362 .

Jevons MP., 1961. "Celbenin"-resistant staphylococci. Br Med J., 1:124–125. 16.

Klein EY, Van Boeckel TP, Martinez EM, Pant S, Gandra S, Levin SA, Goossens H, Laxminarayan R. 2018. Global increase and geographic convergence in antibiotic consumption between 2000 and 2015. Proc. Natl. Acad. Sci 115, E3463–E3470. https://doi.org/10.1073/pnas.1717295115

Larsson DJ and Flach CF. 2022. Antibiotic resistance in the environment. Nature reviews, Microbiology. 20: 257-269.

Lowy FD., 2003. Antimicrobial resistance: the example of Staphylococcus aureus . J Clin Invest., 111:1265– 1273. 10.1172/JCI18535

Mustafa S, Akbar M, Khan MA, Sunita K, Parveen S, Pawar JS, Massey S, Agarwal NR, Husain SA. 2022. Plant metabolite diosmin as the therapeutic agent in human diseases. Curr. Res. Pharmacol. Drug Discov., 3, 100122.

Salam MA, Al-Amin MY, Salam MT, Pawar JS, Akhter N, Rabaan AA, Alqumber MAA., 2023. Antimicrobial Resistance: A Growing Serious Threat for Global Public Health. Healthcare, 11, 1946. https://doi.org/10.3390/ healthcare11131946

Sophia Inbaraj, VK Sriram, P Thomas, A Verma, P Chaudhuri (2019). Antibiotic Resistance in the Veterinary Perspective: A Major Challenge in Achieving One Health, *In Global Applications of One Health Practice and Care*, 142-157, IGI Global publishers, USA

Velazquez-Meza ME, Galarde-López M, Carrillo-Quiróz B, Alpuche-Aranda CM. 2022 Antimicrobial resistance: One Health approach, Veterinary World, 15(3): 743-749.

Vikesland P, Garner E, Gupta S, Kang S, Maile-Moskowitz A and Zhu N. 2019. Differential Drivers of Antimicrobial Resistance across the World. Acc. Chem. Res., 52, 916–924.

WHO, 2015. Global Action Plan on Antimicrobial Resistance. Available online: https://www.who.int/publications-detail-redirect/97892415 09763.

World Health Organisation. 2017. One health. https://www.who.int/newsroom/q-a-detail/one-health.

Zaman S, Hussain M, Nye R *et al.*, 2017. A Review on Antibiotic Resistance: Alarm Bells are Ringing. Cureus 9(6): e1403. DOI 10.7759/cureus.1403.

2

Antimicrobial Resistance in Europe An Insight

Yanshi

Scientist (GI Surveillance), UK Health Security Agency, United Kingdom

Abstract

Antimicrobial Resistance (AMR) is a major public health concern in the European region. A World Health Organisation (WHO) antimicrobial resistance report of Europe with 2020 data from European Union/ European Economic Area (EU/ EEA) has reported that more than 67000 antibiotics resistant bacterial infections have been seen in the region each year, with nearly 33,000 deaths as a direct consequence (ECDPC-2022). The current chapter details about epidemiology of AMR in EU

Keywords: *European Union; European Economic Area, Antimicrobial Resistance, Epidemiology, Risk factors*

AMR has been prevalent in almost all European countries from past decades. A 2021-2022 report published by the European Food Safety Authority (EFSA) and the European Centre for Disease Prevention and Control (ECDC) on AMR in zoonotic and indicator bacteria from humans, animals and food origin reported vast differences in antimicrobials resistance levels among the European countries, with comparatively higher AMR percentages in the southern and eastern parts of Europe (ECDC, 2022, 2023). The resistance levels ranged from very high for tetracyclines, sulfonamides and ampicillin, moderate for ciprofloxacin to low levels for third-generation cephalosporins (cefotaxime and ceftazidime) in human cases infected with *Salmonella* spp. in 2022 (ECDC, 2023). The trends are dynamic and over a decade of 2013-2022, the human isolates from 12 and 15 countries reported a statistically significant reduction in tetracycline and ampicillin resistance, particularly for *S. typhimurium* (ECDC, 2023). The ciprofloxacin and cefotaxime combination, a highest priority critically important antimicrobials (CIA), had very low and rare resistance levels for *Salmonella* isolates of humans and animal and their derived meat.

Livestock species wise variation was also observed in the resistance pattern in imported meat, being higher in poultry meat isolates compared to pig or cattle meat for *Escherichia coli* (ECDC, 2023). High to extremely high levels of fluoroquinolone resistance from *Campylobacter jejuni* and *C. coli* of both human and animal origin isolates exist, due to which the fluoroquinolones can no more be used as a treatment option for human *Campylobacter* infections (ECDC 2023). The combined occurrence of erythromycin resistance and ciprofloxacin in *Campylobacter* spp is considered of high public health importance, and the report mentioned that the combined resistance for these antimicrobials was higher in *C. coli* compared to *C. jejuni* from food-producing animals and humans. However, while the ciprofloxacin resistance showed an increase in over 13 study countries, seven countries reported reduced erythromycin resistance for *C. jejuni*. Overall, resistance to conventional antimicrobials was frequent in *Campylobacter* and *Salmonella* from humans and animals. Increasing trend in resistance to one of two CIA for treatment in humans has been observed in poultry-originated *Salmonella* serovars and *Campylobacter* while combined resistance was is low in few *Salmonella* serovars and *C. coli* isolates from humans and animals in some countries (ECDC, 2023).

Risk Factors Contributing to AMR

No region of the globe remains unaffected by AMR. Low- and middle-income countries hold the major share owing to socioeconomic inequalities. However, certain major risk factors have a significant contribution in affecting AMR rates in high-income countries. Some of these factors affecting the levels in Europe are described below:

I. Antimicrobial consumption

Increased and improper antimicrobial consumption is one of the biggest risk factors for higher rates of antimicrobial resistance in the population (Prestinaci *et al.*, 2015). Most European countries have stringent regulations to limit unnecessary consumption of antimicrobials. In countries like the United Kingdom, the antimicrobials cannot be bought over the counter without a prescription from a registered professional in human as well as livestock domain. The EU laws also prohibit the routine or nontherapeutic use of antibiotics in farm animals (Simjee and Ippolito, 2022; commonslibrary.parliament.uk/research-briefings, 2023). Antibiotics can only be given to the sick, not entire herds, and they can't be used to compensate for poor hygiene or animal husbandry practices (Nunan, 2022). The EU also bans the use of antibiotics to promote fast growth of animals, and imposes guiltiness for maximum permissible limits of antibiotic residues in the import of animal products.

Although the consumption rates reduced 2019 to 2021 in almost all EU countries, but the ratio of broad to narrow spectrum antibacterials has increased (ESAC-Net, 2022). In 2022, 18 countries had an antibiotic consumption rate of less than 0.01 DDD (defined daily dose) per 1,000 inhabitants per day for oral vancomycin and fidaxomicin, while 23 countries reported consumption rates of oral and rectal metronidazole ranging from 0.005 to 0.032 DDD per 1,000 inhabitants per day (ESAC-Net, 2023). Similarly, as per the antimicrobial consumption in the EU/EEA (ESAC-Net) annual epidemiological report for 2022, the systematic use of antibacterial consumption for EU population has decreased by 2.5% compared to the baseline year of 2019, indicating a slow progress towards the EU 2030 target of reducing the consumption by 20%(ESAC-Net, 2023).

II. Health infrastructure

Water, sanitation and hygiene (WASH) infrastructure, health care systems, GDP per capita, and climate have been found as primary risk factors for AMR emergence and transmission (Allel *et al.*, 2023). Health systems accessibility, performance and quality, and few socio-economic factors including gender, living standards, health awareness / education, can remarkably affect the multidrug resistant microorganism transmission rates, along with the antibiotic utilization etiquette in the European region as well. A recent study for determining the AMR factors among the different European countries have shown that there is a closer, and often significant inverse correlation of AMR related to expenditure on health (Silva, 2021). Environmental like seasonal changes, agriculture and pollution are highly interlinked and complex and play an important role in the resistance genes transmission (Allel *et al.*, 2023). A lower expenditure on public health, leading to worsen healthcare conditions and a higher level of resistance transmission often has a strong correlation with a higher rate of AMR. Each year, the AMR expenditure is around 1.1 billion to the health care systems of EU/EEA countries (Silva *et al.*, 2021). Additionally, the Organisation for Economic Co-operation and Development (OECD) has predicted escalation of the AMR cost in the healthcare system of EU and OECD countries to be approximately $134 billion by 2050 (Anderson *et al.*, 2023).

III. Immigration

Europe hosts the largest number of international migrants. Out of the 20 main destination countries of international migrants, seven are in Europe, with approximately 2% of the average annual growth rate of migrant populations (UN, 2019). In 2019, it is estimated that more than 2.5 million people migrated to the EU from non-member countries (Eurostat Statistics, 2022). It also has the largest positive net migration, i.e. it also hosts the largest number of foreign-born population after accounting for emigration from Europe with a median age of 42.5years (UN, 2019). India, China and Pakistan constitute the major countries of origin of migrants to Europe (Van Mol and Valk, 2016). All these three countries also have very high rates of AMR (Walsh *et al.*, 2023). A systematic review and meta-analysis has found that migrants have higher AMR rates with more prevalence in high-migrant community settings than in hospitals (Nellums *et al.*, 2018). The review also reported higher rates in refugees and asylum seekers than other migrant groups in Europe (Nellums *et al.*, 2018). The results are supported by another research which mentioned that people who are forced to migrate and experience exclusionary living conditions are more likely to have AMR compared to other migrant groups (Yıldız *et al.*, 2023; Yusuff *et al.*, 2023). The study further states that the migration journey itself may be a factor in AMR, rather than just the countries they come from (Yıldız *et al.*, 2023). This is specifically important for countries like Russia and Ukraine where vast displacement of individuals and communities have occurred due to conflicts, as these might extensively result in increased AMR transmission rates among the population.

Strategies to Combat AMR in Europe

A holistic approach is essential to effectively combat antibiotic resistance in Europe and ensure the continued efficacy of antibiotics for future generations. Some of the methods which can be used to combat the issue of AMR in Europe are:

I. Research and Product Development

Encouraging the development of new antimicrobial agents, alternative treatments and vaccines (like phage therapy), and rapid diagnostic and susceptibility tests can be one of the ways to tackle AMR in European countries. With the recent advancements in medical and technology field, nanomedicine-based drugs are also a focus of attention due to their favourable physicochemical characteristics (Patra *et al.*, 2018). This can be supported by providing incentives such as grants, tax breaks or public-private partnership.

Further, in depth knowledge about the socio-economic factors which influence the emergence and transmission of AMR genes is needed (Silva, 2021). Moreover, using big data and artificial intelligence to analyse prescribing patterns can help in predicting resistant infections outbreaks (Ali *et al.*, 2023).

II. Rational use of Antimicrobials

Inappropriate use of antimicrobials contributes to the emergence and spread of AMR. Combination therapy, meaning prescribing two or more antibiotics simultaneously may be more beneficial for treating AMR suspected cases (Ahmed *et al.*, 2014). Secondly, regulating the prophylactic use of antibiotic may be helpful to curtail the chances of AMR development. The European Association of Urology recommends antibiotic prophylaxis as a first-line strategy for preventing recurrent urinary tract infections (Cruz *et al.*, 2009). However, more uropathogens have become resistant to urinary antimicrobials, thereby decreasing the successful treatment probability (Cruz *et al.*, 2009). Therefore, limiting the use of antimicrobials is important. Additionally, limiting the use of antibiotics for growth promotion and limit their use in veterinary medicine to cases where they are necessary for animal health, ideally under veterinary supervision, which is already in force by the EU for farmed animals is a good method to ensure AMR gene circulation in the food chain (6,7). Further, encouraging the adoption of alternative farming practices, including improved biosecurity measures, good husbandry practices and vaccination to decrease antibiotics need can also be helpful (Dhaka *et al.*, 2023).

III. Improving Healthcare Facilities

Implementing Stewardship programs in hospitals, which includes educating, monitoring and guiding healthcare professionals on antibiotic prescribing practices can largely help in regulating antimicrobial consumption in hospitals. Secondly, using rapid diagnostic tests for accurate identification of bacterial infections and subsequently determining the appropriate antibiotic can largely reduce the unnecessary use of broad-spectrum antibiotics (Kaprou *et al.*, 2021). Thirdly, developing and maintaining robust surveillance systems to actively monitor AMR patterns and outbreaks across Europe will allow for timely interventions. Promoting the use of vaccinations for infections such as influenza and pneumococcal vaccines, especially in migrants (including refugees and asylum seekers) can be a measure to reduce incidence of infections which else might require antibiotic treatment (van Heuvel *et al.*, 2023). Collaboration between EU member states and international organisations (including World Health Organisation, World Organisation for Animal Health, Food and Agriculture Organisation) and the ECDC to coordinate efforts, share data, and implement unified policies, and developing and implementing comprehensive national action plans with the 'One-Health' approach can be used to combat the issue (Cella *et al.*, 2023).

Conclusion

AMR represents a significant and emerging challenge to the health sector in Europe, posing a threat to public health, economic stability, and the effectiveness of modern medicine. Addressing this challenge requires a multi-faceted approach, combining improved stewardship of existing antibiotics, stringent infection control measures, investment in research and innovation, and global collaboration. Effective implementation of these strategies is essential to mitigate the impact of AMR and ensure sustainable health outcomes for future generations.

References

Ahmed A, Azim A, Gurjar M, Baronia AK. Current concepts in combination antibiotic therapy for critically ill patients. Indian J Crit Care Med. 2014 May;18(5):310-4.

Ali T, Ahmed S, Aslam M. Artificial intelligence for antimicrobial resistance prediction: challenges and opportunities towards practical implementation. Antibiotics. 2023 Mar 6;12(3):523.

Allel K, Day L, Hamilton A, Lin L, Furuya-Kanamori L, Moore CE, Van Boeckel T, Laxminarayan R, Yakob L. Global antimicrobial-resistance drivers: an ecological country-level study at the human–animal interface. The Lancet Planetary Health. 2023 Apr 1;7(4):e291-303.

Anderson M, Panteli D, Mossialos E. How can the EU support sustainable innovation and access to effective antibiotics? Policy options for existing and new medicines [Internet]. Copenhagen (Denmark): European Observatory on Health Systems and Policies; 2023. (Policy Brief, No. 51.) Policy brief. Available from: https://www.ncbi.nlm.nih.gov/books/NBK594074/

Cella E, Giovanetti M, Benedetti F, Scarpa F, Johnston C, Borsetti A, Ceccarelli G, Azarian T, Zella D, Ciccozzi M. Joining Forces against Antibiotic Resistance: The One Health Solution. Pathogens. 2023 Aug 23;12(9):1074.

Cruz F, Dambros M, Naber KG, Bauer HW, Cozma G. Recurrent urinary tract infections: Uro-Vaxom®, a new alternative. European Urology Supplements. 2009 Sep 1;8(9):762-8.

Dhaka P, Chantziaras I, Vijay D, Bedi JS, Makovska I, Biebaut E, Dewulf J. Can Improved Farm Biosecurity Reduce the Need for Antimicrobials in Food Animals? A Scoping Review. Antibiotics (Basel). 2023 May 11;12(5):893.

European Centre for Disease Prevention and Control. Antimicrobial consumption in the EU/EEA (ESAC-Net) - Annual Epidemiological Report for 2021. [Internet]. 2022. Available from: https://www.ecdc.europa.eu/en/publications-data/surveillance-antimicrobial-consumption-europe-2021

European Centre for Disease Prevention and Control. Antimicrobial consumption in the EU/EEA (ESAC-Net) - Annual Epidemiological Report for 2022. [Internet]. 2023. Available from: https://www.ecdc.europa.eu/en/publications-data/surveillance-antimicrobial-consumption-europe-2022

European Centre for Disease Prevention and Control. Antimicrobial resistance surveillance in Europe 2022 - 2020 data. [Internet]. 2022. Available from: https://www.ecdc.europa.eu/en/publications-data/antimicrobial-resistance-surveillance-europe-2022-2020-data

European Centre for Disease Prevention and Control. Antimicrobial resistance surveillance in Europe 2023 - 2021 data.[Internet]. 2023. Available from: https://www.ecdc.europa.eu/en/publications-data/antimicrobial-resistance-surveillance-europe-2023-2021-data

Eurostat Statistics. Migration and migrant population statistics. [Internet]. 2022 [cited 2022 May 14]. Available from: https://ec.europa.eu/eurostat/statistics-explained/index.php?title=Migration_and_migrant_population_statistics

House of Commons Library. The use of antibiotics on healthy farm animals and antimicrobial resistance. 2023. Available from: https://commonslibrary.parliament.uk/research-briefings/cdp-2023-0012/#:~:text=Antibiotics%20can%20also%20no%20longer,must%20comply%20with%20its%20requirements.

Kaprou GD, Bergšpica I, Alexa EA, Alvarez-Ordóñez A, Prieto M. Rapid Methods for Antimicrobial Resistance Diagnostics. Antibiotics (Basel). 2021 Feb 20;10(2):209.

Nellums LB, Thompson H, Holmes A, Castro-Sánchez E, Otter JA, Norredam M, Friedland JS, Hargreaves S. Antimicrobial resistance among migrants in Europe: a systematic review and meta-analysis. Lancet Infect Dis. 2018 Jul;18(7):796-811.

Nunan C. Ending routine farm antibiotic use in Europe. Achieving responsible farm antibiotic use through improving animal health and welfare in pig and poultry production. 2022 Jan.

Patra JK, Das G, Fraceto LF, Campos EV, Rodriguez-Torres MD, Acosta-Torres LS, Diaz-Torres LA, Grillo R, Swamy MK, Sharma S, Habtemariam S. Nano based drug delivery systems: recent developments and future prospects. Journal of Nanobiotechnology. 2018 Dec;16:1-33.

Prestinaci F, Pezzotti P, Pantosti A. Antimicrobial resistance: a global multifaceted phenomenon. Pathog Glob Health. 2015; 109(7):309-18.

Silva AC, Nogueira PJ, Paiva JA. Determinants of antimicrobial resistance among the different European countries: more than human and animal antimicrobial consumption. Antibiotics. 2021 Jul 9;10(7):834.

Simjee S, Ippolito G. European regulations on prevention use of antimicrobials from january 2022. Braz J Vet Med. 2022 Oct 5;44:e000822.

United Nations. Department of Economic and Social Affairs. International Migration 2019. [Internet]. 2019 [cited 2022 May 14]. Available from: https://www.un.org/en/development/desa/population/migration/publications/migrationreport/docs/InternationalMigration2019_Report.pdf

van Heuvel L, Paget J, Dückers M, Caini S. The impact of influenza and pneumococcal vaccination on antibiotic use: an updated systematic review and meta-analysis. Antimicrob Resist Infect Control. 2023 Jul 14;12(1):70.

Van Mol C, Valk HD. Migration and immigrants in Europe: A historical and demographic perspective. InIntegration processes and policies in Europe 2016 (pp. 31-55). Springer, Cham.

Walsh TR, Gales AC, Laxminarayan R, Dodd PC. Antimicrobial Resistance: Addressing a Global Threat to Humanity. PLoS Med. 2023 Jul 3;20(7):e1004264.

Yusuff SI, Tajudeen YA, Oladunjoye IO, Oladipo HJ, Bolarinwa OV, Popoola OT, Ahmed AF, Olana MD. The need to increase antimicrobial resistance surveillance among forcibly displaced persons (FDPs). Tropical Diseases, Travel Medicine and Vaccines. 2023 Sep 1;9(1):12.

Yıldız SS, Hekimoğlu CH, Sucaklı MB, Bakkaloğlu Z, Çevik YN, Ünaldı Ö, Arslantürk H, Zikusooka M, Keçik M, Nellums L, Elci OC. Community-acquired antimicrobial resistance among Syrian refugees and the local population in Türkiye. European Journal of Public Health. 2023 Oct 1;33(5):809-14.

3

Antimicrobial Resistance
A Threat to Public Health

***Sundus Gazal*[1]*, Sabahat Gazal*[2] *and Paviter Kaur*[3]**

[1,2]*Division of Veterinary Microbiology and Immunology, SKUAST Jammu, Jammu and Kashmir, India*

[3]*Department of Veterinary Microbiology, GADVASU, Ludhiana, Punjab, India*

Abstract

Antimicrobial resistance is the process by which microorganisms become resistant to a drug to which they were earlier susceptible. Antimicrobial resistant bacterial infections have few therapeutic choices, leading to severe morbidity and mortality with a large financial cost. The unnecessary use of antibiotics globally especially in the livestock sector as growth promoter further helps in selective enrichment of AMR pathogens which further increases health risks. Bacteria may become resistant to one antimicrobial class or may become resistant to more antimicrobial classes termed as Multiple drug resistance (MDR). Various terms like extensively drug-resistance (XDR) and pandrug-resistance (PDR) have been introduced after recognizing different degrees of MDR in bacteria. Bacteria develop resistance to antibiotics by various mechanisms which include limiting drug uptake, altering a drug target, inactivating a drug, and increasing active efflux of the drug. Antibiotic resistant bacteria can spread in the environment by many routes and various factors like poor hygienic measures and poor sanitation may lead to the dissemination of resistant bacteria in hospitals, in animal farms and in the community. Some important factors that may help in combatting the problem of AMR includes improvement and strengthening of hygiene measures, use of antibiotics rationally in exact doses as required for an adequate time, complete ban on the sale of over-the-counter pharmaceuticals, reduction on the overall use of antibiotics for growth promotion and disease prevention and use of good hygienic practices as well as use of good animal husbandry techniques to promote animal health. This chapter describes the different types of resistance, the mechanisms of its origin, development and dissemination as well as various strategies being adopted at the global level for its mitigation.

Keywords: Antimicrobial Resistance, Antimicrobial Stewardship, One Health, AMR Mitigation.

Antimicrobial Resistance abbreviated as AMR is defined as the process by which microorganisms like bacteria, fungi, viruses, and parasites change over a period and become resistant to a drug to which they were earlier susceptible to. This makes the medicines ineffective for treatment overtime, thus making infections difficult to treat thereby increasing the risk of spread of diseases caused by them and severe illness which may lead to death. This in turn necessitates the need for development of newer antibiotics. However, there has been a sharp decline in the development and manufacture of new antibiotics in the recent years resulting in development of only few antibiotics in the past two decades. The increase in emergence of antibiotic resistance concurrent with decline in development of newer antibiotics poses a serious threat to health of both humans and animals. Every year about 700,000 deaths have been reported to occur due to resistant infections and this rate is likely to increase further with estimated infections due to resistant pathogens expected to reach over 50 million globally by 2050 (O'Neill, 2016). The worrisome trends of increasing antimicrobial resistance across the globe poses a serious threat to both animal and human health as AMR not only increases the morbidity and mortality rates but also increases the economic burden on health care (Zhu *et al.*, 2022). This presents an extremely grave situation as the supply of new antibiotics is inadequate to cope with the increase of AMR pathogens. The unnecessary use of antibiotics globally especially in the livestock sector as growth promoter further helps in selective enrichment of AMR pathogens which further increases health risks. It is well known that resistant pathogenic and commensal bacteria can persist and spread within and between premises despite zero antimicrobial drug use. This may be explained due to maintenance, replication, and further dissemination of resistance genes by horizontal transfer of genes via natural ecosystem and can occur either by conjugation, transformation and transduction; and these mechanisms can rapidly spread AMR genes among microbial community in natural environment and human microbiome, where these resistant bacterial species may be selected due to presence of antimicrobial drugs (Zhu *et al.*, 2022). The physical transfer of bacteria via movement of animals, workers, and equipment and ineffective cleaning and disinfection may also be responsible for increasing the AMR pathogens in the natural environments.

The bacterial resistance to a specific antimicrobial agent is measured by minimum inhibitory concentration (MIC) of that antibiotic. MIC is defined as the minimal concentration of a drug which inhibits growth of bacteria. Bacteria may be resistant to one antimicrobial class or may become resistant to more antimicrobial classes. The growing rate of Multiple drug resistance (MDR) in bacteria is another serious threat and is defined as antimicrobial resistance shown by a species of microorganism to at least one antimicrobial drug in three or more antimicrobial categories. Various terms like extensively drug-resistance (XDR) and pandrug-resistance (PDR) have been introduced after recognizing different degrees of MDR in bacteria. The extensively drug-resistant (XDR) pathogens are those that exhibit non-susceptibility to all antimicrobial agents except in two or less antimicrobial categories. The pandrug-resistant (PDR) pathogens represent non-susceptibility of bacteria to all antimicrobial agents in all antimicrobial categories (Magiorakos *et al.*, 2012).

Origin of Resistance

The antibiotic resistance is often described as an evolutionary response of bacteria against a challenge of antibiotics. So, all targeted pathogens theoretically remain susceptible to an antibiotic when it is first used against it, but with continuous use, the bacteria develop resistance to it. Bacteria may acquire resistance to the action of antibiotics either by chromosomal gene mutations or by acquisition of resistance gene by horizontal gene transfer. Gene mutations that lead to development of antibiotic resistance can be categorized into three types viz. 1) mutations in the gene which encodes for the antibiotic target leading to antibiotic target modification; 2) mutations in genes involved in transporting the antibiotic, and 3) mutations in genes that regulate the expression of antibiotic transporters (e.g., the antibiotic-modifying enzymes and multidrug efflux pumps). The second mechanism of acquisition of antibiotic resistance involves when bacteria acquire resistance genes through horizontal gene transfer (HGT) by conjugation, transformation, and transduction. It has been well known that commensal or environmental bacteria are regarded as the source and reservoir of antibiotic-resistance gene(s) that are transmitted to pathogenic bacteria through HGT (Davies & Davies, 2010). Since, many environmental bacteria are natural synthesizers of antibiotics, it is argued that they must also possess certain resistant genes that provide protection against the effects of their own synthesized antibiotics (Koch *et al.*, 2021).

Types of Antibiotic Resistance

The bacteria exhibiting antibiotic resistance may contain resistance gene(s) from intrinsic, acquired, or adaptive sources (Lee, 2019). Intrinsic resistance is defined as bacteria's inherent natural capacity to exhibit resistance to certain classes of antibiotics due to the existence of their own chromosomal genes without mutation or gain of further genes. Such intrinsic resistance in bacteria will allow them to show inevitable resistance against certain antibiotics if they are used to treat infections caused by them.

Acquired resistance is described as acquisition of resistance by a previously sensitive bacterium to an antimicrobial agent due to chromosomal gene mutation or by acquisition of resistance determinant by HGT; and this type of resistance is mostly mediated by plasmids (Holmes *et al.*, 2016 and Munita *et al.*, 2016)

Adaptive resistance involves a metabolic adaptation of bacteria that limit the bactericidal capability of antimicrobials. It seems to be due to modulations in gene expression and is observed when bacterial growth is influenced by subinhibitory antibiotic concentration as well as in response to environmental changes. In contrast to resistance caused due to genetic alterations which produce irreversible phenotypes, adaptive resistance may be due to epigenetic changes, and DNA methylation by DAM methylase enzymes have been thought to cause differential expression of genes in bacterial population which provide the heterogeneity of gene expression required for adaptive resistance to occur (Motta *et al.* 2015; Salimiyan Rizi *et al.* 2018). Particularly, modulation in genes responsible for the expression genes encoding for efflux pumps and porins have been implicated in its emergence. Adaptive resistance usually develops transiently and is seen to revert to the original state when the inducing signals are removed (Christaki *et al.*, 2019).

Mechanism of Antibiotic Resistance

Bacteria develop resistance to antibiotics by acting on one of the four essential targets of antibiotics in a bacterial cell viz. cell wall, protein synthesis, or nucleic acid synthesis. There are various primary mechanisms by which bacteria develop the ability to resist the action of antimicrobials and include limiting drug uptake, altering a drug target, inactivating a drug, and increasing active efflux of the drug.

1. Limiting drug uptake: Gram negative bacteria possess a lipopolysaccharide which is a highly acylated glycolipid that serves as permeability barrier for several antibiotics. Thus, the presence of lipopolysaccharide layer in Gram negative bacteria limits the uptake of various different drugs by these bacteria. This is a form of intrinsic resistance exhibited by Gram-negative bacteria which enables the bacteria to lower the permeability for several antibiotics leading to resistance. Apart from this, modifications observed in the permeability of outer-membrane proteins viz. porins, can give rise to acquired resistance. Porin proteins are the primary entry point for hydrophilic antibiotics like Beta-lactams, fluoroquinolones, tetracyclines, and chloramphenicol and the quantity and type of porin proteins affect the entry of such antibiotics inside the bacteria which in

turn affects the susceptibility of the bacteria to such antibiotics (Choi and Lee, 2019). Additionally, mutations that result in impairment in the expression of porin proteins or its function in combination with various other mechanisms of resistance like drug efflux or enzymatic degradation of antibiotics can further lead to resistance (Ghai and Ghai, 2018).

2. Modification of targets for the drug: Another important antibiotic resistance mechanism observed in bacteria is their ability to modify the drug targets so that the drug cannot bind to or binds poorly to the modified target and hence antibiotic action is compromised. This drug target modification usually results from spontaneous mutations observed in the gene or genes which encode the protein that serves as the drug target. For example, mutations of the quinolone-resistance-determining region (QRDR) in the gene which codes for DNA gyrase enzyme results in fluoroquinolone resistance which can develop in both Gram-positive as well as in Gram-negative bacteria (Ashley *et al.*, 2017). Another example includes drug target modification by methylation in the erm methylase enzymes which leads to development of antibiotic resistance against macrolides, lincosamides, and streptogramin B in both gram-positive and gram-negative bacteria. In *Staphylococcus* spp. the *mec*A and other *mec* genes like *mec*C have been seen to encode for an alternative penicillin binding protein, that leads to significant reduction in its affinity to the B-lactam antibiotics (Foster, 2017 and Wendlandt *et al.*, 2015).

3. Inactivation of drug: Antibiotic resistance can also occur due to production of various enzymes by bacteria that inactivate the antibiotic in one of two ways: by either degradation of the antibiotic, or by addition of a chemical group to the antibiotic after it has entered bacteria. The most common example includes the production of hydrolyzing enzymes like B-lactamases which are efficient at inactivating the B-lactam antibiotics. These B-lactamases inactivate the B-lactam ring structure and thus render it ineffective to bind to its target, the penicillin-binding proteins in the bacterial cell wall. Various members of the *Enterobacteriaceae* family and many Gram-positive bacteria like *Staphylococcus aureus* harbour B-lactamase genes that are transmitted by HGT. Additionally, tetracycline resistance can be mediated by hydrolysis of tetracycline by an enzyme which is expressed by *tet*X gene present in some bacteria (Blair *et al.*, 2015). The resistance can also be mediated by transfer of acetyl, phosphoryl, or adenyl group to an antibiotic for its inactivation. For instance, aminoglycoside resistance is mediated by phosphorylation

and adenylation of the drug whereas acetylation is the mostly utilized mechanism against aminoglycosides, chloramphenicol, streptogramins, and fluoroquinolone resistance (Reygaert, 2018).

4. Efflux of drug: Another efficient way by virtue of which bacteria may acquire resistance is by employing an energy-dependent efflux pump located on the cytoplasmic membrane which enables the bacteria to reduce the accumulation of antibiotic inside the bacterial cell. By this mechanism, the bacteria can efficiently control its internal environment such that the bactericidal drug concentration is not achieved inside the bacteria. The first efflux pump was discovered in 1980 in *E. coli* which was plasmid encoded and was engaged in tetracycline efflux out of the bacterial cell. Most efflux systems provide multidrug efflux and are mostly chromosomally encoded (Nikaido and Pagès, 2012). Also, genes involved in substrate-specific efflux pump viz., efflux pumps for chloramphenicol, tetracyclines, and macrolides, may also be found on mobile genetic elements (Reygaert, 2018; Poole, 2005).

Methods of Dissemination of Antibiotic Resistant Bacteria

Antibiotic resistant bacteria can spread in the environment by many routes. Different factors affect bacterial spread which is facilitated by poor hygienic measures and poor sanitation. These interconnected factors may lead to the dissemination of resistant bacteria in hospitals, in animal farms and in the community.

Person to Person Spread

Bacterial spread from between people may occur via direct contact or by indirect contact with a contaminating surface. It has been observed that AMR bacteria are frequently transmitted to humans in public settings like buses (Conceicao *et al.*, 2013), railway stations (Lin *et al.*, 2017), on subway trains (Mason *et al.*, 2016) and in University classrooms (Li *et al.*, 2015) where high population movement is observed (Batista e Silva *et al.*, 2020). As the surfaces in public places are frequently touched and contaminated by many people, this can accelerate the spread of AMR bacteria. For preventing the transmission of AMR spread, measures must be taken to educate general public about hand hygiene and for undertaking cleaning/infection control practices that may ultimately help to stop the transmission of infections caused by antibiotic resistant bacteria (Cave *et al.*, 2021).

Spread Between Animals and Humans

Antibiotics are often used in farm animals at a very high level and it was estimated that the global usage of antimicrobials in food animals was more than 93,000 tonnes in 2017 (Tiseo *et al.*, 2020), accounting for more than 70% of the global antimicrobial production. And because the same bacterial species infect/colonize humans and farm animals, this leads to exchange of resistant bacteria among humans and animals. Bacteria readily spread between animals and humans and vice versa and the spread of such antibiotic resistant bacteria lead to diseases in target population which complicates treatment. As such, the livestock farmers and veterinarians are occupationally considered at a higher risk of getting infected with such strains, which then act as spreaders of such bacteria in society.

Food

Antibiotics have been invariably used in food animals for prevention and control of bacterial diseases and for growth promotion. The commensal bacteria in the gut experience high antibiotic pressure which leads to development of resistance in them. Thus, these antibiotic resistant bacteria colonizing the gut of the animals can spread among other animals. These resistant bacteria can also get transferred to meat at the time of processing which may prove as a human health hazard and resistant bacteria have most frequently been detected in chicken and meat. Consumption of such food may cause infection e.g., diarrhoea caused by *Salmonella*, *Campylobacter* and enterohaemorrhagic *E. coli* (EHEC). These resistant strains can transfer the resistance genes to the normal flora present in the gut of consumers which may lead to resistance in human consumers. So, following proper control measures can help reduce the risk of spread of antibiotic resistance by food and this includes disease prevention in farms, and use of appropriate hygienic practices from farm to fork. The consumers can protect themselves by ensuring food is properly cooked and handled which can significantly decrease the spread of resistant strains as well as the diseases caused by them.

Water

Resistant bacteria may readily spread through drinking water or by water supplies used for various agricultural and farm activities like irrigation, drinking water, farm washing and cleaning as well in human activities like cooking, washing utensils or other hygienic purposes. These resistant bacterial strains may enter drinking water wells and rivers from different sources like effluents from industries and wastewater treatment plants and release of untreated waste water from animals and humans get discharged in these water reservoirs and serve as a source of spread of various disease like typhoid and cholera.

Spread of Antibiotic Resistant Bacteria in Health Care Settings

Health care settings like hospitals are considered as hotspots for emergence and dispersal of resistant bacteria as many diseased patients are housed in close proximity to each other and since the usage of antibiotics is quite high in such patients, this results in selection of resistant bacterial strains and their spread. Another critical factor which facilitates their spread is poor hygienic practices adopted by hospital staff, patients, or their visitors and improper cleaning of instruments and hospital facilities. Moreover, overcrowding in hospital wards and isolation rooms may further facilitate the spread of resistant bacteria.

Travel

Resistant bacteria can also be spread by international travellers across the world. It has been estimated that at any point of time, millions of people travel by public transport like flights or trains and a person that carries a resistant bacterial strain also spread it along. Many travellers may also acquire the resistant bacterial strains during travel if they visit areas that have a high percentage of resistant bacteria. This may also lead to spread of resistance in environment and population.

Driving Forces to AMR

AMR is a multi-factorial problem which is caused by various factors. While the emergence of resistance is a natural process, overuse of antibiotics both in humans as well as animals has hastened this process. Unfortunately, despite constant warnings from health organisations, antibiotic abuse and overuse persist at a disproportionate rate around the world. The abuse involves administering antibiotics in incorrect doses and durations, as well as overuse in the form of administering antibiotics in inappropriate indications. The accessibility of antibiotics as over-the-counter (OTC) medications for both human and animal usage further contributes to the creation and spread of drug-resistant bacteria. AMR has gotten worse in many developing nations because of substandard or low-quality antibiotics in the supply chain. Additionally, doctors may prescribe antibiotics for longer periods of time than necessary or administer them at incorrect dosage, which can subsequently lead to antibacterial resistance. Even though unethical in nature, some doctors, particularly in underdeveloped nations, provide antibiotics without a prescription in order to meet patient expectations and receive financial incentives from pharmaceutical firms (Chokshi *et al.*, 2019 and Klein *et al.*, 2018).

Another important factor leading to antibiotic resistance is the usage of antibiotics in Veterinary medicine and agriculture. Most developing nations have seen a significant rise in the usage of antibiotics in animal husbandry for a number of reasons, including a rise in the demand for animal protein in recent years. Antibiotics are often used for growth promotion and prevention of diseases in food animals. Antibiotic usage for growth promotion in animals involves the antibiotic administration at subtherapeutic doses which targets multiple organs and affects various physiological processes. These result in an improved net energy balance and better animal performance by causing reduced number of harmful bacteria and increased biosynthesis of vitamins at intestinal level. But this use of sublethal dosage of antibiotics has been seen to work as selective pressure that stimulate bacterial evolutionary machinery to adapt to the environmental stressors and allows the survival of more resistant bacteria which propagate and further spread the AMR genes to other non-resistant bacteria. Thus, usage of antibiotics for growth promotion acts as a fuelling agent for antimicrobial resistance as animal-derived products such as meat, milk and eggs have been found to contain certain antibiotic residues. Many a times, the livestock farmers do not follow the required withdrawal period guidelines which may pose a significant health risk to the consumers.

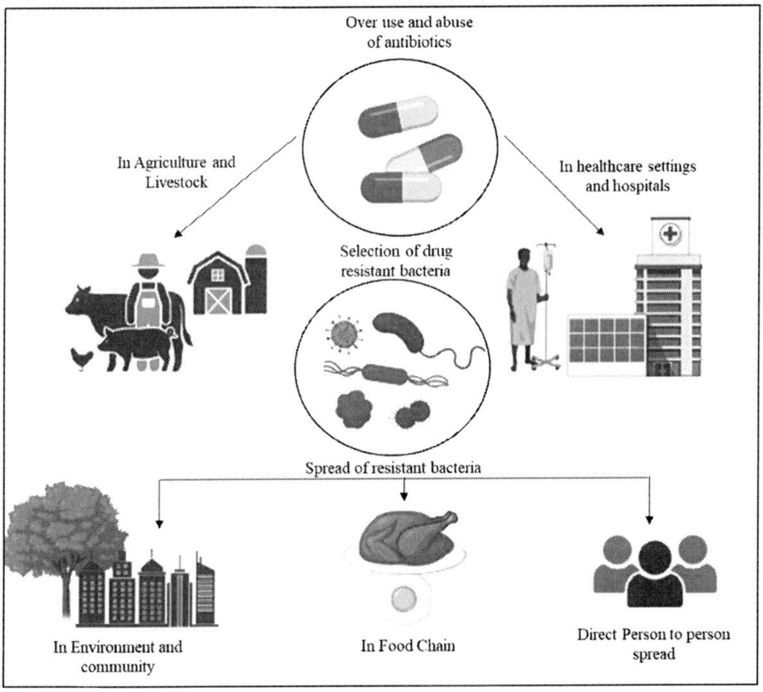

Fig. 1: Mechanism of development and spread of Antibiotic resistance.

Current Scenario and importance

The mainstay of contemporary medicine is the use of antibiotics. Our capacity to treat common illnesses and carry out life-saving operations in animals and humans is under tremendous risk due to introduction and dissemination of drug-resistant microorganisms. Moreover, infections caused by drug-resistant pathogens endanger food security, have an adverse effect on plant and animal health, and lower farm productivity. Both health systems and national economies bear heavy costs because of AMR as it increases the need for more costly and intensive care, reduces agricultural productivity, and impairs the productivity of patients or their carers during extended hospital stays. The increase in prevalence of antibiotic resistance worldwide presents a serious risk since it reduces the efficacy of common medicines in treating common bacterial diseases. Alarming rates of resistance among common infections of bacterial etiology have been highlighted in the 2022 Global Antimicrobial Resistance and Use Surveillance System (GLASS) report. A significant concern is the median reported resistance rate of 35% in methicillin-resistant *Staphylococcus aureus* and 42% in third-generation cephalosporin-resistant *E. coli* across 76 nations. In 2020, 1 in 5 cases of *E. coli* urinary tract infections showed reduced susceptibility to common antibiotics like ampicillin, co-trimoxazole, and fluoroquinolones (Antimicrobial Resistance Collaborators, 2022). Common gut bacteria like *Klebsiella pneumoniae* have also displayed increased level of resistance to important drugs. This may lead to more people using last resort antibiotics like carbapenems, against which resistance has been on rise. The Organisation for Economic Cooperation and Development (OECD) has projected that by 2035, resistance to antibiotics used as a last resort will have doubled from the levels observed in 2005. This highlights the critical need for strong antimicrobial stewardship protocols and increased global surveillance coverage.

A recent study showed that bacterial AMR was associated with nearly 5 million deaths in 2019 (Murray *et al*., 2022). In addition, the AMR has been associated with significant economic costs and the World Bank has estimated that by 2050, AMR may result in an additional loss of $1 trillion in healthcare costs, and by 2030, it may cause annual losses in GDP ranging from $1 trillion to $3.4 trillion (Anonymous, 2024).

India is one of the world's largest consumers of antibiotics owing to widespread availability of over-the-counter antibiotics as well as their indiscriminate use and misuse. In fact, according to WHO (2021) data, India was the fifth-largest user of antibiotic drugs in food animals (cattle, pigs, and poultry) in 2010. Given the present trends and increased demand for animal protein, the country's antimicrobial usage is expected to rise by 312% by 2030. The most significant threat to public health, food safety, and the economy is antimicrobial resistance (AMR). To reduce the establishment and spread of AMR, concerted efforts are being made at international, national, and local levels. The Department of Biotechnology and the WHO Country Office for India worked together to develop the Indian Pathogen Priority List (IPPL), which is in line with the WHO's Global Priority Pathogen List of antibiotic-resistant bacteria. This list consists of bacteria that have been published and for which research and medication are urgently needed. To promote investments in containing the spread of AMR, the IPPL divides bacterial pathogens into three priority groups based on species and resistance: critical, high, and medium as depicted in Table 1. Thus, with the serious threat of antimicrobial resistance as well as its possible spread in animals and humans, the timely detection of multidrug-resistant pathogens becomes utmost important.

Table 1: Indian pathogen priority list adapted from WHO.

Level of Priority	Bacteria	Antibiotics resistant
Critical	Enterobacteriaceae (*Klebsiella pneumoniae* and *Escherichia coli*)	Carbapenem – R Tigecycline – R Colistin – R
	Non-fermenting bacteria (*Acinetobacter baumannii* and *Pseudomonas aeruginosa*)	Carbapenem – R Colistin – R
High	*Staphylococcus aureus*	MRSA, hVISA Daptomycin – NS Linezolid – R
	Enterococcus species	Vancomycin – R Linezolid – R Daptomycin – NS
	Salmonella species (Typhoidal and Non-typhoidal)	Azithromycin – NS Third generation cephalosporins – NS Carbapenem – NS
Medium	*Streptococcus pneumoniae*	Cephalosporin – R Fluoroquinolones – R Linezolid – R
	Staphylococcus, coagulase-negative	Vancomycin – R Linezolid – R
	Shigella species	Third generation cephalosporins – R Azithromycin – R
	Haemophilus influenzae	Third generation cephalosporin – NS Carbapenem – NS
	Neisseria meningitidis	Fluoroquinolones – NS Third generation cephalosporins – NS

(R: resistant; NS: non-susceptible; MRSA: methicillin resistant *S. aureus*; hVISA: heterogenous vancomycin-intermediate *S. aureus*)

Combatting AMR

The successful prevention as well as treatment of a variety of illnesses remain at risk due to emergence of AMR. Some important factors that may help in combatting the problem of AMR have been highlighted below:

- Improvement and strengthening of hygiene measures can help to prevent the spread of infections and hence reduce the demand for antimicrobial usage. This will reduce the likelihood of development and spread of such resistant strains.
- Antibiotic usage rationally in exact doses as required for an adequate time can decrease the development of resistance.
- The sale of over-the-counter pharmaceuticals, which is regrettably still a widespread practice in many poor and impoverished nations, should be subjected to strict regulation.
- There should be stringent legislation on use of important antibiotics to be used in animals so as to minimize the emergence of resistance. Further, the overall use of antibiotics for growth promotion and prevention of diseases should be reduced. As an alternative, it is advised to practise good hygiene, provide probiotics or nutritional supplements in feed, and use vaccinations and other animal husbandry techniques to promote animal health.
- An integrated approach that encompasses the development of vaccines and novel antibiotics is crucial, given the speed at which resistance to each new class of antibiotic is developing and the difficulties in creating new, potent medications. Increased funding for operational research and for the development and commercialization of novel antibiotics through industry and academic collaboration at the national and international levels is needed to address AMR.
- Global public awareness and education is crucial to inform the population about the dangers dur to overuse and misuse of antimicrobials so that such practices can be discouraged.
- Promotion of new and rapid diagnostic tests for proper disease diagnosis will enable the doctors to use the most effective antimicrobials for use in patients.

International Efforts to Control AMR

Antimicrobial resistance poses a severe threat to the ecosystem, harming not just humans but also animals, plants, and other living things. AMR affects all nations, regardless of wealth and its expansion transcends national boundaries. Thus, concerted efforts which includes the efforts of several sectors like the healthcare, pharmacy, finance, trade, education, and nongovernmental organisations at the national and international level, are required to contain and control the menace of AMR.

One Health Approach

It has been established that humans and animals can harbour the same bacteria, contract the same illnesses, and share common medicines used for treatment of infectious diseases. This makes AMR as a major "One Health" concern due to its capacity to spread quickly throughout the population, the food chain, healthcare facilities, and the environment. This makes managing numerous infectious diseases in humans and animals more difficult.

The term "One Health" describes a comprehensive, unified strategy that seeks to promote the best health outcomes for people, animals, and ecosystems. It acknowledges the connections and interdependencies between the health of people, domestic and wild animals, plants, and the larger ecosystem. The One Health strategy for prevention and control of AMR brings together relevant stakeholders to collaborate on the development, execution, and oversight of policies, laws, programmes, and research aimed at reducing AMR and improving health and economic outcomes. A coordinated strategy across many sectors, as well as sector-specific activities in the animal, food production, human health, as well as environmental domains are necessary for addressing the complex issue of AMR.

The concept of One Health involves three Cs: Communication, Coordination, and Collaboration of human health professionals, animal health experts and environmentalists so that they share their expertise and help in mitigation of AMR. This also involves participation of pharmacists, physicians, patients, epidemiologists, veterinarians, agriculturalists, ecologists and wildlife experts (CDC, 2023). AMR prevention would be aided by the worldwide evaluation of the One Health strategy and the committed efforts of the FAO, OIE, and WHO through awareness campaigns, instruction on the use of antibiotics, political activism, and antimicrobial stewardship.

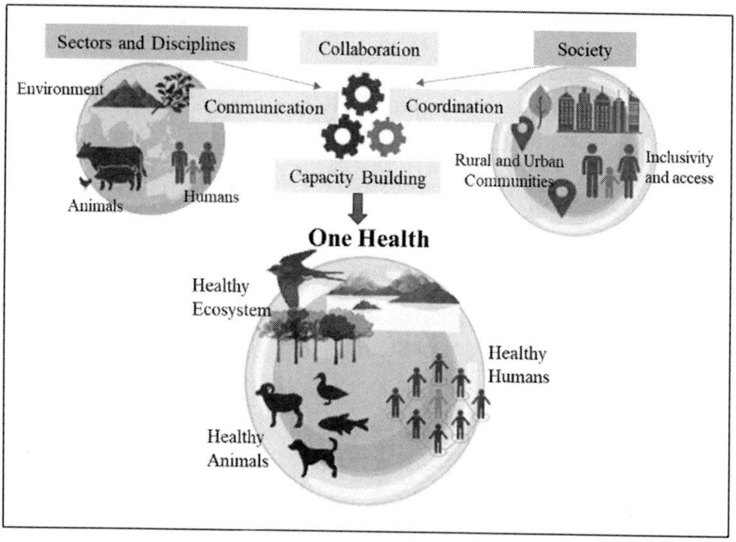

Fig. 2: One Health for AMR mitigation

Antimicrobial Stewardship and AWaRe Programs

Antimicrobial stewardship is a concerted effort to stop the emergence of microbial resistance by educating the prescribers to use antimicrobial drugs according to the appropriate selection, dosage, and duration for better patient outcomes. Ensuring that healthcare providers prescribe the best antibiotic at the right dose and duration for each patient is the primary objective of antimicrobial stewardship. The other objectives include the minimization of overuse, exploitation, and abuse of antibiotics as well as to diminish the establishment of resistance. The development and implementation of Antimicrobial Stewardship Programmes as guided by World Health Organisation is among the most affordable and effective strategy to maximise antimicrobial usage and reduce AMR and infections linked to it.

The WHO has also created the AWaRe (Access, Watch, Reserve) classification system for antibiotics to decrease improper antibiotic usage and increase the access to suitable treatment. This antibiotic book offers brief, scientifically supported recommendations on antibiotic selection, dosage, delivery method, and course of therapy for over thirty of the most prevalent clinical illnesses in adults and children in primary care and hospital settings.

GAP and GLASS

Various countries have agreed to develop and implement a multisectoral national action plan using a One Health approach for addressing the issue of

AMR. For this, several countries have adopted the Global Action Plan (GAP) on AMR during the 2015 World Health Assembly. This approach attempts to guarantee that antimicrobials are preserved responsibly, with proper accessibility and quality inspections, so that infectious diseases can always be properly treated and avoided. The major goal is to improve the effectiveness of antimicrobial drugs used for the health of humans and animals.

To close knowledge gaps and provide guidance for initiatives at all levels, WHO introduced the Global Antimicrobial Resistance and Use Surveillance System (GLASS) in 2015. It aims to support AMR surveillance worldwide and promotes identification of AMR causes. It involves using a standardised method for data collecting, analysis, interpretation, and exchange among nations and territories. Additionally, it keeps an eye on the state of both new and old national surveillance systems and offers counsel and direction to countries for putting corrective measures into place as needed.

World AMR Awareness Week (WAAW)

World AMR Awareness Week (WAAW) is an international initiative aimed at increasing public knowledge, comprehension, and best practices among One Health stakeholders, other policymakers, and general public. WAAW, which has been an official WHO health campaign since 2015, is observed annually from November 18 to November 24.

Conclusion

Antimicrobial resistance is a serious threat and it is imperative to acknowledge the effects of all four domains—agriculture, livestock, humans, and the ecosystem—in the fight against AMR. The global prevalence of antimicrobial resistant bacteria has reached an unsettling level, posing a silent pandemic threat to public health and demands immediate action. Antimicrobial resistant bacterial infections have few therapeutic choices, leading to severe morbidity and mortality with a large financial cost. To address this perilous scenario, further study on the manufacture of antibiotics is desperately needed, and new medicines need to be produced. Unless a coordinated and forceful global response is launched, the world will move close to a post-antibiotic era where ordinary illnesses could once again prove to be fatal to humans and animals.

References

Anonymous. (2024). Drug-Resistant Infections: A Threat to Our Economic future (March 2027) https://www.worldbank.org/en/topic/health/publication/drug-resistant-infections-a-threat-to-our-economic-future

Antimicrobial Resistance Collaborators. (2022). Global burden of bacterial antimicrobial resistance in 2019: a systematic analysis. The Lancet; 399(10325): P629-655. DOI: https://doi.org/10.1016/S0140-6736(21)02724-0

Ashley, R. E., Dittmore, A., McPherson, S. A., Turnbough Jr, C. L., Neuman, K. C., & Osheroff, N. (2017). Activities of gyrase and topoisomerase IV on positively supercoiled DNA. Nucleic acids research, 45(16), 9611-9624.

Batista e Silva F., Freire S., Schiavina M., et al. Uncovering temporal changes in Europe's population density patterns using a data fusion approach. Nat. Commun. 2020;11:4631.

Blair, J. M., Webber, M. A., Baylay, A. J., Ogbolu, D. O., & Piddock, L. J. (2015). Molecular mechanisms of antibiotic resistance. Nature reviews microbiology, 13(1), 42-51.

Cave, R., Cole, J., & Mkrtchyan, H. V. (2021). Surveillance and prevalence of antimicrobial resistant bacteria from public settings within urban built environments: Challenges and opportunities for hygiene and infection control. Environment international, 157, 106836. https://doi.org/10.1016/j.envint.2021.106836.

CDC (Centers for Disease Control and Prevention), 2023. One health basics. Centers for Disease Control and Prevention. https://www.cdc.gov/onehealth/basics/index.html

Choi, U., & Lee, C. R. (2019). Distinct roles of outer membrane porins in antibiotic resistance and membrane integrity in Escherichia coli. Frontiers in microbiology, 10, 953.

Chokshi, A., Sifri, Z., Cennimo, D., & Horng, H. (2019). Global contributors to antibiotic resistance. Journal of global infectious diseases, 11(1), 36.

Christaki, E., Marcou, M., & Tofarides, A. (2019). Antimicrobial resistance in bacteria: Mechanisms, evolution, and persistence. Journal of Molecular Evolution, 88(1), 26–40. https://doi.org/10.1007/s00239-019-09914-3.

Conceicao, T., Diamantino, F., Coelho, C., de Lencastre, H., & Aires-de-Sousa, M. (2013). Contamination of public buses with MRSA in Lisbon, Portugal: a possible transmission route of major MRSA clones within the community. PLoS One, 8(11), e77812.

Davies, J., & Davies, D. (2010). Origins and evolution of antibiotic resistance. Microbiology and molecular biology reviews, 74(3), 417-433.

Foster, T. J. (2017). Antibiotic resistance in Staphylococcus aureus. Current status and future prospects. FEMS microbiology reviews, 41(3), 430-449.

Ghai, I., & Ghai, S. (2018). Understanding antibiotic resistance via outer membrane permeability. Infection and drug resistance, 523-530.

Holmes, A. H., Moore, L. S., Sundsfjord, A., Steinbakk, M., Regmi, S., Karkey, A., Guerin, P.J.& Piddock, L. J. (2016). Understanding the mechanisms and drivers of antimicrobial resistance. The Lancet, 387(10014), 176-187.

Klein, E. Y., Van Boeckel, T. P., Martinez, E. M., Pant, S., Gandra, S., Levin, S. A., ... & Laxminarayan, R. (2018). Global increase and geographic convergence in antibiotic consumption between 2000 and 2015. Proceedings of the National Academy of Sciences, 115(15), E3463-E3470.

Koch, N., Islam, N. F., Sonowal, S., Prasad, R., & Sarma, H. (2021). Environmental antibiotics and resistance genes as emerging contaminants: methods of detection and bioremediation. Current research in microbial sciences, 2, 100027.

Lee, J. H. (2019). Perspectives towards antibiotic resistance: from molecules to population. Journal of Microbiology, 57, 181-184.

Li, X., Qiu, Y., Yu, A., Shi, W., Chen, G., Zhang, Z., & Liu, D. (2015). Characteristics of airborne Staphylococcus aureus (including MRSA) in Chinese public buildings. Aerobiologia, 31, 11-19.

Lin, J.L., Peng, Y., Ou, Q.T., Lin, D.X., Li, Y., Ye, X.H., & Yao, Z.J. (2017). A molecular epidemiological study of methicillin□resistant Staphylococci environmental contamination in railway stations and coach stations in Guangzhou of China. Letters in applied microbiology, 64(2), 131-137.

Magiorakos, A.-P., Srinivasan, A., Carey, R. B., Carmeli, Y., Falagas, M. E., Giske, C. G., Harbarth, S., Hindler, J. F., Kahlmeter, G., Olsson-Liljequist, B., Paterson, D. L., Rice, L. B., Stelling, J., Struelens, M. J., Vatopoulos, A., Weber, J. T., & Monnet, D. L. (2012). Multidrug-resistant, extensively drug-resistant and Pandrug-resistant bacteria: An international expert proposal for interim standard definitions for acquired resistance. Clinical Microbiology and Infection, 18(3), 268–281. https://doi.org/10.1111/j.1469-0691.2011.03570.x.

Mason C., Afshinnekoo E., Ahsannudin S., et al. (2016). The Metagenomics and Metadesign of the Subways and Urban Biomes (MetaSUB) International Consortium inaugural meeting report. Microbiome, 4: 24.

Motta, S. S., Cluzel, P., & Aldana, M. (2015). Adaptive resistance in bacteria requires epigenetic inheritance, genetic noise, and cost of efflux pumps. PLOS ONE, 10(3). https://doi.org/10.1371/journal.pone.0118464.

Munita, J. M., & Arias, C. A. (2016). Mechanisms of antibiotic resistance. Virulence mechanisms of bacterial pathogens, 481-511.

Murray C.JL., Ikuta K.S., Sharara F., Swetschinski L., Robles Aguilar G., Gray A., et al. (2022). Global burden of bacterial antimicrobial resistance in 2019: a systematic analysis. Lancet, 399(10325): 629–655.

Nikaido, H., & Pagès, J. M. (2012). Broad-specificity efflux pumps and their role in multidrug resistance of Gram-negative bacteria. FEMS microbiology reviews, 36(2), 340-363.

O'Neill, J. (2016). Tackling drug-resistant infections globally: final report and recommendations.

Poole, K. (2005). Efflux-mediated antimicrobial resistance. Journal of Antimicrobial Chemotherapy, 56(1), 20-51.

Reygaert, W. C. (2018). An overview of the antimicrobial resistance mechanisms of bacteria. AIMS microbiology, 4(3), 482.

Salimiyan Rizi, K., Ghazvini, K., & Noghondar, M. kouhi. (2018). Adaptive antibiotic resistance: Overview and perspectives. Journal of Infectious Diseases & Therapy, 06(03). https://doi.org/10.4172/2332-0877.1000363.

Tiseo K., Huber L., Gilbert M., Robinson T.P., van Boeckel T.P. Global trends in antimicrobial use in food animals from 2017 to 2030. Antibiotics. 2020;9(12):918–934.

Wendlandt, S., Shen, J., Kadlec, K., Wang, Y., Li, B., Zhang, W. J., ... & Schwarz, S. (2015). Multidrug resistance genes in staphylococci from animals that confer resistance to critically and highly important antimicrobial agents in human medicine. Trends in microbiology, 23(1), 44-54.

WHO. (2021). New Indian Priority Pathogen List to guide discovery of effective antibiotics. World Health Organization. Retrieved from https://www.who.int/india/news/detail/09-03-2021-new-indian-priority-pathogen-list-to-guide-discovery-of-effective-and-affordable-antibiotics

Zhu, Y., Huang, W. E., & Yang, Q. (2022). Clinical perspective of antimicrobial resistance in bacteria. Infection and Drug Resistance, 15, 735.

4

Emerging Antimicrobial Resistance (AMR): Mechanisms, Strategies, and Future Directions

Chayanika Das[1], Ashok Kumar[2], Ram Kumar[3], Vikas Gupta[4], Ranjana Singh[5], Vinod Kumar Singh[5*]

[1]CADRAD, Indian Veterinary Research Institute, Izatnagar, Bareilly (U.P.), India
[2]Animal Disease Research Centre, Guru Angad Dev veterinary and Animal Sciences University, Ludhiana (Punjab), India
[3]Department of Veterinary Microbiology, Rajasthan University of Veterinary and Animal Sciences, Bikaner (Rajasthan), India
[4]CCS-National Institute of Animal Health, Baghpat (U.P.), India
[5]Department of Veterinary Microbiology, College of Veterinary and Animal Sciences, Datia, Rani Lakshmi Bai Central Agricultural University, Jhnasi (U.P.), India

Abstract

Antimicrobial resistance is a major public health problem of today's world. The emergence of resistant microorganisms is a natural phenomenon, but the indiscriminate use of antimicrobials in healthcare and animal production sector has greatly increase the pace and magnitude of AMR development. The issue needs to be addressed and judicious use of antimicrobial should be followed to reverse the resistance trend otherwise we are on a course towards a post-antibiotic era. This chapter provides a comprehensive overview of the information on the discovery of antimicrobials and the mechanisms of antimicrobial resistance developments. It highlights the biomarkers for AMR and strategies or methods for AMR detection. Finally, it reviews ongoing efforts in research, policy, and international collaboration aimed at mitigating the spread of AMR, emphasizing the importance of stewardship programs, alternative therapies, and public awareness campaigns. This chapter underscores the urgency of coordinated global action to address AMR and safeguard the effectiveness of antimicrobial agents for future generations.

Keywords: AMR, Emergence, Mechanism, One health, Control

Introduction

The antibiotics are low molecular weight natural, semi-synthetic, or synthetic substance that kills or slows the growth of germs while causing little or no harm to the host is considered an antimicrobial (Walsh, 2000). Antibiotics are the type of medicine produced by some microorganisms that kill or slow the growth of other microorganisms. It includes any of a large group of chemical substances, as penicillin or streptomycin, produced by various microorganisms and fungi, having the capacity in dilute solutions to inhibit the growth of or to destroy bacteria and other microorganisms, used chiefly in the treatment of infectious diseases (De Vetten *et al.,* 2003). However today, a large number of bacteria are resistant to various antibiotics. Antibiotic resistance occurs when a bacterium becomes able to survive and multiply despite the presence of an antibiotic that would normally control or kill it. In other words, the bacteria become "resistant" and continue to grow even at therapeutic levels of the antibiotic. While antibiotic resistance is a natural phenomenon, it is accelerated by the selective pressure exerted when an antibiotic is used. Bacteria that are naturally resistant to the antibiotic have a better chance of survival compared to those that are susceptible. As the susceptible bacteria are killed or inhibited, resistant strains are favored and continue to thrive (Holme *et al.*, 2006). Some resistance arises without human influence, as bacteria can naturally produce antibiotics against other microorganisms, resulting in a low-level, natural selection for antibiotic resistance. However, the current surge in antibiotic-resistant bacteria is largely attributed to the overuse and misuse of antibiotics. One of the main issues facing public health is antimicrobial resistance, particularly in developing nations where access to and use of medications are easier than in developed nations, leading to a disproportionately higher rate of inappropriate antibiotic use and higher resistance levels (Ganguly *et al.,* 2011). Antimicrobial resistance will make it more difficult to control infections in the community and make health care services less effective (Bhatia *et al.,* 2010). It is well known that India has one of the highest rates of infectious disease burdens in the world, and that the country's high rates of malnutrition and inadequate sanitation make these circumstances worse (http://www.resistancestrategies.org/wpcontent/uploads/2011/03/Indiareport). There are currently specific policies or guidelines for the appropriate use of antibiotics under various national health programs, such as the Integrated Management of Neonatal and Childhood Illness (IMNCI) for respiratory infections and diarrheal diseases, but these are not available for other diseases of public health importance, such as enteric fever. National guidelines were developed and put into effect regulating the restricted use and sale of oseltamivir and remdesivir in the nation during the most recent H1N1 pandemic and unusual pandemic COVID-19 respectively (Sharma *et al.,* 2023). For the treatment of syphilis, Paul Ehrlich developed the first antimicrobial medication, salvarsan (arsphenaminesan arsenic-based medicines), in 1909 (Gould, 2016). He viewed salvarsan as a panacea that specifically attacked germs that caused sickness while also having no negative effects on the host (Liebenau, 1990). Alexander Fleming's discovery of penicillin (β-Lactams) in 1928 marked the beginning of the antibiotic era. After that several synthetic, semi-synthetic, and natural classes of antibiotics/antimicrobials were discovered viz. Sulphonamides (1935); Polypeptides (1939); Aminoglycosides (1943); Tetracyclines (1945); Amphenicols (1947); Lipopeptides (1947); Macrolides (1950); Oxazolidinones (1952); Glycopeptides (1953); Streptogramins (1953); Ansamycinsin (1957); Quinolones (1962); and Lincosamidesin (1963). Consequently, the years from 1930 to 1970 were regarded as the "golden era" (Aminov, 2017). Since the discovery of the first antibiotic, there has been a positive outlook that the spread of infectious diseases is almost at an end. But today, antimicrobial medication resistance is rising at an alarming rate and is becoming a worldwide scourge (Zaman *et al.,* 2017). When microorganisms are exposed to antibiotics, their first priority is to figure out how to survive. Antibiotic overuse leads to the development of bacteria that are resistant to drugs (Levy and Marshall, 2004). Treatment failure and persistent infections are brought on by antibiotic-resistant bacteria. Currently, it is become more difficult to treat a variety of common illnesses include hospital-acquired ventilator-associated pneumonia, urinary tract infections, diarrhea, gonorrhea, tuberculosis, and malaria (Barbosa and Levy, 2000). The current situation makes it difficult and time-consuming to identify or develop new antibiotics, while the emergence of drug resistance in bacteria to all already available antibiotics complicates and challenges the condition (Roca *et al.,* 2015). In order to propose a potential approach to stop the spread of drug resistance, we thus explored the emergence of drug resistance against several classes of antibiotics from a molecular and phenotypic perspective in this chapter.

Historical Perspective of Antimicrobial Discovery

Antimicrobials are the natural, semi-synthetic or synthetic used to treat microbial infections in medicals and veterinary practices. In post antibiotics era, infectious diseases were the most devastating and one of the leading cause of mortality. More than 2000 years ago antibiotics producing microbes were usually used for treating infectious disease in Serbia, China, Greece, and Egypt. The use of moldy bread and medicinal soils to treat infections is mentioned in the ancient text The Ebers Papyrus, an Egyptian medical document dating back to 1550 BC.. Trances of antibiotics (tetracycline) were found in human skeletons from ancient Sudanes Nubia dating back 350-550 CE, and in histological samples of femoral midshafts of the late Roman period skeletons from the Dakhleh Oasis, Egypt. Antibiotics exposures in ancient time were also evidence in anectodal about antibiotic like properties in red soil of Jordan. The red soil of Jordan is still used as inexpensive alternative to modern day's antimicrobial products for treating skin infection. This anectodal was instrumental for discovery of soil dwelling actinomycetals as source of many natural antibiotics. Many medicinal herbs reconsidering to have antimicrobial activity were used as remedies for treating disease since long time in traditional Chinese medicine. The discovery of potent anti-malarial drugs qinghaosu (artemisinin) from Artemisia plants were the best known example of Chinese herbalist which was used for thousands of year as remedy to treat many disease. The credit for foundation of modern era of antibiotics is usually associated with mainly two researchers; Paul Ehrlich and Alexander Fleming. The Paul Ehrlich's idea of magic bullet, means highly selective and targeted killing of disease causing micro-organism, led to development of first synthetic anti-infective arsenic-based pro-drugs salvarsan and neosalvarsan circa to treat syphilis, that is caused by *Treponema pallidum* (Aminov, 2010). In later years, Gerhard Domagk, a bacteriologist at Bayer discovered sulfonamide pro-drug; prontosil, to save his daughter's arm from amputation (Domagk, 1935). Sulfonamides were the first truly effective broad-spectrum antimicrobials in clinical use and are still relevant. Sulfonamides groups of antibiotics were superseded by Penicillin, the first natural antibiotics discovered by Alexander Fleming in 1928 (Fleming, 1929). The protocol developed by Oxford team led by Howard Florey and Ernest Chain for purification of penicillin led to its mass production and distribution in 1945 (Chain *et al.*, 2005) and Penicillin was successfully used to treat bacterial infections in soldiers during World war-II. The discovery of the first three antimicrobials—salvarsan, prontosil, and penicillin—was groundbreaking, as these drugs established the foundation for future research in drug discovery (Aminov, 2010). The period from the 1930s to the 1970s is often referred to as the "golden era" of antibiotics, during which numerous new classes of antibiotics were discovered. However, after this period, no entirely new classes of antibiotics were developed, and subsequent advancements were limited to modifications of existing antibiotics (Chopra *et al.*, 2002).

Emergence of Antimicrobial Resistance

Antimicrobials and antimicrobials resistance coexisted since long as evolutionary and regulatory mechanism of many microbial communities. Trend of inappropriate and in-discriminated use and administration of antimicrobials to treat infection, and to get production in commercial livestock and poultry industry resulted generation and transfer of antimicrobial resistance gene (ARG). Micro-organism of anthropogenic, commensal and environmental origins collectively acts as antibiotic resistome and contributes in transfer of antimicrobial resistance gene. he widespread use and misuse of antimicrobials in human medicine, as well as in disease prevention, control, treatment, and to promote growth in food-producing animals, has significantly contributed to the rise of antimicrobial resistance (AMR). This has led to the transmission of resistant microbes both between individuals and from environmental sources, facilitating the spread of resistance. Alexander Fleming himself warned about the prudent use of penicillin, cautioning that resistance could develop if the drug was used in insufficient doses or for too short a duration during treatment. The first penicillin resistance *Staphylococcus* strain was described in 1940 even before use of penicillin. To encounter penicillinase producing characteristic of penicillin resistance *Staphylococcus aureus* (*S. aureus*), methicillin was introduced as an alternative of penicillin but unfortunately within a year, Methicillin Resistance *S. aureus* (MRSA) was identified in year 1960 (Sengupta *et al.* 2013). Today, MRSA have become a challenge to treat due to resistance against all classes of antibiotics. Further, Vancomycin was introduced for treatment of MRSA, and after two decades in 1979 coagulase-negative *Staphylococci* resistant to vancomycin were described and one decade later vancomycin resistant *Enterococci* (vancomycin-intermediate *S. aureus*, VISA) was identified (Courvalin, 2006) and in the year 1997 vancomycin less sensitive *S. aureus* was reported from Japan (Levine, 2005). Tetracycline antibiotic was first introduced in 1950 and with in the span of 9 year tetracycline resistant *Shigella* strains was indentified. Levofloxacin was become effective against *Pneumoccocus* infection in the year of its introduction for clinical use (Sengupta *et al.*, 2013). With the time and inappropriate use of antibiotics, many mirco-organisms got resistance to multi-drugs and multi-drugs resistance mirco-organisms were evolved.

Molecular Basis of Antimicrobial Drug Resistance

The antibiotic resistance achieved by following two mechanisms viz. (i) Intrinsic resistance (Cox and Wright, 2013) and (ii) Acquired resistance (Van Hoek *et al.*, 2011).

Intrinsic Resistance

Bacterial genome encodes for specific protein that allows innate resistance to some group of antibiotic. This resistance may include (i) have permeability barrier (which restricts antimicrobial access to target sites) (ii) altered cell structure (iii) altered cell metabolism and (iv) detoxification of antibiotic (mediated by drug inactivating enzyme) (Munita and Arias, 2016).

Permeability Barrier

The Gram-negative bacteria's cell wall is made up of a single layer of peptidoglycan that is encircled by an outer membrane with a membranous structure. Lipopolysaccharide (LPS), in addition to porin proteins and phospholipids, is a distinctive component of the outer membrane of Gram-negative bacteria (Shetty *et al.,* 2009). For hydrophobic antibiotics, the LPS acts as a substantial permeability barrier. Porin proteins, however, permit non-specific transport of tiny hydrophilic medicines (Nikaido, 1989; 2003; 2005). Porin levels in bacterial cells can reach 10^6 copies per cell (Vergalli *et al.,* 2020), however cells can control to some extent how permeable their membrane is by controlling how porin expression is regulated in response to environmental cues. Since, porins typically have exclusion limits that are close to the sizes of many antibiotics, they tend to slow down the pace at which these molecules diffuse, which helps to create intrinsic resistance (Mathur *et al.,* 2004). As a result, the type and number of porins a cell has will affect its permeability and, in turn, whether or not it is susceptible to or resistant to antibiotics. But multidrug efflux transporters (efflux pump) further fight this gradual entry of medicines across the outer membrane (Li *et al.,* 1994). Their widespread occurrence in both pathogenic and non-pathogenic bacteria shows that their evolution and spread happened independently of the widespread use of antimicrobials by humans (Sykes *et al.,* 2010). Due to decreased permeability, sulfonamides, ampicillin, first- and second-generation cephalosporins, chloramphenicol, and tetracycline are less effective against *Pseudomonas aeruginosa* (Li *et al.,* 1994). In addition, the sugar-functionalized phospholipids (LPSs) that make up the outer half of the outer membrane have a net negative charge that attracts cationic aminoglycosides (Garneau-Tsodikova and Labby, 2016). Drug transportation is hampered by the modification in net charge, for example, when the positively charged 4-amino-4-deoxy-L-arabinose sugar is incorporated into the LPS layer, thus reducing the net negative charge of the LPS layer and decreasing the affinity for aminoglycosides (Delcour, 2009). In order to develop microbial defense against environmental contaminants, efflux pumps are crucial. For instance, the RND pump "AcrAB-TolC" in the gastrointestinal *Escherichia coli* (*E. coli*) gives protection from bile salt (Koirala *et al.,* 2023).

Efflux pumps

Efflux pumps are transporter proteins that contribute to antibiotic resistance by helping export of harmful or numerous drugs from their cells (Marquez, 2005). When compared to non-specific multi drug resistance systems, which are chromosomally encoded, specific efflux pumps (active against a specific class of drugs) are typically found on mobile elements, contributing to both acquired and intrinsic resistance in both Gram-negative and Gram-positive bacteria (Poole, 2007). The Gram-negative and mycobacterial microorganisms with low permeable envelopes co-operate with the efflux pump. Gram-positive bacteria have a single polypeptide in their cytoplasmic membrane that is part of their efflux system, but Gram-negative bacteria can have a tripartite organization with components in their inner membrane, outer membrane, and periplasm (Hajiagha *et al.*, 2023). Antibiotics can act as inducers and regulators of the expression of certain efflux pumps. Efflux pumps are currently known to confer resistance to practically all antibiotic classes (Lee *et al.*, 2000). Based on the sequence comparison efflux pumps are grouped into five major categories: (i) Adenosine triphosphate (ATP)-binding cassette (ABC) family, (ii) Multidrug and toxic compound extrusion family (MATE), (iii) Major facilitator super-family (MFS) family, (iv) Small multidrug resistance (SMR) family, and (v) Resistance-nodulation-division (RND) family (Webber and Piddock, 2003). Only the ABC-type systems among them uses ATP hydrolysis as a source of energy while other four use proton motive force.

Adenosine Triphosphate (ATP)-binding Cassette (ABC) Family

ABC super-family is the primary transporters. Transporters from the ABC family are involved in the uptake and efflux of a variety of substrates, including proteins, carbohydrates, amino acids, ions, medicines, and polysaccharides (Gupta *et al.*, 2021). This family's proteins or permeases typically have six trans-membrane regions (Akhtar *et al.*, 2022). Many transporters of this type play a role in antibiotic resistance, including the very recently discovered MacAB pump in *E. coli* macrolide-specific resistance (Tabrizi *et al.*, 2021).

Multidrug and Toxic Compound Extrusion Family (MATE)

Gram-positive microbes have mostly been linked to the MATE family when it comes to resistance. The member proteins have 12 trans-membrane regions which utilize sodium gradients to export of toxic compounds like Fluoroquinolones, Aminoglycosides, and cationic dyes (de Morais *et al.*, 2023), for instance, NorM of *Vibrio parahaemolyticus* is a type of MATE transporters for efflux of norfloxacin (Haque *et al.*, 2023).

Major facilitator super-family (MFS) family

The MFS family (chromosome or mobile genetic element) is thought to be the most varied family among the secondary transporters and is primarily connected to Gram-positive bacteria. The member proteins have 12–14 transmembrane areas that they can use for uniport, symport, or antiport functions (Wang *et al.*, 2020). Uniport is the transport of a substrate without associated ion movement. Symport is connected to ion movement in the same direction. Antibiotic efflux is connected to the drug/proton (H^+ or Na^+) antiporters (DHAs) transporter proteins. There are three subfamilies of DHAs transporters: DHA1, DHA2, and DHA3. Only DHA3 has been associated to antibiotic extrusion from Gram-negative and Gram-positive bacteria, including macrolides and tetracycline (Laudy *et al.*, 2018). QacA of *S. aureus*, Bmr of *Bacillus subtilis* and EmrB from *E. coli* come under DHA3 subfamilies.

Small Multidrug Resistance (SMR) family

SMR family proteins often form tetramers in the cytoplasmic membrane and have four trans-membrane regions (Poulsen, 2012). Only a small number of SMR transporter proteins have been linked to antibiotics (Bay *et al.,* 2009). For instance, AbeS of A.baumannii and EmrEof,E. coli (Lalaurie *et al.*, 2018)

Resistance-nodulation-division (RND) family

Several members of Gram-negative bacteria have genes linked with RND multidrug efflux pumps that are primarily chromosomally encoded and primarily offer intrinsic resistance, in contrast to other well-known horizontally acquired antibiotic resistance determinants (Alvarez-Ortega *et al.*, 2013). The RND transporters consist of three components: two sizable periplasmic loop proteins, an outer membrane protein known as a channel-tunnel, and an inner membrane pump protein or membrane fusion protein with 12 transmembrane domains. Individual subunits appear to engage and then disengage substrate molecules in a rotatory manner as the entire system is alternatively protonated. Numerous classes of antibiotics, biocides, poisonous fatty acids, bile salts, aromatic hydrocarbons, inhibitors of fatty acid biosynthesis, detergents, homoserine lactones, and dyes are among the many substrates that the RND pumps are known to export (Scoffone *et al.*, 2021). AcrAB-TolC from E. coli and MexAB-OprM from *Pseudomonas aeruginosa* (*P. aeruginosa*) are the two RND pumps with the best characterization (Poole *et al.*, 2001)

Altered Cell Structure

Because *Mycoplasma* lacks a cell wall, they are naturally resistant to penicillin (Bebear and Pereyre, 2005). Aztreonam (monobactam) binds poorly to the penicillin binding protein (PBP) sites of Gram-positive bacteria and so has relatively ineffective inhibitory effects against these bacteria. However, it has a high affinity for the protein-binding protein 3 (PBP-3) of Gram-negative bacteria (Lo et al., 2008). *Listeria monocytogenes* is inherently resistant to broad spectrum cephalosporin antibiotics and proteins involved in the formation and modification of peptidoglycans, cell-envelope proteins with structural or general detoxifying functions, cytoplasmic proteins with unknown functions, and regulatory proteins (Bierne and Cossart, 2007; Krawczyk-Balska and Markiewicz, 2016). Due to the v*anC* gene, Gram-negative bacteria are resistant to glycopeptides (vancomycin). The outcome is that Gram-negative bacteria become resistant to the action of vancomycin because the peptidoglycan tetra-peptide has an altered tail with D-ala-D-ser instead of D-ala-D-ala (Courvalin, 2006).

Cell Metabolism (Lack of Synthetic Pathways Targeted by drug)

As a result of their dietary dependence on purines and pyrimidines rather than folic acid, M*ycoplasma* and *Chlamydia* are resistant to sulphonamide and trimethoprim (Wehelie, 2006). Also, naturally resistant to trimethoprim are *Neisseria, Brucella, Bacteroides, Clostridium*, and *Moraxella* species (Schwarz and Noble, 1999; LaPlante *et al*., 2016).

Detoxification of Antibiotic

Beta lactamase in *Entrobacteriacae* and AmpC in *Pseudomonas,* both provide inherent resistance to beta-lactam drugs (Livermore and Woodford, 2006; Jacoby, 2009). Goat and cow rumen microbes have the ability to inactivate numerous classes of antibiotics. But neither the name of the accountable bacteria nor the make-up of the goods are known (Chaucheyras-Durand *et al*., 2008; Hungate, 2013).

Acquired Resistance

Bacteria acquired drug resistance subsequent exposure of drug (Grkovic *et al*., 2002). These types of resistance fall into two categories: drug resistance in bacteria owing to mutation (changes to the target site and existing bacterial proteins that result in reduced permeability) (Sahare *et al*., 2013; Sharma *et al*., 2014) and drug resistance acquired through horizontal gene transfer and the acquisition of new genetic material in bacteria of the same or different species or genera (mediated by the acquisition of mobile genetic elements by conjugation, transformation, and transduction) include the acquisition of drug detoxification enzymes (enzymatic modification or degradation of the antibiotic), target site protection enzymes (modification of antibiotic targets) and efflux pumpproteins (Kelly *et al.,* 2009).

Acquired drug resistance by mutational changes in microbes

a. Reduced Permeability (mutation in porins and over-expression of efflux pump)

Antibiotics are known to be transported through a size-selective channel by porins, which are found in the outer membrane of Gram-negative and *Mycobacterium* bacteria. The bulk of porin proteins are so-called universal porins, which permit non-specific diffusion of hydrophilic medicines based on size (up to 600 Da) (Ziervogel, 2012). However, some porin proteins (special porins) have a binding site that is only moderately selective for a particular class of chemicals, and they only express under specific growth-restraining circumstances (Welte *et al*., 1995). As a result, generic porins play a significant role in defining the permeability characteristics of Gram-negative bacteria's outer membranes. While bigger antibiotics like erythromycin or novobiocin are thought to enter the outer membrane through lipid bilayer by diffusion, which is expected to be slow, most hydrophilic and amphiphilic antibiotics reach the periplasm through porins (Fernández and Hancock, 2012; Zgurskaya *et al.,* 2015). Antibiotic diffusion is slowed down by mutations that affect porin selectivity, porin down-regulation, or porin deletion. For instance, point muatation in *E. coli* reduces the expression of PorinOprD makes *P. aeruginosa* carbapenem-resistant, whereas porinOmpF causes resistance to β-lactams (Majewski *et al*., 2020). OmpFporine of an isolate of *Enterobacter cloacae* is ertapenem resistant (Pal et al., 2019). The G-to-D mutation in loop 3 of the OmpF/OmpC-like protein in Enterobacter aerogenes leads to a loss of pore conductance, which in turn reduces the bacteria's susceptibility to β-lactams (Wang *et al*., 2020). Additionally, due to changes in loop 3 of the porin PIB, *Neisseria gonorrhoeae* develop resistance to penicillin and tetracycline (Laudy *et al.,* 2018). While a D116A mutation in OmpU causes less cephalosporin binding in *Vibrio cholerae.* Several resistant *E. coli* isolates have constriction zone mutations that restricted the passage of cefotaxime and other β-lactams through the OmpC channel (Haque *et al*., 2023). Additionally, occasionally, drug resistance against particular antibiotic classes may result from mutations in porinc regulatory proteins. For instance, a mutation in the ompB operon, which contains the genes *ompR* and *envZ* and is known to control OmpC and OmpF production in *E. coli,* results in cefoxitin resistance (Miller *et al*., 2016). Along with porins, efflux pumps over expression is linked to altered cell membrane permeability. Occasionally, changes to regulatory proteins may increase a pump's effectiveness in pushing antibiotics out of the cell. An RND transporter of *P. aeruginosa* with the mutation F1018L substitution enhanced resistance to aminoglycosides, fluoroquinolones, and the β-lactam cefepime. Similar to this, *Salmonella enterica* serovar Typhimurium acquired fluoroquinolone resistance due to the IS1 or IS10 insertion element in the promoter region of the AcrEF coding genes.

b. Alteration in Target Site (mutation on drug binding site)

As a results of mutation there is alteration in amino acid sequence of target site results in either complete loss or reduction of binding affinity of target site with antimicrobials (Lambert, 2005).

Acquired drug resistance by new gene by horizontal gene transfer

Mobile genetic elements are associated with capture, accumulation and dissemination of resistance genes among same species and different microbial species (Partridge *et al.,* 2018). They also known to promote intracellular DNA mobility (e.g., from chromosome to a plasmid or plasmid to plasmid). There are several genetic mobile elements are known that are associated with horizontal gene transfer among same species or different species of bacteria (Stokes and Gillings, 2011).

Drug Detoxification

The drug detoxification is achieved by either modification of drug by transfer of new group or by destruction of chemical structure of antimicrobials (Wright, 2005). The modification is carried out by transfer of different groups on antibiotics such as acetic acid, nucleotide, phosphate etc with the help of wide varieties of antimicrobials modifying enzymes (Kimura and Bugg, 2003). Whereas the disruption of chemical structure is take place by de-cyclization, hydrolysis and esterase activity of enzymes.

Target Site Protection

There are two class of target protecting enzyme were identified. Enzyme hinder the binding affinity of target site by transfer of certain groups such as methylate in order to protect target site from binding with antimicrobials (Dessen *et al.,* 2001) whereas, an another class of target protecting enzyme that are known to catalyze the GTP-dependent release of drug from the target site eg. Tetracycline release from ribosome by tetO, tetM and tetP. The tetP of *Clostridium perfringens* have overlapping genetic unit act for both ribosomal protection and efflux mechanism (Vester and Ntokou, 2017).

Drug Insensitive Target

Some of microbes known to carry drug insensitive target having similar biological function. Thereby, on exposure of antimicrobials they ensure survivability. For example sulphonamide drug resistance reported in several bacterial families such as *Staphylococci* and *Enterobacteriacae* due to acquisition of drug insensitive enzyme dihydrophoratesynthatase (Sul1, Sul2 and Sul3 encoded) (Wang et al., 2014; Gong et al., 2018). Similarly β-lactum resistance reported by acquisition of drug insensitive enzyme PBP2a (mecA encoded) in MRSA (Kim et al., 2012; Müller *et al.*, 2015). The phenotypic foundation of antimicrobial drug resistance (also known as antibiotic tolerance) which is temporary and often reverts once the environmental trigger factor is removed (Corona and Martinez, 2013). The over expression and activation of multidrug transporters (efflux pump), over production of drug target enzymes, and biofilm development is included tolerance (Kvist *et al.*, 2008; Blair *et al.*, 2014). Biofilm provides a multilayered resistance for microbes by allowing poor antibiotic penetration and the production of persister cells (Olsen, 2015). *Neisseria* and *S. aureus* have a hyper production of p-aminobenzoic acid and over production of chromosomal DHFR in *E. coli* and TMP-resistant *Hemophilus influenza* (Then, 1982). Microbes can alter their transcriptome very rapidly in response to changes in the surrounding environment or may exposure of nonlethal doses of antimicrobials, which eventually leads to greater ability of survival of microbes via temporary acquisition of resistance to a given antibiotic.

Antimicrobial Resistance Markers (ARM)

The use of antimicrobial resistance markers plays a crucial role in genetic engineering by facilitating the selection of recombinant clones through artificial screening methods. This not only saves time but also ensures high accuracy in identifying appropriate recombinants. The advantages of using antimicrobial resistance markers include:

- **Differentiation of transformed and untransformed cells:** Transformed cells can be distinguished from untransformed ones based on their ability to grow in the presence of an antibiotic.
- **Reduction in untransformed cells:** The use of resistance markers significantly decreases the number of untransformed cells.
- **Time-saving in selection:** The markers help expedite the process of identifying transformed cells.

- **Molecular detection of resistance:** Techniques such as PCR can be used to detect antibiotic resistance at the molecular level.

Classification of Antibiotic Resistance Genes by their Biological Distribution

If the transfer of an antibiotic resistance gene from the genome of a transgenic organism to that of a bacterium should occur at all, the risk associated with this very rare event should be viewed against the presence of antibiotic resistance genes in soil, plant, water and enteric bacteria. Furthermore, consideration must be given to the importance of specific antibiotics in therapeutic use. On the basis of these two criteria for evaluation, the antibiotic resistance genes have been assigned to three groups:

Group I

Group I contains antibiotic resistance genes which are already widely distributed among soil and enteric bacteria and confer resistance to antibiotics which have no or only minor therapeutic relevance in human medicine and only restricted use in defined areas of veterinary medicine. It is therefore extremely unlikely (if at all) that the presence of these antibiotic resistance genes in the genome of transgenic organisms will change the already existing bulk spread of these antibiotic resistance genes in the environment or will impact significantly on human and animal health. This refers to the following two antibiotic resistance genes.

nptII gene

The substrates of the APH (3′)II enzymes include the antibiotics, kanamycin, neomycin, paromycin, butirosin, gentamicin B and geneticin (G 418). The antibiotics of this category which are relevant for human therapy, amikacin, gentamicin (predominantly C1, C1a and C2) and other aminoglycosides and aminocyclitoles, are not substrates for the APH (3′)-II enzymes. The *npt*II gene is widely spread in micro-organisms in the environment.

hph gene

Hygromycin is not used in human therapy, and there is no cross-resistance with other antibiotics used for human therapy. The antibiotic was originally developed for veterinary use and is still added in some parts of the world to animal feed as an anthelmintic.

Group II

Group II includes antibiotic resistance genes that are commonly found in microorganisms in various environmental settings such as soil, plants, water, and the mammalian gut. These genes confer resistance to antibiotics that are used in human and veterinary medicine. The presence of these resistance genes in the genomes of transgenic organisms is unlikely to significantly contribute to the spread of these genes in the environment, and therefore should have minimal impact on human or animal health, if any. As a result, these genes in genetically modified organisms (GMOs) do not contribute to the emergence or spread of antibiotic resistance in bacteria. This category includes the following antibiotic resistance genes:

CmR gene

Chloramphenicol-resistant micro-organisms are widely distributed in the environment, and many of these carry the *CmR* gene. In the EU, chloramphenicol is rarely used for medical purposes because of the risk of causing aplastic anaemia and has not been authorized for use in food-producing animals.

ampr gene

It is reasonable to assume that almost every person on earth harbours or has harboured *Escherichia coli* cells containing the *ampr* gene in their intestinal tract, even without exposure to β-lactam antibiotics. This is supported by the finding that approximately 35% of all clinical E. coli isolates are resistant to ampicillin (Kresken *et al.*, 1999), with 90% of these resistances being attributed to the presence of TEM-1 β-lactamases (Livermore, 1995). Studies have also demonstrated that approximately 74% of all *E. coli* isolates from cattle and swine are ampicillin resistant. Thus, even in the light of the clinical relevance of ampicillin, the presence of *ampR* (bla gene) in transgenes is not seen to siginificantly alter the existing pool of already resistant bacteria.

Group III

Group III includes antibiotic resistance genes that confer resistance to antibiotics highly relevant for human therapy. Regardless of the perceived risk, these genes should be avoided in the genomes of transgenic plants to maintain the highest standards of preventive health care. This category includes the following antibiotic resistance genes:

nptIII gene

This gene is most frequently used antibiotic resistant marker in plant gene technology. *npt* III inactivate the aminoglycoside groups of antibiotics very easily. Aminoglycoside group of antibiotics such as neomycin, kanamycin, amikacin etc are important reserve antibiotic for human medicine and veterinary medicine. The bacteria may take this gene resistance from waste of these genetically modified plants and may become resistance to Aminoglycoside group of antibiotics. Therefore, inclusion of the *nptIII* gene in the establishment of genetically modified plants may impair medicinal relevance of aminoglycoside group of antibiotics.

tetA gene

Tetracyclines are characterized by their wide spectrum of action and continue to be of therapeutic importance in human medicine; they are used to control *Brucella, Chlamydia, Mycoplasma, Rickettsia, Vibrio,* etc.

Antimicrobial Resistance and One Health

The rapid emergence of antimicrobial-resistant (AMR) pathogens has been a growing threat for decades, endangering global health systems and the environment. Key contributors to this rise in resistance include the misuse and overuse of antimicrobials in both human and veterinary medicine, as well as environmental pollution from hospital and pharmaceutical waste (UNEP, 2022). Additionally, the shift from extensive to intensive farming practices has increased the reliance on antimicrobial growth promoters. Contaminated water used for irrigation, plant spraying, and washing vegetables and fruits can further spread resistant pathogens. Similar to humans, animals can also become infected by pathogens resistant to multiple antibiotics, which would otherwise be effective for treatment. Wildlife, plants, and the environment are equally impacted by this growing threat. The emergence of AMR is therefore deeply interconnected with the relationships between animals, humans, and the environment, highlighting the need for a One Health approach to effectively combat AMR. Since 2010, organizations such as the World Health Organization (WHO), the World Organization for Animal Health (WOAH), and the UN Food and Agriculture Organization (FAO) have taken leadership roles in raising awareness, coordinating efforts, and driving responses to AMR. This increased focus culminated in the World Health Assembly's endorsement of the Global Action Plan (GAP) on AMR in May 2015, urging member states to develop National Action Plans (NAPs) to tackle AMR. The UN General Assembly's adoption of the Political Declaration on AMR in September 2016 marked another major step in the global fight. Subsequently, the Interagency Coordination Group on Antimicrobial Resistance was formed, and the One Health Global Leadership Group was established. In May 2022, the Tripartite Alliance became the Quadripartite Alliance on One Health with the addition of the United Nations Environment Programme (UNEP), emphasizing the need for a One Health approach to preserve antimicrobial efficacy and ensure equitable, responsible access to antimicrobials in human, animal, and plant health. At the national level, many countries have joined the global effort against AMR (Table 1). For instance, during its G7 Presidency in 2015, the German government committed to a One Health approach and pledged support for the WHO's GAP and NAPs on AMR. In 2017, Germany instigated the creation of the Global Antimicrobial Resistance Research and Development Hub, and continued to address AMR during its G7 Presidency in 2022. India has made significant progress in addressing AMR and can serve as a model for other low-resource countries. Since 2007, the Bureau of Indian Standards has banned the use of antibiotics for growth promotion in poultry, following the European Union's example. The Indian Ministry of Health and Family Welfare developed a national policy on the judicious use of antibiotics in human medicine, and the National Livestock Policy has promoted cautious antibiotic use in livestock. Additionally, the Drug Controller General of India has specified withdrawal periods for antibiotics in poultry, livestock, and seafood, while the Food Safety and Standards Authority of India (FSSAI) has issued guidelines on antibiotic residue limits in meat and meat products. India's National Action Plan (NAP) for AMR, a five-year strategy (2017–2021) developed by the Union Ministry of Health and Family Welfare and led by the National Centre for Disease Control (NCDC), was launched in April 2017. Following the NAP's guidelines, various states in India have initiated their own State Action Plans (Dasgupta *et al.*, 2021). India has also strengthened its AMR surveillance network and joined the WHO Global Antimicrobial Resistance Surveillance System (GLASS). The WHO-ESBL-E. coli Tricycle project, adopted by India, bridges the research gap on AMR prevalence across human, animal, and environmental sectors, employing a true One Health approach. Several recent initiatives have further promoted the One Health concept in India: (i) the establishment of a National Expert Group on One Health, (ii) the creation of the National Institute of One Health in Nagpur, Maharashtra, and (iii) the development of Integrated Public Health Laboratories (Dasgupta *et al.*, 2021). Both central and state governments are increasingly adopting One Health approaches to address the rapid rise of AMR, zoonoses, and food safety concerns (Ranjalkar and Chandy, 2019). However, India still faces significant challenges in implementing mitigation strategies for AMR in the wildlife and agriculture sectors.

Table 1: Integrated antimicrobial resistance surveillance program (reproduced from Biswas et al., 2022).

Year	Name of the programme	Aims of the programme	Nodal authority
1994	WHONET	To provide free software and training to the laboratories for enabling standardized data collection and analysis	WHO
1995	Danish Integrated Antimicrobial Resistance Monitoring and Research Program (DANMAP)	I. AMR surveillance in human and animal clinical cases, healthy animals, locally produced and imported meat products at wholesale and retail outlets II. Antibiotic consumption surveillance in human and animal hospitals, primary healthcare centers and pharmacies	Ministry of Health and the Ministry of Food, Agriculture and Fisheries, Denmark
1995	Swedish Strategic Programme Against Antibiotic Resistance (STRAMA)	AMR and antibiotic consumption surveillance in human	Sweden
1996	Latin American network for antimicrobial resistance surveillance (ReLAVRA)	Surveillance of resistance in the pathogens isolated from community and hospitals	Pan American Health Organization
1996	Asian network for surveillance of resistant pathogens (ANSORP)	Surveillance of resistance in human hospital associated pathogens (pneumococcus) in Asia	Asia Pacific Foundation for Infectious Diseases
1996	National Antimicrobial Resistance Monitoring System (NARMS)	Monitoring antimicrobial resistance in enteric bacteria from human, retail meat, and food animals	USA
1997	The European Committee on Antimicrobial Susceptibility Testing (EUCAST)	To provide technical aspects of phenotypic *in vitro* antimicrobial susceptibility testing	ECDC, European Society of Clinical Microbiology and Infectious Diseases (ESCMID)
1998	European Antimicrobial Resistance Surveillance Network(EARS-Net)	Data collection from public health laboratories in European Union countries, data management, analysis and validation	European Centre for Disease Prevention and Control (ECDC)
1998	Monitoring of Antimicrobial Resistance and Antimicrobial Use in Animals in Netherlands (MARAN)	AMR and antibiotic consumption surveillance in animals, crops, fruits, vegetables, herbs	Netherlands

Year	Name of the programme	Aims of the programme	Nodal authority
1999	Central Asian and Eastern European Surveillance of Antimicrobial Resistance (CAESAR)	Network of national AMR surveillance systems and it comprises all countries of the WHO European Region that are not part of the EARS-Net	WHO
1999	The European Centre for the Study of Animal Health (CEESA)	Surveillance of AMR in healthy livestock at slaughter, clinically sick food and companion animals	ECDC
1999	Japanese Veterinary Antimicrobial Resistance Monitoring System (JVARM)	AMR and antibiotic consumption surveillance in food animals Japan	Japan
1999	National Observatory of the Epidemiology of Bacterial Resistance to Antibiotics (ONERBA)	AMR and antibiotic consumption surveillance in human, food animals, food	France
2000	Global Foodborne Infections Network (GNF)	I. Integrated AMR surveillance. II. Interdivisional coordination among human health, veterinary and food-related disciplines through training courses and events.	WHO
2000	Swedish Veterinary Antimicrobial Resistance Monitoring Programme (SVARM)	AMR and antibiotic consumption surveillance in animals	Sweden
2001	European Surveillance of Antimicrobial Consumption Network (ESAC-Net)	Collection of data on systemic use of antibiotics, antifungals and antivirals in hospital and community in EU countries	ECDC
2001	GermVet	AMR and antibiotic consumption surveillance in food animals	Germany
2003	Italian Veterinary Antimicrobial Resistance Monitoring (ITAVARM)	AMR and antibiotic consumption surveillance in food animals	Italy
2005	CODEX Alimentarius, (CXC 61–2005)	AMR surveillance in humans, food animals, crops and food	FAO & WHO
2005	The Healthcare Associated Infection Network (HAI-Net)	Surveillance of AMR and antimicrobial use in acute and long-term care services	ECDC
2006	Canadian integrated program for antimicrobial resistance surveillance (CIPARS)	AMR and antibiotic consumption surveillance in human, food animals, food items	Canada

Year	Name of the programme	Aims of the programme	Nodal authority
2008	Advisory Group on Integrated Surveillance of Antimicrobial Resistance (AGISAR)	I. To establish uniform sampling techniques and methodology for isolation of bacteria and detection of antibiotic resistance II. To afford expert advice III. To stimulate information sharing and supporting capacity-building for AMR surveillance and antimicrobial practice in member country.	WHO
2009	Transatlantic Taskforce on Antimicrobial Resistance (TATFAR)	I. To sponsor appropriate use of antimicrobials in human and veterinary medicine. II. To stop resistant infections in hospital and communities. III. To advance development of new antimicrobials	CDC (USA) and European Union
2010	European Surveillance of Veterinary Antimicrobial Consumption (ESVAC)	Collection of harmonized data on the sales of veterinary antimicrobials (wholesalers, veterinarians, pharmacies)	ECDC
2011	Joint Programming Initiative on Antimicrobial Resistance (JPIAMR)	To assist transnational research and activities in the selected areas such as therapeutics, diagnostics, surveillance, transmission, environment and interventions	European Commission
2012	Viet Nam resistance project (VINARES)	Monitoring antimicrobial resistance in enteric bacteria from human	Viet Nam
2012	Indian network for surveillance of antimicrobial resistance (INSAR)	Monitoring antimicrobial resistance in human	India
2013	Anti-microbial resistance surveillance and research network (AMRSN)	Effective development of a stewardship program	India (ICMR)
2015	Global Antimicrobial Resistance Surveillance System (GLASS)	To give support worldwide surveillance and research in order to reinforce the evidence base on antimicrobial resistance (AMR)	WHO
2017	Indian network for fishery and animals antimicrobial resistance (INFAAR)	Monitoring antimicrobial resistance in livestock, poultry and fishery	ICAR. India
2018	FINRES-Vet	AMR and antibiotic consumption surveillance in food animals	Finland
2020	NethMap	AMR and antibiotic consumption surveillance in human	Netherlands

Methods to Identify AMR

Antibiotic resistance has become a critical global health issue, and unless we can reverse the current trajectory, we risk entering a post-antibiotic era. Diagnostic testing plays a key role in managing this challenge by helping to optimize the use of antibiotics. At a high level, rapid diagnostic assays that can differentiate between viral and bacterial infections are crucial, as they can prevent unnecessary antibiotic treatments. For bacterial infections, accurately identifying the pathogen and its antibiotic susceptibility is vital for tailoring treatment and avoiding the misuse of broad-spectrum drugs. Traditional diagnostic methods used in clinical microbiology can take up to 48 hours or more to yield conclusive results, but newer rapid tests can provide valuable information within hours. While rapid tests benefit individual patients, diagnostics have a much broader role in combating antimicrobial resistance (AMR) by supporting antimicrobial stewardship, surveillance, and epidemiological research. For instance, rapid susceptibility testing is essential for the development of new anti-infective agents, while real-time data on local AMR trends is crucial for guiding appropriate therapy and guiding public health efforts.

Traditional Methods of AMR Detection

Traditional methods for detecting antimicrobial resistance (AMR) primarily rely on identifying the morphological and biochemical characteristics of bacterial colonies. This often begins with culturing samples on non-selective or enriched media to detect the presence of bacterial growth. Subsequently, selective media are used to favor the growth of the target bacteria while inhibiting the growth of others. Phenotypic methods such as microscopy, enzymatic activity tests, and antibiotic susceptibility assays, including the Minimum Inhibitory Concentration (MIC), disk diffusion, and E-test, are then employed to assess the resistance profile.

Minimum Inhibitory Concentration (MIC)

The MIC test is one of the most widely used techniques to determine antimicrobial susceptibility. This method involves inoculating an agar or broth with a defined bacterial concentration and exposing it to varying concentrations of an antimicrobial agent. The MIC is the lowest concentration of the drug that visibly inhibits bacterial growth. This straightforward and low-cost approach does not require specialized equipment, making it accessible for many laboratories. Once the MIC is determined, clinicians can adjust treatment protocols to ensure effective therapy, using the drug concentration that effectively controls bacterial growth.

Disk Diffusion Method

In the disk diffusion method, a paper disc impregnated with an antimicrobial agent is placed on an agar plate inoculated with bacteria. As the drug diffuses from the disc, it creates a zone of inhibition where bacterial growth is prevented. The size of this zone indicates the susceptibility of the bacteria to the drug. This method is qualitative, categorizing bacterial samples as resistant, intermediate, or susceptible. It's particularly effective for rapidly growing bacteria and is simple to perform, which makes it widely used in routine clinical settings.

E-test

The E-test is a hybrid between the disk diffusion and MIC methods. This test involves placing a plastic strip with a continuous gradient of antimicrobial concentrations onto an inoculated agar plate. The point where bacterial growth intersects the gradient indicates the MIC. Although it shares some limitations with the previous methods, such as requiring time for bacterial growth, the E-test offers a simpler and more direct way to measure antimicrobial susceptibility, especially for pathogens that are difficult to culture.

Molecular Methods

Polymerase Chain Ceaction (PCR)

PCR is an essential molecular technique used to detect bacteria and antimicrobial resistance (AMR) genes. Unlike traditional cultivation methods, PCR can identify microorganisms that are non-culturable or dead, enabling detection of genetic material from a broader range of pathogens. This ability to amplify genes from viable or non-viable organisms makes PCR especially valuable for investigating infections caused by difficult-to-culture bacteria or those present in low numbers. PCR can be multiplexed, allowing simultaneous detection of multiple pathogens or resistance genes in a single test. For example, a multiplex PCR assay can target several AMR genes in one run, providing a comprehensive snapshot of the resistance profile.

PCR Combined with Restriction Fragment Length Polymorphism (PCR–RFLP)

PCR–RFLP involves using restriction enzymes to digest amplified DNA into fragments based on nucleotide sequence patterns. These fragments are then analyzed to identify specific AMR genes. This method is highly effective for confirming the presence of resistance genes, although it can be time-consuming and expensive due to the need for multiple steps and specialized reagents.

Despite these drawbacks, PCR–RFLP remains a valuable tool for studying resistance at the genetic level.

Real-Time PCR (qPCR)

Real-time PCR, or quantitative PCR (qPCR), improves on traditional PCR by providing faster results and the ability to quantify the amount of target DNA or RNA present in a sample. Unlike standard PCR, qPCR monitors the amplification process in real-time, allowing for a more precise measurement of microbial load and resistance gene expression. While qPCR is more expensive than conventional PCR, it can provide important insights into the relative abundance of resistance genes. However, challenges such as microbial inhibitors in environmental or food samples, as well as the need for precise interpretation of gene expression data, must be considered when using qPCR in AMR diagnostics.

Microarray

Microarray technology enables the simultaneous detection of thousands of genes by hybridizing DNA or RNA from a sample with specific probes on a solid surface. This method is particularly useful for studying gene expression related to AMR. It can detect resistance genes directly from the DNA sample without the need for prior bacterial culture, making it faster than traditional methods. Although microarrays were once the gold standard for genomic studies, they have been largely superseded by next-generation sequencing (NGS) technologies, which offer even greater sensitivity and resolution.

Whole-Genome Sequencing (WGS) and Metagenomics

The advent of next-generation sequencing (NGS) technologies has revolutionized our ability to study AMR at the genetic level. WGS involves sequencing the entire genome of an organism, enabling researchers to identify not only resistance genes but also the broader genetic context, including potential virulence factors. The ability to assemble sequenced DNA into contigs using computational tools allows researchers to pinpoint resistance markers and trace their transmission across populations. Moreover, metagenomics allows for the study of entire microbial communities, providing insights into resistance dynamics within complex environments, such as hospitals or the human microbiome. Although NGS is more costly and requires specialized equipment, its unparalleled accuracy and ability to detect novel resistance genes make it an invaluable tool for comprehensive AMR surveillance.

Preventive Strategy to Minimize AMR

Antimicrobial resistance (AMR) is a global challenge, and addressing it requires urgent and coordinated action from both the scientific community and governments worldwide (Michael *et al.*, 2014). As a result, various strategies have emerged from researchers to combat AMR, including: (i) minimizing or banning the use of antibiotics, (ii) exploring alternative therapies (such as bacteriophage therapy, biological response modifiers (BMRs), antibacterial peptides from natural sources, and new antibiotic discovery, though the latter is time-consuming and costly), (iii) host-based therapies (like immune therapy, vaccination, and targeting host factors that are essential for both the host and bacteria), and (iv) repurposing existing drugs (to enhance drug entry into target cells, block efflux pumps, or protect drugs from inactivation through combination therapies) (Organization, 2001).

Minimize the use of Antibiotics

While minimizing or even banning the use of antibiotics might seem like a solution to reduce antibiotic resistance, it is not a permanent fix. Even without antibiotic use, resistant bacteria can persist due to beneficial mutations or gene acquisition, leading to the continued presence of resistant clones (Johnsen *et al.*, 2009). Additionally, phenotypic mutations, such as overexpression of efflux pumps or biofilm formation, may temporarily subside but could re-emerge upon re-exposure to antibiotics. For example, resistance to sulphamethoxazole and streptomycin in E. coli remained stable even without the use of these antibiotics (Maertens *et al.*, 2006). Thus, while reducing antibiotic use may slow the spread of resistance, it is not a long-term solution on its own.

Alternative Therapies

(a) Bacteriophage therapy

Bacteriophages, viruses that infect and kill specific bacteria, present a promising alternative treatment for bacterial infections. These phages are selective, meaning they cause minimal toxicity to humans and animals (Viertel *et al.*, 2014). However, while this approach is theoretically sound, it still requires extensive clinical trials and further research before it can be widely adopted in animal or human therapies.

(b) Biological Response Modifiers (BMRs)

Biological response modifiers (BMRs) play a crucial role in optimizing the microbial flora of the intestines, which can, in turn, improve overall health and reduce the incidence of infectious diseases in animals (Ashraf *et al.*, 2019).

For example, antibacterial peptides derived from natural sources, such as beta-defensins found in cow's milk, may offer potential for combating infections (Brogden *et al.*, 2003; Goldammer *et al.*, 2004; Jarczak *et al.*, 2013).

Discovery of New Antibiotics

The discovery of new antibiotics has been a slow and costly process. From the 1970s to the 2000s, the development of new antibiotic classes stagnated. However, some new candidates are emerging through wide-scale screening efforts. For example, Iclaprim, a dihydrofolate reductase inhibitor, is currently in Phase III clinical trials (Hawser *et al.*, 2006). Similarly, new chimeric peptidomimetic antibiotics, such as OMPTA (Outer Membrane Protein Targeting Antibiotics), are currently undergoing preclinical toxicology studies.

Use of Phytochemicals

In light of the growing prevalence of drug-resistant pathogens, there has been increasing interest in the antimicrobial properties of plant-derived compounds, which have long been used in traditional medicine. These plant-based substances are a rich source of secondary metabolites with antimicrobial activity, particularly against bacteria and fungi. The pharmaceutical and scientific communities are investigating these natural products for their potential to combat infectious diseases. Many of these compounds are becoming valuable resources in the search for new antimicrobial agents, and with advances in technology, these plant-derived molecules may soon be developed into therapeutic tools (Jouany and Morgavi, 2007; Savoia, 2012).

Host-Based Therapies

(a) Immuno-stimulators

Stress can compromise the immune system, leading to an increased susceptibility to infections due to elevated cortisol levels. In such cases, using immuno-stimulators, such as vitamins A, C, and E, can help bolster the immune response and reduce the risk of infectious diseases (Buford and Willoughby, 2008).

(b) Vaccination

Vaccination plays a crucial role in preventing infections and improving resistance to major pathogens. For instance, vaccination with outer membrane complexes has been shown to provide rapid protection against multidrug-resistant Acinetobacter baumannii (McConnell *et al.*, 2011). Additionally, combining vaccination with antibiotic therapy, such as hyperimmune sera, has proven effective in treating certain infectious diseases.

(c) Targeting Host Factors

Some drugs target host factors that are indispensable for both the host and bacteria. For example, phosphodiesterase inhibitors like verdenafil have been explored for their ability to modulate the inflammatory response during *Mycobacterium tuberculosis* infection (Schepers *et al.*, 2019). Such host-targeting approaches offer alternative avenues for treating infections without directly targeting the pathogen.

Repurposing Existing Antibiotics

Many bacteria resist existing antibiotics through mechanisms such as efflux pump overexpression, biofilm formation, antimicrobial inactivating enzymes, and mutations in carrier porin proteins (Wright, 2007; Schweizer, 2012). To restore the effectiveness of these antibiotics, it is essential to target and disrupt these protective mechanisms. Several natural bioactive compounds derived from plants, animals, and microbes have shown promise in restoring the potency of antibiotics. For example, beta-lactamase inhibitors, which are commonly used in conjunction with beta-lactam antibiotics, help combat infections caused by beta-lactam-resistant microbes (Bush and Bradford, 2019). This approach of repurposing existing drugs, either alone or in combination with other agents, is a promising strategy for overcoming antibiotic resistance.

Conclusion

Antimicrobial resistance (AMR) represents one of the most urgent and complex global health challenges, with significant implications for human, animal, and environmental health. The mechanisms of AMR, ranging from genetic mutations in microbes to the spread of resistance genes through horizontal gene transfer, highlight the adaptability of bacteria and other pathogens. As resistance to critical antibiotics continues to increase, the need for innovative strategies to mitigate this threat has never been more critical. Preventive strategies aimed at minimizing antibiotic use, developing alternative therapies, and enhancing host-based immune responses are essential components of the global fight against AMR. While reducing the use of antibiotics can slow resistance, it is not a panacea. The persistence of resistant strains, even in the absence of antibiotic pressure, underscores the necessity for integrated approaches that include the development of new antibiotics, alternative therapies such as bacteriophage therapy, and the use of biological response modifiers and natural compounds. In addition to exploring alternative therapeutic options, repurposing existing antibiotics through strategies like combination therapies and overcoming bacterial protective mechanisms (such as efflux pumps and biofilms) offers a practical approach to restoring the effectiveness of older drugs. Immuno-stimulants, vaccination, and targeting host factors provide promising avenues for boosting the body's natural defense systems without directly targeting pathogens. Ultimately, the battle against AMR requires a global, coordinated effort that integrates the principles of the One Health approach, addressing the interconnectedness of human, animal, and environmental health. The ongoing work of international organizations like the WHO, FAO, and WOAH, along with national and regional initiatives, is critical in shaping policies and action plans that curb the rise of resistant pathogens. While the road ahead is challenging, the continued development of innovative treatments and preventive measures, alongside more responsible antibiotic use, provides hope for safeguarding public health and preserving the effectiveness of antimicrobials for future generations.

References

Alvarez-Ortega, C., et al. (2013). Role of Resistance-nodulation-division (RND) Efflux Pumps in Antibiotic Resistance in Gram-negative Bacteria. FEMS Microbiology Reviews, 37(3), 708-734.

Aminov, R. I. (2010). History of Antibiotics and Their Role in Public Health. In Antibiotics: A Key to Bacterial Pathogenesis (pp. 9-20). Springer.

Aminov, R. I. (2017). History of Antimicrobials and Antimicrobial Resistance. In Antimicrobial Resistance in the Environment (pp. 3-17). Springer.

Ashraf, S., Hassan, S. A., & Ahmed, R. (2019). "Role of biological response modifiers in optimizing microbial flora and reducing infections in animals." Frontiers in Veterinary Science, 6, 98-105.

Barbosa, T. M., & Levy, S. B. (2000). The Impact of Antibiotic Use on Resistance and the Need for Alternative Strategies. Drug Resistance Updates, 3(4), 224-231.

Bay, D. C., et al. (2009). SMR Transporters and Antibiotic Resistance. FEMS Microbiology Reviews, 33(3), 450-472.

Bébéar, C., & Pereyre, S. (2005). Mycoplasma Antibiotic Resistance. Clinical Microbiology and Infection, 11(8), 520-522.

Bhatia, R., et al. (2010). Antimicrobial Resistance and Its Impact on Public Health in Developing Countries. Clinical Microbiology and Infection, 16(5), 517-520.

Bierne, H., & Cossart, P. (2007). Listeria monocytogenes: Resistance to Antibiotics. In Listeria monocytogenes: Methods and Protocols (pp. 287-300). Springer.

Blair, J. M., Webber, M. A., Baylay, A. J., & Piddock, L. J. (2014). "Molecular mechanisms of antibiotic resistance." Nature Reviews Microbiology, 13(1), 42-51.

Brogden, K. A., Slade, M. B., & Brogden, R. N. (2003). "Antibacterial peptides from natural sources as potential therapeutic agents." Current Pharmaceutical Design, 9(3), 187-202.

Buford, T. W., & Willoughby, D. S. (2008). "Immuno-stimulants in reducing infection risks: The role of vitamins in the immune response." Journal of Clinical Immunology, 28(1), 47-53.

Bush, K., & Bradford, P. A. (2019). "Beta-lactamase inhibitors in the fight against antibiotic resistance." Journal of Clinical Microbiology, 57(1), e01394-18.

Chain, E., et al. (2005). Penicillin: Its Role in the Treatment of Infectious Diseases. The Oxford Dictionary of National Biography.

Chopra, I., et al. (2002). Antibiotics: From Discovery to Resistance. Nature Reviews Microbiology, 4(7), 535-547.

Corona, F., & Martinez, J. L. (2013). "Phenotypic resistance to antibiotics in biofilm-associated bacteria." Frontiers in Microbiology, 4, 145.

Courvalin, P. (2006). Antimicrobial Resistance in Gram-positive Cocci. Clinical Infectious Diseases, 42(4), 556-561.

Cox, G., & Wright, G. D. (2013). Intrinsic Antibiotic Resistance: Mechanisms, Exploitation, and Therapy. Nature Reviews Microbiology, 11(5), 350-359.

Dasgupta, S., Sahu, K. K., & Patra, S. (2021). "India's initiatives for One Health approach to combat antimicrobial resistance (AMR)." Indian Journal of Medical Research, 154(6), 675-682.

de Morais, M. A., et al. (2023). Multidrug and Toxic Compound Extrusion (MATE) Transporters: Mechanisms and Role in Antibiotic Resistance. Frontiers in Microbiology, 14, 618232.

De Vetten, N., et al. (2003). Antibiotics: Classification and Mechanisms of Action. Annual Review of Microbiology, 57, 609-630.

Delcour, A. H. (2009). The Barrier of the Outer Membrane of Gram-negative Bacteria. The Journal of General Physiology, 133(6), 671-680.

Dessen, A., Mandi, M., & Morais, M. (2001). "Target protection enzymes as antibiotic resistance determinants." Trends in Microbiology, 9(3), 99-106.

FAO (Food and Agriculture Organization). (2022). "Antimicrobial Resistance and One Health." FAO Report, 2022.

Fernández, L., & Hancock, R. E. (2012). "Adaptive and mutational resistance: Role of porins and efflux pumps in drug resistance." Clinical Microbiology Reviews, 25(4), 657-681.

Fleming, A. (1929). On the Antibacterial Action of Cultures of Penicillium, with Special Reference to Their Use in the Isolation of B. influenzae. British Journal of Experimental Pathology, 10(3), 226-236.

Ganguly, N. K., et al. (2011). The Growing Threat of Antimicrobial Resistance in India. International Journal of Infectious Diseases, 15(11), e794-e797.

Garneau-Tsodikova, S., & Labby, K. J. (2016). Mechanisms of Resistance to Aminoglycosides. In Antimicrobial Resistance: From Molecular Mechanisms to Clinical Applications (pp. 229-259). Springer.

Gong, Y., Zhao, Y., & Wang, Y. (2018). "Sulfonamide resistance in bacteria: Mechanisms and clinical consequences." Journal of Clinical Microbiology, 56(5), e01726-17.

Gould, K. (2016). The History of Antibiotics and the Discovery of Salvarsan. The Lancet Infectious Diseases, 16(3), 309-312.

Grkovic, S., et al. (2002). Acquisition of Antibiotic Resistance by Horizontal Gene Transfer. In Antibiotic Resistance: The Case for Action (pp. 133-150). Cambridge University Press.

Gupta, P., et al. (2021). ABC Transporters in Antibiotic Resistance: Mechanisms and Approaches for Overcoming Resistance. Frontiers in Pharmacology, 12, 571235.

Hajiagha, M., et al. (2023). Efflux Pumps and Antibiotic Resistance in Mycobacterial and Gram-negative Bacteria. Journal of Antimicrobial Chemotherapy, 78(3), 657-670.

Haque, M., Awal, S., & Alam, M. (2023). "Resistance mechanisms in Gram-negative bacteria against β-lactam antibiotics." Antimicrobial Agents and Chemotherapy, 67(3), e01654-23.

Haque, M., et al. (2023). Characterization of MATE Efflux Transporters in Vibrio parahaemolyticus. Journal of Antimicrobial Chemotherapy, 78(2), 435-446.

Hawser, S. P., & Hsueh, P. R. (2006). "Iclaprim, a new antibiotic, in Phase III clinical trials: A review of its pharmacology and clinical potential." International Journal of Antimicrobial Agents, 28(3), 203-210.

Holme, T. W., et al. (2006). Antibiotic Resistance: Causes, Mechanisms, and Prevention. Journal of Antimicrobial Chemotherapy, 58(3), 448-453.

Johnsen, P. J., et al. (2009). "Persistence of resistant bacteria even without antibiotic use." Environmental Microbiology Reports, 1(4), 227-234.

Jouany, J. P., & Morgavi, D. P. (2007). "Antimicrobial activity of plant-derived compounds: Emerging alternatives in the search for new antibiotics." Animal Feed Science and Technology, 137(1-2), 135-141.

Kelly, L. A., et al. (2009). Gene Transfer and Antibiotic Resistance in Bacteria. Journal of Medical Microbiology, 58

Kim, H. S., Lee, S. H., & Lee, S. (2012). "PBP2a-mediated methicillin resistance in Staphylococcus aureus." Microbial Drug Resistance, 18(4), 348-356.

Kimura, K., & Bugg, T. D. (2003). "Antibiotic-modifying enzymes in bacteria." Natural Product Reports, 20(3), 270-287.

Koirala, A., et al. (2023). Role of Efflux Pumps in Antimicrobial Resistance in Escherichia coli. Microorganisms, 11(2), 314.

Krawczyk-Balska, A., & Markiewicz, Z. (2016). Antibiotic Resistance in Listeria monocytogenes. Microbial Drug Resistance, 22(5), 598-608.

Kresken, M., Resch, A., & Gottfried, J. (1999). "E. coli ampicillin resistance in clinical isolates: Role of TEM-1 β-lactamases." Journal of Antimicrobial Chemotherapy, 44(3), 277-282.

Kvist, T., Frier, H., & Dalgaard, L. (2008). "Antibiotic tolerance in bacterial biofilms." Nature Reviews Microbiology, 6(5), 295-301.

Lambert, P. A. (2005). "Mechanisms of bacterial resistance to antibiotics." Journal of the Royal Society of Medicine, 98(5), 222-227.

Laudy, A. E., et al. (2018). DHA Family Transporters in Antibiotic Resistance. Molecular Microbiology, 108(3), 301-317.

Laudy, A., Balandin, M., & Drzewiecki, M. (2018). "Neisseria gonorrhoeae mutations leading to resistance to penicillin and tetracycline." Antimicrobial Resistance and Infection Control, 7, 71.

Lee, C. R., et al. (2000). Antibiotic Efflux Pumps and Their Role in Resistance. Microbiology and Molecular Biology Reviews, 64(4), 901-938.

Levine, D. P. (2005). Vancomycin Resistance in Gram-positive Bacteria. Clinical Infectious Diseases, 41(6), 918-924.

Levy, S. B., & Marshall, B. (2004). Antibacterial Resistance Worldwide: Causes, Challenges, and Responses. Nature Medicine, 10(12), 122-129.

Li, X.-Z., et al. (1994). Efflux Pump-Mediated Resistance to Antimicrobial Agents in Pseudomonas aeruginosa. Antimicrobial Agents and Chemotherapy, 38(3), 542-552.

Liebenau, J. (1990). Ehrlich's Magic Bullet and the Evolution of Chemotherapy. Journal of the History of Medicine and Allied Sciences, 45(3), 309-325.

Livermore, D. M. (1995). "The emergence of β-lactam resistance in Escherichia coli: Role of TEM-1 β-lactamases." Journal of Antimicrobial Chemotherapy, 36(4), 419-429.

Lo, W. U., et al. (2008). Aztreonam Resistance in Gram-negative Bacteria. International Journal of Antimicrobial Agents, 32(1), 6-11.

Maertens, L., et al. (2006). "Stable resistance to sulphamethoxazole and streptomycin in E. coli in the absence of antibiotic use." Antimicrobial Agents and Chemotherapy, 50(10), 3323-3329.

Majewski, P., Vance, L., & Tschetter, R. (2020). "Porin mutations and antibiotic resistance in Pseudomonas aeruginosa." Antimicrobial Agents and Chemotherapy, 64(3), e01628-19.

Marquez, B. (2005). Bacterial Efflux Systems and Their Role in Antibiotic Resistance. Drug Resistance Updates, 8(3), 146-158.

Mathur, S., et al. (2004). The Role of Porins in Antibiotic Resistance. FEMS Microbiology Reviews, 28(2), 261-273.

McConnell, M. J., et al. (2011). "Vaccination with outer membrane complexes protects against multidrug-resistant Acinetobacter baumannii." Journal of Infectious Diseases, 203(4), 564-570.

Michael, C. A., et al. (2014). "The global antimicrobial resistance crisis: A One Health perspective." Lancet, 383(9919), 438-448.

Miller, V., & Choo, Y. (2016). "Mutations in regulatory proteins contribute to cefoxitin resistance in Escherichia coli." Journal of Antimicrobial Chemotherapy, 71(12), 3526-3532.

Müller, A., Nagel, J., & Hegemann, J. (2015). "β-lactam resistance in methicillin-resistant Staphylococcus aureus (MRSA)." International Journal of Antimicrobial Agents, 45(6), 596-601.

Munita, J. M., & Arias, C. A. (2016). Mechanisms of Antibiotic Resistance. Microbiology Spectrum, 4(2), 1-26.

Nikaido, H. (1989). Porins and Permeability Barriers in Bacteria. Annual Review of Microbiology, 43(1), 309-338.

Nikaido, H. (2003). Molecular Basis of Bacterial Outer Membrane Permeability Revisited. Microbiology and Molecular Biology Reviews, 67(4), 593-656.

Nikaido, H. (2005). Multidrug Efflux Pumps of Gram-negative Bacteria. Journal of Bacteriology, 187(3), 719-725.

Olsen, I. (2015). "Biofilm formation and antibiotic resistance." Journal of Clinical Periodontology, 42(S16), S58-S68.

Partridge, S. R., Tsafnat, G., & Iredell, J. R. (2018). "Mobile genetic elements and antimicrobial resistance." FEMS Microbiology Reviews, 42(2), 263-278.

Poole, K. (2007). Efflux Pumps as Antimicrobial Resistance Mechanisms. In Antibiotic Resistance Protocols (pp. 119-133). Springer.

Poole, K., et al. (2001). The RND Efflux Pump of Pseudomonas aeruginosa: Characterization and Role in Antibiotic Resistance. Antimicrobial Agents and Chemotherapy, 45(3), 637-646.

Poulsen, L. (2012). Small Multidrug Resistance (SMR) Efflux Pumps: A Role in Antibiotic Resistance. In Antimicrobial Resistance: A Global Threat (pp. 131-148). Springer.

Ranjalkar, J., & Chandy, S. J. (2019). "Antimicrobial resistance surveillance in India: A One Health approach." Journal of Global Antimicrobial Resistance, 18, 158-160.

Roca, I., et al. (2015). The Global Threat of Antibiotic Resistance: A One Health Perspective. In Antimicrobial Resistance: The Many Facets of a Growing Problem (pp. 9-21). Springer.

Sahare, S., et al. (2013). Antimicrobial Resistance Due to Mutation in Bacterial Target Sites. Microbial Pathogenesis, 64, 111-118.

Savoia, D. (2012). "Plant-derived antimicrobial compounds: An alternative source of natural therapeutics." Microorganisms, 1(1), 28-39.

Schepers, R., et al. (2019). "Phosphodiesterase inhibitors and their role in modulating the inflammatory response during Mycobacterium tuberculosis infection." Journal of Infectious Diseases, 219(4), 574-584.

Schweizer, H. P. (2012). "Efflux pump overexpression and antibiotic resistance." Antimicrobial Agents and Chemotherapy, 56(2), 648-654.

Scoffone, V. C., et al. (2021). The RND Efflux Pump Family: Mechanisms of Drug Export and Their Role in Antibiotic Resistance. Journal of Medicinal Chemistry, 64(5), 2895-2910.

Sengupta, S., et al. (2013). Emergence of Antimicrobial Resistance and Its Consequences. International Journal of Microbial Resistance, 5(2), 189-203.

Sharma, A., et al. (2023). Antibiotic Stewardship in the Context of H1N1 and COVID-19: A Policy Perspective. Journal of Global Health, 13(4), 045204.

Sharma, P., et al. (2014). Mechanisms of Drug Resistance in Bacteria: Target Site Modifications and Reduced Permeability. In Antimicrobial Resistance in Bacteria (pp. 251-269). Springer.

Shetty, N., et al. (2009). Permeability Barriers in Gram-negative Bacteria. Antimicrobial Agents and Chemotherapy, 53(7), 3155-3166.

Stokes, H. W., & Gillings, M. R. (2011). "Gene flow, mobile genetic elements, and the evolution of bacterial antimicrobial resistance." Frontiers in Microbiology, 2, 167.

Sykes, R. W., et al. (2010). Efflux Pumps and Antibiotic Resistance. Current Opinion in Microbiology, 13(5), 594-600.

Tabrizi, M. H., et al. (2021). MacAB Efflux Pump: A Major Contributor to Antibiotic Resistance in Escherichia coli. Antimicrobial Agents and Chemotherapy, 65(8), e01209-21.

UNEP (United Nations Environment Programme). (2022). "The role of environmental pollution in antimicrobial resistance." UNEP Report, 2022.

Van Hoek, A. H. A. M., et al. (2011). Antimicrobial Resistance in Aquatic Environments. Emerging Infectious Diseases, 17(7), 1224-1230.

Vergalli, J., et al. (2020). Porin Expression and Its Regulation in Bacteria. Microbial Drug Resistance, 26(1), 19-27.

Vester, B., & Ntokou, E. (2017). "Ribosomal protection proteins and their role in tetracycline resistance." Antimicrobial Agents and Chemotherapy, 61(6), e00155-17.

Viertel, T. M., et al. (2014). "Bacteriophage therapy: A promising treatment for multidrug-resistant bacterial infections." International Journal of Antimicrobial Agents, 44(5), 421-426.

Walsh, C. (2000). Antibiotics: Actions, Origins, Resistance. ASM Press.

Wang, Y., et al. (2020). Major Facilitator Superfamily (MFS) Transporters in Antibiotic Resistance. In Multidrug Efflux Pumps in Microbial Resistance (pp. 189-210). Springer.

Wang, Y., Li, J., & Zhang, L. (2014). "Sulfonamide resistance genes in bacteria." Microbial Drug Resistance, 20(3), 240-247.

Wang, Z., Sun, S., & Zhang, H. (2020). "Porin mutations in Enterobacter aerogenes leading to β-lactam resistance." Antimicrobial Agents and Chemotherapy, 64(10), e01548-20.

Webber, M. A., & Piddock, L. J. V. (2003). Structure and Mechanism of Efflux Pumps that Mediate Multidrug Resistance in Bacteria. Journal of Antimicrobial Chemotherapy, 51(1), 9-21.

Welte, T., Wolf, T., & Falk, W. (1995). "Porins of Pseudomonas aeruginosa: Mechanisms of antibiotic resistance." Antimicrobial Agents and Chemotherapy, 39(2), 372-379.

WHO (World Health Organization). (2015). "Global Action Plan on Antimicrobial Resistance." World Health Organization. https://www.who.int/publications/i/item/global-action-plan-on-antimicrobial-resistance

WHO (World Health Organization). (2022). "AMR and One Health: Advancing our understanding and responses." WHO Report, 2022.

World Organization for Animal Health (WOAH). (2022). "One Health and Antimicrobial Resistance." WOAH Report, 2022.

Wright, G. D. (2005). "The antibiotic resistance crisis: A call to action." Antimicrobial Agents and Chemotherapy, 49(2), 1-4.

Wright, G. D. (2007). "The antibiotic resistome: The nexus of microbial evolution and human medicine." Nature Reviews Microbiology, 5(3), 175-186.

Zaman, S., et al. (2017). The Global Threat of Antimicrobial Resistance: Science and Surveillance. Journal of Global Health, 7(1), 010406.

Ziervogel, B. K. (2012). "Porins in Gram-negative bacteria and their role in drug permeability." Nature Reviews Microbiology, 10(8), 542-548.

5

Current Scenario of Antimicrobial Resistance in Extended-spectrum β-lactamase Producing Zoonotic Bacterial Species

***Vibha Yadav*[1], *R.K. Joshi*,[2] *and Namita Joshi*[3]**

[1&2]*Department of Veterinery Microbiology*
[3]*Department of VPH & Epidemiology; College of Veterinary Science & Animal Husbandry, Acharya Narendra Deva University of Agriculture and Technology, Kumarganj, Ayodhya, Uttar Pradesh, India*

Abstract

Emergence of antimicrobial resistance in animal husbandry is of utmost concern as it has resulted in therapeutic failure. It is a complex phenomenon due to triangular interplay of the host, pathogens and antimicrobial agents. Nowadays resistance to antibiotics of β -lactum groups expanding rapidly worldwide and threatening the public health care due to limited treatment options. However their inappropriate use or even their unnecessary use leads to the development of multidrug resistant bacteria. Members of Enterobacteriaceae, are most commonly implicated food borne pathogens as they are generally commensal in GIT of human and animal. Among them Escherichia coli and Klebsiella pneumoneae strains have been found resistant to most of the common antimicrobials which may be alarming for human health. Resistance may be intrinsic, may be acquired through spontaneous mutations or may occur due to horizontal gene transfer. Due to horizontal gene transfer, even non-pathogenic microbial species may become pathogenic and serve as an ecological reservoir of resistant genes.

Introduction

Today, antimicrobial resistance (AMR) has become a global issue, contributing to rise in mortality and cost of treatment. Antimicrobial resistance (AMR) is the resistance of a microorganism against an antimicrobial agent to which it was originally sensitive (WHO, 2013). Dispersion of antibiotics is done at large scale, in India even sometimes without any proper prescription. Animal Husbandry is not untouched and antibiotics are used to a great extent, which needs enforcement of strict government rules and regulations for their use in field conditions (PHFI, 2011).

Extended-spectrum β-lactamases (ESBLs) are enzymes that hydrolyse most of the β-lactam antibiotics and thus mediate resistance to penicillins, 3rd and 4th generation cephalosporins (Saravanan *et al.*, 2018). Beta-lactamase inhibitors, inhibit these ESBLs such as clavulanic acid, sulbactam and tazobactam (Trott, 2013). The genes encoding for these enzymes are commonly found both on the chromosomes and plasmids among *Enterobacteriaceae* family (Kotsoana *et al.*, 2019).

Among *Enterobacteriacae*, *E. coli* and *Klebsiella* species are main environmental pathogens associated with various illnesses such as acute bovine mastitis (Koovapra, 2015), pathogenic *E. coli* with diarrhoea and extra intestinal infections in humans and animals (Levine *et al.*, 1987), *K. pneumoniae* with respiratory and urinary tract as well as bloodstream infections (Daehre *et al.*, 2018). Resistance to extended-spectrum β-lactams occurs mainly in members of *Enterobacteriaceae* family through plasmids encoded ESBL genes. (Sharma *et al.*, 2010).

Antimicrobial Resistance and Modes of Transmission

Antimicrobial resistance (AMR) is not limited to only specific area but has also been considered as worldwide global health issue for both human and veterinary field (WHO, 2013). It is a complex phenomenon due to triangular interaction of the host, pathogens and antimicrobial agents. There is an estimate that up to 2050, approximately 10 million per year deaths will occur due to infections with resistant bacteria (O'Neill, 2014). Development of antibiotic resistance in animal pathogens is due to use of antibiotics in agriculture and animal husbandry practices which has emerged as major threat for animal health and their welfare aspect (O'Neill, 2015). Most of the time antibiotics are used in livestock at sub-therapeutic levels for growth promotion, prophylaxis and treatment. The development of AMR has been attributed with prolong and indiscriminate use of antimicrobials in food animal production and in the treatment of bacterial infections (Boonyasiri *et al.*, 2014). In U. K. a study was carried out from 2006 to 2011 and it was found that use of antibiotic in treatment of food-producing animals was more than the amount used in humans (Wellington *et al.*, 2013). Resistant bacteria cover both pathogens and commensal organisms, as later serving as a potential reservoir for mobile resistance elements. The high occurrence of resistance has been predicted in large population of the animals, which are probably treated with antimicrobial drugs (de Verdier *et al.*, 2012). Causes of resistance are many sometimes; it may be intrinsic, may be acquired through spontaneous mutations or may occur due to horizontal gene transfer (Dodd, 2012). Even non-pathogenic microbial species may become pathogenic due to horizontal gene transfer and act as an ecological reservoir of resistant genes. For survival the bacteria rely on adaptation to the ever changing environmental conditions. Genetic variability is necessary for the evolution of any living organism and it also occur in bacteria by three different mechanisms (Mandell *et al.*, 2010). The mechanisms vary from a micro evolutionary change which is due to point mutation that can occur in nucleotide base pair; the second one is a macro evolutionary change which is the rearrangement of large segments of deoxyribonucleic acid (DNA) as a single event to the thirdly by acquiring foreign DNA that is acquired by plasmids, bacteriophages, naked sequence of DNA or transposable genetic elements from other bacteria. Thus the unlimited capacity to develop antibiotic resistance in bacteria comes by these above mentioned three mechanisms.

Genes encoding bacterial resistance are either intrinsic as a result of vertical transmission or acquired as a result of horizontal gene transmission (HGT) or arises from de novo mutations (Versalovic, 2011). ESBL encoding genes are mostly carried on plasmids, which can easily be transferred between isolates, bearing additional resistance determinants for other classes of antimicrobial agents, mainly fluoroquinolones, aminoglycosides and sulphonamides, which are attributed to the multidrug resistant phenotype (Jiang *et al.*, 2012).

Enteropathogens- *Escherichia Coli* and *Klebsiella Pneumoniae*

Escherichia coli and *Klebsiella pneumoniae,* are normal inhabitant of intestinal microbiota of animals and human and may be involved in various infections. Both are an opportunistic pathogen of which *E. coli* serves as a sentinel organism for antimicrobial resistance development in different types of animals, because it is a common enteric pathogen, can easily acquires resistance and therefore can act as a reservoir and play a potent role in transmission of resistance to other species/pathogens (Ashbolt *et al.*, 2013). Nowadays, ESBL producing *E. coli* have been become very common in veterinary medicine, especially in livestock, companion animals and wildlife, while ESBL producing *Klebsiella pneumoniae* have been detected rarely in healthy broiler (Mahanti *et al.*, 2018), diseased horses (Vo *et al.*, 2007), dairy cows (Locatelli *et al.*, 2010) and companion animals (Ewers *et al.*, 2014). Among *Enterobacteriaceae* family, *Klebsiella* pneumoniae are the most common bacteria which is found among ICU's patients (Custovic *et al.*, 2014). ESBL producing *E. coli* and *Klebsiella pneumoniae* represents a serious clinical threat both in community settings and healthcare acquired infection because it has been linked to the consumption of contaminated meat (Daehrae *et al.*, 2018). That's why ESBL producing *Klebsiella pneumoniae* and *E. coli* have been listed as pathogen of critical priority for the development of new antibiotics and research by the world health organization (WHO, 2017).

Exteded-spectrum β-lactamases and its Mechanism of Action

In India, β-lactam antibiotics are most commonly prescribed drug against bacterial infections. This is the one of the most important group of antibiotics which are most commonly used in veterinary field and animal food production accounting for more than 50% of all systemic antibiotics (Bronson and Barrett, 2001). Extended-spectrum β-lactamases (ESBLs) are the economically and clinically most important enzymes which are able to hydrolyze and inactivate β-lactam antibiotics. This group of enzymes hydrolyze most of the *β*-lactam antibiotics including penicillins, oxyimino-cephalosporines (third generation cephalosporines) and monobactam (aztreonam) but are inhibited by *β*-lactamase inhibitors viz. clavulanic acid, sulbactam and tazobactam (Trott, 2013). These enzymes catalyse and hydrolyze *β*-lactam ring of antibiotics and finally destroy their antimicrobial property. On genetic basis, the presence of ESBLs is associated with resistance to other classes of non-*β*-lactam antibiotics, including fluoroquinolones, aminoglycosides, and trimethoprim-sulfamethoxazole. In this context, therapeutic options are limited in infections caused by these bacteria (Nobrega and Brocchi, 2014). The most commonly found ESBL genes such as TEM, SHV and CTX-M belong to Ambler class A (1980) and Bush-Jacoby (2010) group 2be. The OXA- type ESBL belongs to Ambler class D and Bush-Jacoby groups 2d, 2de and 2df.

Resistance against the *β*-lactams is mainly mediated by a structural change in the penicillin binding proteins (leading to lower affinity of the drug) or by the production of bacterial enzyme which causes cleavage of *β*-lactam ring. Bacterial cell wall synthesis is disrupted by *β*-lactams which link covalently to enzymes i.e penicillin-binding protein (PBPs), located in the cell wall. The bacterial cell wall consist of peptidoglycan which is made up of a polysaccharide backbone consisting of alternating N-Acetylmuramic acid (NAM) and N-Acetylglucosamine (NAG) and final step in cell wall biosynthesis is a transamidase (CWT), also known as penicillin binding protein-1 (PBP-1) (Hashizume *et al.*, 1984). Variety of effects are produced by various penicillins which bind differently to different PBPs. Binding to PBP-1 (a transpeptidases or transamidases) produces cell lysis, while binding to PBP-2 (also a transpeptidase) also produces cell lysis, while binding with PBP-4, 6 which are carboxypeptidases, has no lethal effects (Yasmin, 2012).

Prevalence of ESBLs in *Escherichia coli* and *Klebsiella* Specices

Extended spectrum β-lactamase producing *Enterobacteriaceae* organisms have become a great concern both in medical and veterinary science, since the first description of ESBL producing *Enterobacteriaceae* isolated from hospitalized humans (Knothe *et al.,* 1983). Prevalence of ESBL producing *E. coli* in animal has been reported to be 35% in Assam, India (Borah *et al.,* 2014), 42.8% in Egypt (Braun *et al.,* 2016), 13.7% in Switzerland (Geser *et al.,* 2012), 4.1% in France (Madec *et al.,* 2008) and 44.3% in Great Britain (Horton *et al.,* 2011) and 10.2% in Denmark (DANMAP, 2012). The first report of CTX-M producing *Enterobacteriaceae* organisms in New Delhi was published in 2001 (Karim *et al.,* 2001). Later, in 2006, 66% of third generation cephalosporin-resistant *E. coli* and *K. pneumoniae* were reported from three medical centres in India, while other 10 centres showed 70% with CTX-M being dominant enzymes among ESBL- producing *Enterobacteriaceae* organisms (Rao *et al.,* 2014). Due to sharing of common habitat, prevalence of ESBLs has been increasing among animals in last few years and they are being reported from different parts of the country including abroad and India.

Reports on Prevalence of ESBL Producing *E. coli* and *Klebsiella pneumoniae* from Abroad

Ewers *et al.*, (2014) studied on clinical samples from Germany and European countries mainly from companion animals and horses. They reported 29.3% ESBLs producers in soft tissue infections and 14.9 % in urinary tract infections. The major ESBL type was *bla*-$_{\text{CTX-M-15}}$ (85.4%) followed by *bla*-$_{\text{CTX-M-1}}$ (5.6%), *bla*-$_{\text{CTX-M-9,}}$ *bla*-$_{\text{SHV-2}}$ and *bla*-$_{\text{SHV-12}}$ (1.1%) each.

Olowe *et al.* (2015) studied the phenotypic and molecular characterization of ESBL producing *E. coli* from animal faecal samples in Ado Ekiti, Nigeria and reported, 71.0% isolates were ESBL positive.

Braun *et al.*, (2016) studied on the surveillance of ESBL producing *Escherichia coli* in dairy cattle farms in Nile Delta, Egypt and found 42.8% *E. coli* were ESBL positive and revealed *bla*-$_{\text{CTX-M}^{-}15}$ was present in highest number followed by *bla*-$_{\text{CTX-M-9'}}$ *bla*-$_{\text{TEM}}$ and *bla*-$_{\text{SHV}}$ respectively.

Badri *et al.*, (2017) studied in Sudan on raw milk of cow and found that 29.3% isolates *E. coli* and 44.8% isolates *K. pneumoniae* were ESBL positive. Prevalence of ESBL *bla*-$_{\text{CTX-M}}$ genes was 61% followed by 23% *bla*-$_{\text{SHV}}$ and 16% *bla*-$_{\text{TEM}}$ gene.

Chen *et al.*, (2017) carried out a study on ESBL producing *E. coli* in beef carcasses of Taiwan and found 42.2% *E. coli* isolates were ESBL producers with *bla*-$_{CTM-M}$ gp 1 and *bla*-$_{CTX-M}$ gp 9 as the most commonly identified ESBL genotypes.

Ibrahim *et al.*, (2018), studied the prevalence of ESBL producing *Enterobacteriaceae* isolated from bovine mastitic milk, in Egypt, 70% isolates were found ESBL positive. All ESBL positive isolates were found to be *E .coli.* of which 42.1% belongs to *bla*-$_{CTX-M}$ group, 29.4% *bla*-$_{TEM}$ group and 11.8% *bla*-$_{SHV}$ group respectively.

Kotsoana *et al.*, (2019) conducted a study on antimicrobial resistance factors of ESBLs producing *E. coli* and *Klebsiella pneumoniae* from cattle farms and raw beef in North- West Provinces, South Africa and reported 51.3% prevalence of ESBL producing *E. coli* and *Klebsiella pneumoniae. E. coli* isolates harboured (85.0%) *bla*-$_{TEM}$, followed by *bla*-$_{SHV}$ (69.6%) and 58% *bla*-$_{CTX-M}$ while *Klebsiella pneumoniae* isolates harboured 40% *bla*-$_{CTX-M}$ and 42.9% *bla*-$_{OXA}$ genes.

Reports on Prevalence of ESBL Producing *E. coli* and *Klebsiella pneumoniae* from India: Das *et al.*, (2017) studied on the prevalence of ESBL producing gram negative isolates from subclinical mastitic milk of cattle in West Bengal and found that 42% isolates were ESBL producers. Major ESBL producing genes were *bla*-$_{TEM}$, *bla*-$_{SHV}$ and *bla*-$_{CTX-M}$.

Dewangal *et al.*, (2017) conducted a study on prevalence and molecular characterization of ESBL (*bla*-$_{TEM}$) producing *E. coli* isolated from humans and food of animal origin in Chhattisgarh, India and found that (6.25%) isolates were ESBL positive in chevon meat and (7.69%) in raw milk.

Batabyal *et al.*, (2018) conducted a study to isolate and characterize ESBL producing *E. coli* from milk samples of bovine from different parts of West Bengal, (India) and found that more than 50% *E. coli* isolates were ESBL positive with *bla*-$_{CTX-M}$ gene.

Rawat *et al.*, (2018) studied the detection and characterization of ESBLs genes among β-lactam-resistant faecal coliforms of dairy cattle from Chhattisgarh, India and found 40% isolates were ESBL positive of which, 20% isolates were positive for *bla*-$_{TEM}$ and 13.6% positive for *bla*-$_{SHV}$.

Gupta *et al.*, (2019) conducted a study to isolate and characterize ESBL producing *E. coli* from faecal samples of healthy and diarrhoeic neonatal calves and found, 32.9%, and 71.43% ESBL positive *E. coli* in healthy and diarrhoeic calves respectively.

Tiwari *et al.*, (2019) studied the ESBL, AmpC- lactamase and MBL-producing *E. coli* variants circulating in livestock of Meghalaya and Assam and reported 75% prevalence of ESBL in isolates of faecal samples.

Kuralayanapalya *et al.*, (2019) have statistically analysed the overall prevalence of ESBLs among animals in India and found that total prevalence rate was 9%. The pooled prevalence of ESBLs in animals was 26%, 11%, 6% and 8% for North, East, South and Central zones respectively. The results showed a predominance of ESBLs producing *Klebsiella pneumoniae* strains, *E. coli* and *Pseudomonas* spp. 11%, 7% and 5% respectively.

Zoonotic Importance of ESBL-Producing Enteropathogens

Nowadays, food animals and their products have been found as important sources of infectious pathogens for humans (Gundogan and Avci, 2013). Being commensal in GIT of human and animal, members of *Enterobacteriaceae,* are most commonly implicated food borne pathogens. Most common cause of diarrhoea and mastitis in animals are pathogens which belong to family *Enterobacteriaceae* and are of great zoonotic importance for human being (Ibrahim *et al.*, 2018; Athira, 2017). *Escherichia coli* and *Klebsiella pneumoniae* are predominant ESBL- producing bacteria and are often detected as the cause of urinary tract infections, pneumonia and sepsis. In the last decade, transmission and dissemination of ESBLs by animals has become a potential issue of new threats to human. Livestock provide animal protein in the form of meat and milk that are included in the global supply chain of trade and food. Potential source of contaminants are animal waste materials which, play important role for the possible spread of ESBL bacteria to human and the environment (Widodo, 2020). *Escherichia coli* and *Klebsiella pneumoniae* are opportunistic pathogens of humans and animals responsible for a wide range of infections, such as diarrhoea, urinary tract infections, pneumonia, wound infections, septicaemias, haemolytic uremic syndrome and nosocomial infections especially meningitis in infant (Slama *et al.*, 2010).

E. coli is one of the dreadful pathogen, especially the "*Enterohaemorrhagic E. coli*" strains (EHEC) causing infection through meat and milk which has a great effect on human health (Hickey *et al.*, 2015). Ruminants especially cattle are known to be most important reservoir of shiga toxin-producing *E. coli* (STEC) (Irino *et al.*, 2005). *Klebsiella pneumoniae* has also been isolated from bovine mastitis in France by Dahmen *et al.*, 2013. *E. coli* is not only one of the most common cause of neonatal calf diarrhoea but its different strains are responsible to many other human and animal infections also. These infections can be restricted to gastrointestinal tract or the cause of urinary, systemic or meningeal infections (Croxen *et al.,* 2013). Animal faeces are the secondary source of human *E. coli* infection for some DEC (Diarrhoeic *E. coli*) strains, mainly those capable of producing Shiga-like toxin. The incidence of ESBL producing strains among clinical isolates has been steadily increasing over the past years, resulting in limited therapeutic options. Microorganisms responsible for urinary tract infections such as *E. coli* and *Klebsiella* spp have ability to produce ESBL in large quantities. Several nosocomial outbreaks have been reported among patients in intensive care facilities and hospital-acquired infections due to ESBL-producing enterobacteria (Pitout, 2005). In community based studies, *Enterobacteria* specially CTX-M enzyme producing ESBL *Escherichia coli*, have been reported in recent past as a common cause of urinary tract infections (Bradford, 2001). Infections caused by ESBL producing bacteria are associated with prolonged stay, increased cost of treatment and increased mortality.

Conclusion

Overall use of antimicrobial agents has made alarming situation in the treatment of various infectious diseases. The day to day increase in resistance pattern of these agents against different antibiotics leads difficulty to clinicians. The emergence of ESBL producing strains has aggravated this with failure of treatment and thus limiting the treatment options. In addition plasmid with ESBL genes frequently carry a variety of other resistant determinants conferring reduce susceptibility to different other classes of antibiotics, which is alarming animal and human health. High resistance of enteropathogens to antibiotics particularly third generation cephalosporins, for which regular monitoring, appropriate and regulated use of antibiotics after referring antibiogram should be encouraged. It also suggests the need for further investigation and judicious use of antibiotics in animal husbandry practices.

References

Ambler, R.P., (1980). The structure of β-lactamases. Philosophical Transactions of Royal Society of London-Series B: Biological Sciences. 289(1036):321-331.

Ashbolt N J, Amezquita A, Backhaus T (2013). Human health risk assessment (HHRA) for environmental development and transfer of antibiotic resistance. Environ Health Perspect. 121:993–1001.

Athira C.K. (2017). Epedemiology and molecular characterization of selected enteric bacterial zoonotic pathogens associated with neonatal calves. Thesis Ph.D. Deemed University, ICAR-IVRI, Izatnagar, India. pp15-16.

Badri A.M., Ibrahim T. I., Mohamed S.G., Garbi M.I., Kabbashi A.S. and Arbab M. H. (2017). Prevalence of ESBL producing E. coli and Klebsiella pneumoniae isolated from raw milk samples in Al Jazirah State, Sudan. Molecular Biology: Open Access 7;1. DOI:10.4172/2168-9547.1000201.

Batabyal, K., Abhiroop,B. Pal, Samir Dey, Siddhartha Narayan Joardar, Indranil Samanta, Devi Prasad Isore and Abhishek Dharm Singh (2018). Detection, characterization and antibiogram of extended-spectrum β-lactamase Escherichia coli isolated from bovine milk samples in West Bengal, India. Veterinary World. 11(10):1423-1427.

Boonyasiri A, Tangkoskul T, Seenama C, Saiyarin J, Tiengrim S, Thamlikitkul V (2014). Prevalence of antibiotic-resistance in healthy adults, foods, food animals, and the environment in selected areas in Thailand. Pathog. Glob Health.108:235-45.

Borah,V.V., Bora, P., Roy, M. and Saikia K.K. (2014). High prevalence of antibiotic resistance in Escherichia coli isolated from faecal samples of cows and assessment of antibacterial efficacy indigenous medicinal plants from Assam, India. Austin J. Biotechnol. Bioeng. 1:6.

Bradford, P.A. (2001). Extended-spectrum beta-lactamases in the 21st century: characterization, epidemiology and detection of this important resistance threat. Clin. Microbiol. Rev. 14: 933-951.

Braun, S. D., Ahmed, M.F.E., El-Adawy, H., Hotzel, H., Engelmann, I., Daniel Weil, D., Monecke, S. and Ehricht, R. (2016). Surveillance of Extented-Spectrum β-Lactamase-producing Escherichia coli in Dairy Cattle Farms in the Nile Delta, Egypt. Front. Microbial. 7:1020.

Broson, J.J. and Barrett, J.F., (2001). Quinolones, Everninimycin, Glycylcycline, carbapenem, Lipopeptide and Cephem antibacterials in clinical development. Curr. Med. Chem. 8: 1697-1704.

Bush, K. and Jacoby, G.A., (2010). Updated functional classification of β-lactamases. Antimicrob Agents Chemother. 54:969-976.

Chen, CM, Ke SC,Li CR, Wu YC, Chen TH, Lai CH, Wu XX, Wu LT., (2017). High diversity of antimicrobial resistance genes, class 1 Integrons and genotypes of multidrug resistant E. coli in beef carcasses. Microb. Drug Resist. 23(7): 915-924.

Croxen, M.A., Law, R.J., Scholz, R., Keeney, K.M., Wlodarska, M. And finlay, B.B. (2013). Advances in understanding enteric pathogenic Escherichia coli. Clin. Microbial. Rev. 26:822-880.

Custovic, A., Smajlivic, J., Hadzic, S., Ahmetagic, S., Tilic, N. and Hadzagic, H. (2014). Epidemiological surveillance of bacterial nosocomial infections in the surgical intensive care unit. Mater Sociomed. 26:7-11.

Daehre K., projahn M, Friese A., Semmler T., Guenther S., Roesler U.H. (2018). ESBL-Producing Klebsiella pneumonia in the broiler production chain and the first description of ST3128. Front Microbial. 9:2302.

Dahmen, S., Metayer, V., Gay, E., Madec, J.Y. and Haenni, M. (2013). Characterization of extended-spectrum β-lactamase (ESBL) carrying plasmids and clones of Enterobacteriaceae causing cattle mastitis in France. Vet. Microbiol. 162:793-799.

DANMAP, (2012). Use of antimicrobial agents and occurrence of antimicrobial resistance in bacteria from food animals, food and human in Denmark.http:/www.danmap.org.

Das A., Guha C., Biswas U., Jana PS, Chatterjee A., Samanta I., (2017). Detection of emerging antibiotic resistance in bacteria isolated from subclinical mastitis in cattle in West Bengal. Vet World. 10(5):517.

de Verdier, K., Nyman, A., Greko, C. and Bengtsson, B., (2012). Antimicrobial resistance and virulence factors in Escherichia coli from Swedish dairy calves. Acta veterinaria scandinavica, 54(1):2.

Dewangan, P., Shakya, S., Patyal, A., Gade, NE (2016). Prevalence and molecular characterization of ESBL (bla-$_{TEM)}$ producing E. coli isolated from human and foods of animal origin in Chhattisgarh, India. Indian Journal of Animal Research 51(2):310-5.

Dodd, M.C., (2012). Potential impacts of disinfection processes on elimination and deactivation of antibiotic resistance genes during water and waste water treatment. Journal of Environmental Monitoring. 14(7):1754-1771.

Ewers, C., Stamm, I., Pfeifer, Y., Wieler, L. H., Kopp, P. A., Schonning, K. (2014). Clonal spread of highly successful ST15-CTX-M-15 Klebsiella pneumoniae in companion animals and horses. J. Antimicrob. Chemother. 69:2676–2680.

Geser, N., Stephan, R., and Hachler, H. (2012). Occurance and characteristics of extended-spectrum β-lactamase producing Enterobacteriaceae in food producing animals, minced meat and raw milk. B.M.C. Vet. Res. ESBL. pp21-19.

Gundogan, N. and Avci, E., (2013). Prevelance and antibiotic resistance of extended spectrum beta-lactamase (ESBL) producing Escherichia coli and Klebsiella species isolated from foods of animal origin in Turkey. Afr J Microbiol Res. 7:4059-4064.

Gupta, S., Abhishek, Sameer Shrivastava and Asha K. Verma (2019). Isolation, Identification, Molecular characterization and Antibiogram of E. coli isolates from neonatal calves. International Journal of Current microbiology and applied sciences. ISSN: 2319-7706.

Hashizume, T., F. Ishino, J. Nakagawa, S. Tamaki, and M. Matsuhashi., (1984). Studies on the mechanism of action of imipenem (N-formimidoylthienamycin) in vitro: binding to the penicillin-binding proteins (PBPs) in Escherichia coli and Pseudomonas aeruginosa, and inhibition of enzyme activities due to the PBPs in E. coli. J. Antibiot. (Tokyo) 37:394–400.

Hickey, C.D., Sheehan, J.J., Wilkinson, M.G. and Auty, M.A.E. (2015). Growth and location of bacterial colonies within dairy foods using microscopy techniques: A review. Front. Microbiol. 6:99.

Horton, R.A., Randall, L.P., Snary, E.L., Cockrem, H., Lotz S., Wearing, H., Duncan,D., Rabie, A., McLaren, I., Ragione, R.M. and Coldham, N.G. (2011). Faecal carriage and shedding density of CTX-M extended-spectrum β-lactamase producing Escherichia coli in cattle, Chickens and pigs: implication of environmental contamination and food production. App. Environ. Microbial. 77: 3715-9.

Ibrahim El Sayed F.H., Ashraf M. Abd El wahab, Samy A. Khalil and Helmy A. Torky (2018). Prevalence of ESBL producing Enterobacteriaceae isolated from bovine mastitis milk. AJVS. Vol. 58 (1):102-108.

Irino, K., Kato, M.A., Vaj, T.M., Romas, I.I., Souza, M.A., Cruz, A.S., Gomes, T.A., Vieira, M.A. and Guth, B. E. (2005). Serotypes and virulence markers of Shiga toxin producing Escherichia coil (STEC) isolated from dairy cattle in Sao Paulo State, Brazil. Vet. Microbiol. 105:29-36.

Jiang, H.X., Tang, D., Liu, Y.H., Zhang, X., Zeng, Z. L., Xu, L. and Hawkey, P.M.(2012). Prevalence and characteristics of β-lactamase and plasmid-mediated quinolones resistance genes in Escherichia coli isolated from farmed fish in China. The Journal of Antimicrobial Chemotherapy. 67(10):2350-2353.

Karim, A., Poirel, L., Nagarajan, S. and Nordmann, P. (2001) Plasmid mediated extended spectrum β-lactamase (CTX-M3 like) from India and gene association with insertion sequence ISEcp1. FEMS Microbiol Lett. 201:237-241.

Knothe, H., Shah, P.D.P., Krcmery, V., Antal, M. And Mitsuhashi, S. (1983). Transferable resistance to cefotaxime, cefoxitin, cefamandole and cefuroxime in clinical isolates of Klebsiella pneumoniae and Serratia marcescens. Infect. 11(6):315-317.

Koovapra S., (2015). Characterization of extended spectrum β-lactamase (ESBL) producing Klebsiella spp. of bovine mastitis origin. Thesis M.V.Sc. Deemed University, ICAR-IVRI, Izatnagar, India. pp13-14.

Kotsoana, P., Montso, S.B.D., Ajay, K. and Collins, N.A. (2019). Antimicrobial resistance factors of Extented-spectrum β-lactamases producing Escherichia coli and Klebsiella pneumoniae isolated from cattle farms and raw beef in North-west province, South Africa. BioMed Research Internationals.

Kuralayanapalya S. P., Patil S.S., Hamsapriya, S. Shinduja, R. Roy, P. Amanchawadi, R. G., (2019). Prevalence of Extended-spectrum β-lactamase producing bacteria from animal origin: A systemic review and meta-analysis report from India. PLoS ONE 14 (9): e0221771.

Levine, M. M., Kaper, J. B., Blank, R.E. and Clements, M.L. (1987). New knowledge on pathogenesis of bacterial enteric infections as applied to vaccine development. Microbial. Rev. 47:510-550.

Locatelli, C., Scaccabarozzi, L., Pisoni, G., and Moroni, P. (2010). CTX-M1 ESBL-producing Klebsiella pneumoniae subsp. pneumoniae isolated from cases of bovine mastitis. J. Clin. Microbiol. 48:3822–3823.

Lorenz, I., Fagan, J. And More, S.J. (2011). Calf health from birth to weaning. II. Management of diarroea in pre-weaned calves. Irish Vet. J. 64:9.

Madec, J. Y., Lazizzera, C., P., Meunier, D., Martin, S., Lepage, G., Menard, M. F., Lebreton, P. and Rambaud, T. (2008). Prevalence of faecal carriage of acquired extended-spectrum cephalosporin resistance in Enterobacteriaceae strains from cattle in France. J. Clin. Microbiol. 46:1566-1567.

Mahanti, A., Ghosh, P., Samanta, I., Joardar, S. N., Bandyopadhyay, S., Bhattacharyya, D., et al. (2018). Prevalence of CTX-M-Producing Klebsiella spp. in broiler, kuroiler, and indigenous poultry in West Bengal State, India. Microb. Drug Resist. 24: 299–306.

Mandell, G.L., Bennett, J.E., Dolin, R., (2010). Mandell, Douglas and Bennett's principles and practice of infectious diseases. 7th ed. Philadelphia, PA: Churchill Livingstone/Elsevier.

Nobrega, D.B. and Brocchi, M. (2014). An overview of extended-spectum β-lactamases in veterinary medicine and their public health consequences. J. Infect. Dev. Ctries. 8:954-960.

Olowe, O.A., Adewumi, O., Odewale, G., Ojurongbe, O. and Adefioye, O. J. (2015). Phenotypic and molecular characterization of Extended-spectrum β-lactamase producing E. coli obtained from animal faecal samples in Ado Ekiti, Nigeria. Journal of Enviromental and Public health. http://dx.doi.org/10.1155/2015/497980.

O'Neill, J. (2014). Review on Antimicrobial Resistance- Tackling a crisis for the health and wealth of nation [online].

O'Neill J., (2015). Antimicrobials in agriculture and the environment: reducing unnecessary use and waste. Review on Antimicrobial Resistance.

Pitout, JDD, Nordmann, P., Laupland, K.B., Poire, L. (2005). Community-wide outbreak of clonally related CTX-M-14 beta-lactamase-producing Escherichia coli strains in the Calgary health region. J. Clin. Microbiol. Rev 14: 933-951.

Public Health Foundation of India (2011). A report published by PHFI in 2011.

Rao, S.P., Rama, P.S., Gurushanthappa, V., Manipura, R. And Srinivasan, K. (2014). Extended-spectrum β-lactamases producing Escherichia coli and Klebsiella pneumoniae: A multi-centric Study Across Karnataka. J. Lab Physicians. 6(1):7.

Saravanan, M., Ramachandran, B., and Barabadi, H. (2018). The prevalence and drug resistance pattern of extended-spectrum β-lactamases (ESBLs) producing Enterobacteriaceae in Africa. Microbial Pathogenesis, 114 :180-192.

Sharma, J., Ray, P., Sharma, M. (2010). Plasmid profile of ESBL producing Gram-negative bacteria and correlation with susceptibility ti β-lactams drugs. Indian J Pathol Microbiol, 53:83-6.

Slama, K. B., Jouini, A., Sallem, R. S., Somalo, S., Saenz, Y. (2010). Prevalence of broad-spectrum cephalosporin-resistant Escherichia coli isolates in food samples Tunisia and characterization of integrons and antimicrobial resistance mechanisms implicated. Int. J. Food Microbiol 137: 281286.

Tewari R., Mitra, S., Ganaie, f., Das, S., Chakraborty, A., Venugopal, N., Shome, R., Rahman, H., Shome BR., (2019). Dissemination and characterization of ESBL, AmpC β-lactamase and mettalo- β-lactamase producing E. coli isolated from livestocks and poultry in Northeastern India: A Molecular surveillance approach. J. Global Antimicrob. Res.17:209-215.

Trott. D. (2013). B-lactam resistance in gram-negative pathogens isolated from animals. Curr. Pharm. Des. 19:239-249.

Versalovic, J., (2011). Mechanism of resistance to antimicrobial agents' pp. 1085 by Rice abd Bonomo. Manual of clin microbial. Washington, DC:ASM Press.113.

Vo, A. T., van Duijkeren, E., Fluit, A. C., and Gaastra, W. (2007). Characteristics of extended-spectrum cephalosporin-resistant Escherichia coli and Klebsiella pneumoniae isolates from horses. Veterinary Microbiol. 124:248–255.

Wellington, EMH, Boxall, ABA, Cross P (2013). The role of the natural environment in the emergence of antibiotic resistance in Gram-negative bacteria. Lancet Infect. Dis. 13:155–65.

Widodo, A., Effendi, M. H., Khairullah, A. R. (2020). Extended-spectrum beta-lactamase (ESBL)- producing E. coli from livestock. Sys. Rev. Pharm. 11(7): 382-392.

World Health Organization (2017). Global Priority list of Antibiotic-resistant bacteria to Guide, Research, Discovery and Development of New Antibiotics. (World Health Organization, Geneva).

World Health Organization. (2013). Critically important antimicrobials for human medicine-3rd revision [online]. Geneva Switzerland: (9789241504485).

Yasmin, T., (2012). Prevalence of ESBL among E. coli and Klebsiella spp. in a tertiary care hospital and molecular detection of important ESBL producing genes by multiplex PCR. Department of Microbiology and Immunology, Mymensingh Medicaβl College, Dhaka, Bangladesh.

6

Antimicrobial Resistance: A Menace to Livestock with Special Reference to Eastern India

Siddhartha N. Joardar, Aditya Paul and Rajarshi Bardhan

Department of Veterinary Microbiology, Faculty of Veterinary and Animal Sciences, West Bengal University of Animal and Fishery Sciences, 37, K.B. Sarani, P.O.- Belgachia, Kolkata, West Bengal, India

Abstract

The menace of antimicrobial resistance (AMR) is observed in various pathogenic and non-pathogenic organisms. β- Lactam antibiotics are the most common antibiotics used for antibacterial treatments leading to the development of resistance. Antimicrobial resistance is evolved owing to genetic changes over time. It increases due to the extensive and prolonged use of antimicrobials and sometimes because of application of wrong dosage by the non-professional persons. Production of β-lactamases is the most common form of bacterial resistance. Members of Enterobacteriaceae family possesses genes viz. bla_{CTX-M}, bla_{SHV}, bla_{TEM} *of Extended Spectrum β-lactamases (ESBLs) those can hydrolyse extended spectrum cephalosporin. AmpC is a large group of broad -spectrum β-lactamases mainly encoded by the chromosomal* bla_{AmpC} *gene by various bacteria except E. coli where it is plasmid encoded. The prevalence of bacteria with ESBL-genes vary between 2-3% to more than 50% (in case of* bla_{CTX-M}, bla_{SHV}, bla_{TEM}*) and even more than 90% (in case of* bla_{AmpC}*) in livestock and animal products, poultry and poultry products besides in the environmental samples throughout the globe. Significant differences (*$p<0.01$*) were observed amongst the* bla_{CTX-M} *positive isolates, when studied agro-climatic zone-wise in West Bengal state of India. Statistical differences (*$P<0.05$*) in data were also observed when the positive isolates from two different animal sources i.e. cattle and poultry were compared and between the* bla_{CTX-M} *positive E. coli and Salmonella isolates. The* bla_{AmpC} *gene exhibited the highest prevalence, ranging from 32% to 90%, followed by the genes* bla_{TEM}, bla_{SHV}, *and* bla_{CTX-M} *in the isolates of Escherichia coli, Salmonella spp., and Klebsiella* spp. *sourced from duck and their surrounding environments in West Bengal. Diversity in climate, topography, environmental condition may influence the frequency of occurrence of ESBL positive bacterial species. In conclusion, monitoring and* *reporting antibiotic-use at the farmers' level should be executed and formulation of awareness programmes and alternative strategies are warranted to address the challenges of AMR.*

Keywords: AMR, Antibiotics, Cattle, *Enterobacteriaceae*, ESBL, Livestock, Poultry

Introduction

Antimicrobials, viz. antibiotics, antivirals, antifungals and anthelmintics are substances widely used to prevent and treat infections in humans, fish & prawn, livestock animals, and crops. In a situation where microorganisms such as bacteria, viruses, parasites or fungi become resistant to antimicrobial treatments to which they were previously susceptible, it is apprehended that antimicrobial resistance in the microbes has evolved. In fact, antibiotic-resistant bacteria evade the effects of antibiotics and multiply in their own way leading to severe health consequences in human and animals. The menace is such that antimicrobial resistance (AMR) hinders treatment modalities targeted for infectious diseases. The hazards of antimicrobial resistance is frequently observed in various pathogenic and non-pathogenic organisms, viz. *Salmonella* spp., *Campylobacter* spp., *Yersinia* sp., *E. coli* serotype O157:H7, enterococci, *Pasteurella* sp., *Actinobacillus* sp. with varying severity (McEwen and Fedorka-Cray, 2002). Microorganisms that develop resistance to commonly used antimicrobials are referred to as superbugs. Globally it is a matter of great concern that it spreads rapidly and threatening the ability to treat common infectious diseases, resulting in prolonged illness, disability and death. Without any effective antimicrobial agent, treatment of infectious diseases, many medical procedures like cancer therapy, diabetes management, organ transplantation, and major surgery will not be possible. The microbes showing resistance to multiple antimicrobials are commonly known as multidrug resistance (MDR) organisms (Magiorakos *et al.*, 2012).

Antimicrobial resistance is evolved owing to genetic changes over time. It increases due to the extensive and prolonged use of antimicrobials and sometimes because of application of wrong dosage by the non-professional persons. The bacterial resistance to antibiotics due to genetic changes is of two types – (1) Intrinsic or innate that depends on the biology of the bacteria and (2) Acquired resistance which occurs from (i) Acquisition of external genes by plasmids (conjugation or transformation), transposons (conjugation), integrons and bacteriophage (bacteriophage), (ii) Mutation of cellular genes and (iii) Both of this mechanism combindly (Giedraitienė *et al.*, 2011).

First documentation of antibacterial resistance came into existence in the year 1930. It was against sulphonamides (Zaman *et al.*, 2017). Interestingly, the first β-lactamase was reported in *Escherichia coli* even before the release of penicillin for medical use (Bradford, 2001).

β- Lactam antibiotics are the most common antibiotics used for antibacterial treatments, leading to the development of resistance property mostly in Gram negative bacteria. Extended spectrum β-lactamases (ESBLs) are defined as enzymes produced by certain bacteria that can hydrolyse extended spectrum cephalosporin. So, they are effective against β -lactam antibiotics like Ceftazidime, Ceftriaxone, Cefotaxime and oxyimino-monobactam (Bradford, 2001; Paterson and Bonomo, 2005). Extended spectrum beta lactamases (ESBLs) are mostly plasmid mediated enzymes that efficiently hydrolyze oxyimino cephalosporins and monobactams and are inhibited by beta lactamase inhibitors such as Clavulanic acid or tazobactam (Paterson and Bonomo, 2005).

Extended spectrum β-lactamases (ESBL) providing resistance to broad-spectrum cephalosporin were first detected in *K. pneumoniae* in 1983. The different types of β-lactamases are *TEM, SHV*, and *CTX-M.* The most prevalent β-lactamase is *TEM-1* which is the main cause of 90% ampicillin resistance *E. coli* (Livermore, 1995). Out of 300 β-lactamases, the most important β-lactamases generally produced are by Gram-negative bacteria (Wickens and Wade, 2005). Production of β-lactamases is the most common form of bacterial resistance (Bonnet, 2004).

Based on molecular structure, these enzymes are classified into four major classes (A through D). Class A, C, and D are having serine residue and Class β comprises the metallo-β-lactamases. Class A and D enzymes are plasmid encoded while class B and C are mostly encoded by chromosomal genes. *Escherichia coli* and other *Enterobacteriaceae* are mostly found to be harbouring some genes like bla_{TEM}, bla_{SHV}, and bla_{CTX-M} which encode Class A enzymes whereas Class C enzymes are encoded by bla_{AmpC} gene (Jacoby and Munoz-Price, 2005). Although *TEM*-type β-lactamases are most often found in *E. coli* and *K. pneumoniae*, they are also found in other species of Gram negative bacteria with increasing frequency. The term 'TEM' comes from the name of the Athenian patient (Temoniera) from which the isolate was recovered in 1963 (Ruiz, 2018). The *SHV* enzymes are named after the sulfhydryl variable active site and are commonly associated with *K. pneumoniae* (Samaha-Kfoury and Araj, 2003). The first reported ESBL in Asia was *SHV-2* from *K. pneumoniae* isolates in China, 1988 (Rossi *et al.*, 2006). In 2001, the first *CTX-M* positive strain was reported in New Delhi (Karim *et al.*, 2001). The name CTX is an abbreviation for cefotaximase and refers to the potent hydrolytic activity of this enzyme against cefotaxime (Tzouvelekis *et al.*, 2000). AmpC is a large group of broad-spectrum β-lactamases mainly encoded by the chromosomal bla_{AmpC} gene. However, in *E. coli*, AmpC is found to be encoded by plasmids where the chromosomal component is missing.

The Lateral Gene Transfer (LGT), also known as Horizontal Gene Transfer (HGT) in bacteria, helps in physical movement of DNA containing antibiotic resistant genes and incorporation in the recipient genome with a stable integration irrespective of physical and phylogenic distances between the donor and the recipient bacteria. Bacterial biofilms are important sites of Lateral Gene Transfer (Hall and Mah, 2017).

AMR issue in Livestock: International and National Status

Throughout the globe, in livestock and animal products, poultry and poultry products, prevalence of bacteria with ESBL-genes vary between 2-3% to more than 50% (in case of bla_{CTX-M}, bla_{SHV}, bla_{TEM}) and even more than 90% (in case of bla_{AmpC}). The increasing trend in antibiotic resistance might be correlated to presence of the ESBL-genes in the isolated bacteria through the last two decades. The following year-wise chronology of literature survey reflects the gravity of the AMR threat at the present time.

ESBL producing *Salmonella* were isolated from poultry, poultry products and human patients in Netherlands. The ESBL production was determined genotypically by PCR technique and bla_{TEM-52} gene was found to be most predominant one (Hasman *et al.,* 2005).

A total of 123 antimicrobial resistant *E.coli* were isolated from fecal samples of beef processing plant. Antibiotic disc assay had revealed that 107 *E.coli* isolates were resistant againsttetracycline, 13 against sulfisoxazole, 17 against streptomycin and 25 against ampicillin. PCR study had shown that 13, 11 and 14 *E.coli* isolates showing resistance against tetracycline, streptomycin and ampicillin, respectively, were bla_{TEM} positive and 01 each of tetracycline and ampiciliin resistant *E.coli* were bla_{SHV} positive (Aslam *et al.,* 2009).

ESBL enzymes are found in *Enterobacteriaceae* family members, such as *Escherichia coli* and *Klebsiella pneumoniae*, which have often been isolated in livestock, especially during poultry production (Carattoli, 2009; Li *et al.*, 2014).

In the Baltic Sea Coast of Poland, 65 *E. coli* isolates were detected from mallards (n=86) and six isolates were possessed $bla_{CTX-M-1}$ gene followed by one isolate harboured both the $bla_{CTX-M-9}$ and bla_{TEM-1b} gene while only one isolate carried bla_{SHV-12} gene (Literak *et al.*, 2010).

ESBL producing *E.coli* was isolated from swine and cattle at slaughter in Switzearland. A total of 59 pigs and 64 cattle were investigated for ESBL producing *E.coli.* A total of 21 ESBLproducing strains were isolated, among which, only 1.5% of the isolates harboured the CTXM group 9 gene, and 29.4% of the CTXM positive *E.coli* showed the existence of $bla_{TEM.}$ (Geser *et al.,* 2010).

The bla_{TEM} positive *Salmonella enterica* serovar Typhimurium were isolated from the cattle of Hokkaido, Japan (Tamamura *et al.*, 2010).

The $bla_{CTX\text{-}M}$ positive *E. coli* was detected in the fecal samples of cattle, pig and poultry in U.K. A total of 35, 20 and 32 fecal samples were collected from cattle, pig and poultry, respectively. A total of five *E. coli,* each from pig and chicken were found positive for $bla_{CTXM\text{-}1}$, two *E. coli* isolates from cattle were found to be positive for $bla_{CTXM\text{-}15}$ and three isolates were $bla_{CTXM\text{-}14.}$ These results were confirmed by PCR, followed by gene sequencing (Horton *et al.*, 2011).

ESBL producing *E.coli* was isolated from food producing animals in Japan. Fresh faecal samples were collected from 30 broilers, 17 layers, 16 beef cattle and 33 pigs, derived from 13 farms. From these 96 rectal samples, 109 *E.coli* were isolated. A total of 48 ESBL producing *E.coli* strains were detected by antibiotic disc method. PCR study, followed by gene sequencing had revealed that $bla_{CTXM\text{-}2}$ were present in 24 isolates, $bla_{CTXM\text{-}14}$ were found in 04 isolates, $bla_{SHV\text{-}12}$ in 09 isolates, $bla_{CTXM\text{-}15}$ in 03 and $bla_{TEM\text{-}1}$ in 08 isolates (Hiroi *et al.,* 2011).

A report showed the occurrence of extended spectrum β-lactamase (ESBL) producing *Escherichia coli* in faecal samples of healthy ducks and environmental samples from duck farm in South China and found a total of 68 (55.28%) isolates carrying bla_{TEM} gens out of 123 ceftiofur resistant *E. coli* isolates followed by 108 (87.8%) isolates carrying $bla_{CTX\text{-}M}$ and 5 (4.1%) isolates carrying bla_{SHV} genes (Ma *et al.*, 2012).

Both $bla_{TEM\text{-}52}$ and bla_{CTXM} type ESBL producing *E.coli* were isolated from cattle in France. A total of 204 ESBL producing *E.coli* were collected from sick cattle in France. The study had revealed that 96.6% of the isolates expressed CTXM type ESBL while 3.4% of the isolates expressed TEM-52 type ESBL (Haenni *et al.,* 2012).

A total of 70 bla_{CTXM} positive *E.coli* was obtained from the 747 faecal samples of dairy cattle in Ohio, US (Mollenkopf *et al.,* 2012).

A total of 59 samples, including 41 cloacal swab and 18 fecal samples from broiler chicken were collected from farms in Netherlands. A total of 22 *E.coli* isolates from cloacal swab samples and 06 isolates from fecal samples were found to be positive for *ampC,* confirmed by PCR (Dierikx *et al.,* 2012).

A total of 121 samples from poultry, including 70 carcasses and 51 intestinal samples were collected from broiler chicken flocks in Germany. A total of 76 isolates were confirmed as *E.coli.* PCR analysis had showed that 52.9% of the *E. coli* isolates from carcasses and 56.9% isolates from intestine were positive for *ampC* (Reich *et al.,* 2013).

The *ampC* β- lactamase genes were found in the *E.coli* isolates recovered from chicken meat and Human origin in Netherlands. A total of 98 chicken meat and 479 human fecal samples were collected. The PCR analysis of bla_{AmpC} gene showed that 12 out of 98 chicken samples (12.24%) and 25 out of 479 human samples (5.22%) were confirmed as *ampC* positive (Voets *et al.,* 2013).

The *E.coli* strains, isolated from beef cattle in US, were found to be positive for $bla_{CTXM-32}$, confirmed by PCR (Cottell *et al.,* 2013).

ESBL positive *E.coli,* harbouring the bla_{CTXM} gene, was isolated from cattle in Korea. A total of 1536 samples were collected, including 569 milk samples, 379 faecal samples of cattle, 512 environmental samples and 86 samples from cattle handlers. A total of 84 ESBL producing *E.coli* were confirmed by antibiotic susceptibility test. These isolates were found to be resistant against ampicillin, cephalothin and cefotaxime. PCR analysis had shown that 49 *E.coli* samples were positive for $bla_{CTXM-14}$ followed by $bla_{CTXM-32}$ (n=26) and $bla_{CTXM-15}$ (n=9) (Tamang *et al.,* 2013).

A total of 59 samples, including 41 cloacal swab and 18 fecal samples from broiler chicken were collected from farms in Netherlands. A total of 22 *E. coli* isolates from cloacal swab samples and 06 isolates from fecal samples were found to be positive for *AmpC,* confirmed by PCR (Dierikx *et al.,* 2013).

The *AmpC* β-lactamase genes were found in the *E. coli* isolates recovered from chicken meat and Human origin in Netherlands. A total of 98 chicken meat and 479 human fecal samples were collected. The PCR analysis of bla_{AmpC} gene showed that 12 out of 98 chicken samples (12.24%) and 25 out of 479 human samples (5.22%) were confirmed as *AmpC* positive (Voets *et al.,* 2013).

ESBL producing *E. coli* strains were isolated from the slaughtered animals in Czech Republic. A total of 166 and 140 swabs were taken from pig and cattle carcass surface, respectively. The number of CTXM positive *E. coli* recovered from pig carcasses were 18 and 05 bla_{TEM} positive *E .coli* strains were isolated from 140 cattle samples (Bardon *et al.,* 2013).

Increasing trend of ESBL/ampC type β-lactamase genes were observed in *E.coli,* isolated from calves in Netherlands from 1997 to 2010. The study revealed that the prevalence rate had increased from 4% in 1998 and 1999 to 39% in 2010 (Hordijik *et al.,* 2013).

Zurfluh *et al.* (2014) collected $bla_{CTX\text{-}M}$ gene from meconium of broiler chicks and faeces of broiler breeders and identified similar IncI1/ST3 plasmids harbouring the $bla_{CTX-M-1}$ gene in breeders and broiler suggesting the vertical transmission of gene.

A study was conducted where 100 (49.5%) ESBL producing *E. coli* from faecal samples of poultry (n=202) were isolated. ESBL genes which found in those isolates were $bla_{TEM\text{-}1}$ (n = 49), $bla_{CTX\text{-}M}$ (n = 40) and $bla_{TEM\text{-}206}$ (n = 24), among which $bla_{CTX\text{-}M}$ and $bla_{TEM\text{-}1}$ were co-located in 13 isolates, but no isolates were positive for the bla_{SHV} gene (Li *et al.*, 2014).

Abreu *et al.* (2014) isolated 237 (91.1%) ESBL producing *E. coli* from 260 rectal swabs from healthy broiler, 44 different band patterns were detected in 196 strains and remaining 41 were non-typeable strains. The $bla_{CTX\text{-}M}$ gene was detected in 116 (59.1%) isolates, of which 87 (75.0%) were *CTX-M-9* group, 16 (13.8%) were *CTX-M-1* group, 11 (9.5.0%) were *CTX-M-2* group, and in 2 (1.7%) cases *CTX-M-1* and *CTX-M-2* groups.

ESBL positive *E.coli* samples were found in the cow dung samples of Assam, India. A total of 100 cow dung samples were collected. The number of *E.coli* isolates recovered was 80. Among the *E.coli* isolates, 28 were confirmed as ESBL producers, by double-disc diffusion method. PCR study had shown that 25 out of 80 samples were bla_{CTXM} positive (28.57%), 06 samples were bla_{SHV} positive (21.43%) and 27 samples were bla_{AmpC} positive (96.43%) (Borah *et al.,* 2014).

Carcasses of the broiler chicken were collected from the slaughterhouse in Germany. A total of 81.6% of the *E. coli* samples were recovered from the carcass samples and found positive for *AmpC*, confirmed by PCR (Pacholewicz *et al.,* 2015).

Blaak *et al.* (2015) detected ESBL producing *E. coli* in poultry faeces, environment of the farm and other animals in the same farm of Netherlands. They reported the prevalence of 65% and 81% in faeces of laying hen and broilers, respectively and also reported 81% (21/26) in rinse water and runoff water, 79% (11/14) in other farm animals, 60% (21/35) in dust, 57% (20/35) in surface water adjacent to the farm, 55% (48/87) in soil, 15% (11/73) in flies and 6% (2/33) in barn air. Majority of the isolates were carrying *CTX-M-1* (41%).

In a study conducted in Northeast China and Jiangsu province, 195 isolates were collected from chicken farms and markets to detect ESBL genes, specifically bla_{CTX-M}, bla_{TEM}, and bla_{SHV}. The most frequently observed bla_{CTX-M} variants included *blaCTX-M-15*, *blaCTX-M-65*, *blaCTX-M-55*, and *blaCTX-M-14*. Among the isolates, 7.7% carried both *CTX-M-1* and *CTX-M-9* group genes. Pulsed-field gel electrophoresis analysis revealed 34 distinct genetic types, with the identification of the *blaSHV-5* gene in Chinese chicken *E. coli* for the first time. Conjugation experiments demonstrated the transferability of bla_{CTX-M} and bla_{TEM} genes, while bla_{SHV-5} was not found to be transferable (Tong *et al.*, 2015).

Carcasses of the broiler chicken were collected from the slaughterhouse in Germany. A total of 81.6% of the *E.coli* samples were recovered from the carcass samples and found positive for *ampC*, confirmed by PCR (Pacholewicz *et al.*, 2015).

Antibiotic resistant ESBL producing *E.coli* was isolated from healthy cattle and sheep in Turkey, which were characterized genotypically. A total of 200 fecal samples, each of cattle and poultry were collected, and the isolated *E.coli* species were detected with ESBL genes like bla_{CTXM}, bla_{TEM} and bla_{SHV}, by PCR. The results showed that bla_{CTXM} was the most frequent type of ESBL (87.1%), followed by bla_{TEM}(77.4%) and bla_{SHV}(9.7%) (Faruk *et al.*, 2016).

ESBL positive *E.coli* was found in dairy cattle farms in Nile delta, Egypt. A total of 266 fecal samples were collected from four different dairy farms. Out of 266 samples, 114 (42.8%) ESBL producing *E.coli* was identified, both genotypically and phenotypically. A total of 113 *E.coli* isolates were found to be harbouring atleast one of the resistant genes, confirmed by PCR. The results showed that 105 $bla_{CTXM-15}$, 01 bla_{CTXM-9}, 90 bla_{TEM} and 01 bla_{SHV} genes were obtained from the study (Braun *et al.*, 2016).

ESBL producing *E.coli* was isolated from healthy cattle and sheep in Burdur province of Turkey. A total of 200 faecal samples, each of healthy cattle and sheep were collected, from which, 47 *E.coli* were isolated (45 from cattle and 02 from sheep). Among all the isolates, 34 strains were found to be ESBL producers, characterized by double-disc assay. PCR results revealed that bla_{CTXM} was the most frequent type ESBL gene, found in 27 isolates (79.41%) followed by bla_{TEM}(70.59%) and bla_{SHV}(8.82%) (Faruk *et al.*, 2016).

Prevalence of extended spectrum β- lactamase and ampC producing *E.coli* were observed in dairy farms in Netherlands. Faecal matters were collected from 500 random herds. Further genotypic study revealed that *ampC* positive *E.coli* was found in 41% of the samples (Gonggrijp *et al.*, 2016).

Multi-drug resistant, ESBL producing and *ampC* positive *E.coli* were isolated from slaughterhouses in Bogar, Indonesia. A total of 35 samples were collected from 07 different slaughterhouses. The numbers of ESBL/ampC positive *E.coli* identified were 05 (14.3%). These isolates were found to be resistant against several classes of antibiotics, especially penicillin G (100%), streptomycin (100%), gentamicin (60%) and tetracycline (40%), confirmed by antibiotic sensitivity test (Sudarwanto *et al.,* 2017).

In livestock and animal products, poultry and poultry products showed the highest prevalence of ESBL-producers with *CTX-M-1*, *TEM-52* and *SHV-12* being the most common ESBL-types in poultry (Saliu *et al.,* 2017).

A total of 541 *E. coli* strains were isolated from the poultry samples of different production chains including broiler farms, slaughterhouse and retail. Out of the 541 *E. coli* isolates, 132 were ESBL positive and 122 isolates were found to be carrying the *AmpC* gene, confirmed by antibiotic disc assay and subsequent PCR analysis (Castellanos *et al.,* 2017).

For the analysis of multidrug resistant *E. coli*, a total of 168 positive isolates were collected from the raw meat of broiler and free-range chicken in four different states in India and out of 63 ESBL positive *E. coli*, 50 isolates were found positive for $bla_{CTX\text{-}M}$ gene followed by 40 and 20 isolates carried bla_{TEM} and bla_{SHV} genes, respectively (Hussain *et al*., 2017).

Multi-drug resistant *Escherichia coli* were isolated from the colostrums of cows in the dairy farms of New Brunswick, Canada. Fresh colostrums were collected from 452 cows of 8 separate herds. It was found in the study that 35% of the isolates were bla_{TEM} positive and 45% were bla_{CMY} positive (Awosile *et al*., 2017).

A total of 35 *E.coli* isolates were recovered from fifty fecal samples, collected from diseased cattle suffering from diarrhea, in Diwaniya, Iraq. A total of 32 number of isolates were bla_{AmpC} positive (91.4%), bla_{CTXM} were found in 28 isolates (80%) followed by 22 numbers of bla_{TEM} (62.8%). Lastly, bla_{SHV} were found in 08 isolates (22%). These studies were confirmed byPCR (Ismael *et al.,* 2017).

Beta-lactum resistant *E.coli* was found in the clinical samples of the livestock in Andhra Pradesh, India. A total of 83 clinical samples comprising of faecal samples from 12 cattle, 11 buffaloes and 07 sheep, having clinical diarrhea; 14 cattle and 11 buffaloes having mastitis and 16 cattle and 12 buffaloes with endometritis were collected. A total of 52(62.7%) *E.coli* isolates were recovered. A total of 13 isolates out of 52 were found to be ESBL positive, encompassing 07 bla_{SHV}, 05 bla_{TEM} and 01 bla_{OXA} (Sharif *et al.,* 2017).

A total of 541 *E.coli* strains were isolated from the poultry samples of different production chains including broiler farms, slaughterhouse and retail. Out of the 541 *E.coli*isolates, 132 were ESBL positive and 122 isolates were found to be carrying the *ampC* gene, confirmed by antibiotic disc assay and subsequent PCR analysis (Castellanos *et al.,* 2017).

Antibiotic resistant *E.coli* strains were recovered from the poultry samples from the farms of southern Germany. A total of 438 *E.coli* were recovered. Antibiotic disc assay had confirmed that 45 *E.coli* strains were *amp*C positive (Wieland *et al.,* 2017).

Rahman *et al.* (2018) reported 20 (47.6%) and 14 (38.8%) positive ESBL producing *E. coli* from poultry meat and environment of poultry farm (water, ground, feeding and drinking equipment) and overall prevalence of ESBL *E. coli* was 43.5%. The study results showed that *E. coli* recovered from poultry meat and poultry farm environmental samples were carrying similar type of genes and also showed that $bla_{CTX\text{-}M}$ was a bit prominent gene compared to other ESBL genes.

A total of 101 (50.5%) *E. coli* isolates were recovered from 200 broiler meat samples out of which 29 ESBL producing isolates were found. The major ESBL were $bla_{TEM\text{-}1}$, $bla_{CTX\text{-}M\text{-}14}$, $bla_{CTX\text{-}M\text{-}1}$ (Seo *et al.*, 2018).

Extended spectrum cephalosporin resistant *E.coli* were isolated from fecal matters of pigs in Adelaide, Australia. A total of 219 resistant *E.coli* were determined. These isolates were foundto be resistant against ampicillin (100%), ceftriaxone (99%), trimethoprin (99%), tetracycline (47%) and gentamycin (16.4%). All the isolates were found to be positive for $bla_{CTXM,}$ confirmed by PCR (Abraham *et al.,* 2018).

A total of 318 *E.coli* isolates were recovered from 2897 mastitic milk samples collected from 19 regions in China. Out of these isolates, 73 (22.96%) were identified as ESBL positive. Amongst the ESBL producing *E.coli*, bla_{CTXM} and bla_{TEM} were the most prevalent genes with the occurance rate of 97.26% and 71.23%, respectively. The most predominant CTX-M type ESBL was $bla_{CTXM\text{-}15}$ (65.85%), followed by $bla_{CTXM\text{-}14}$ (10.96%), $bla_{CTXM\text{-}55}$ (9.59%), $bla_{CTXM\text{-}64}$ (5.48%) and $bla_{CTXM\text{-}3}$ (1.37%), confirmed by gene sequencing study. Further, 72 ESBL producing *E.coli* were found to be multidrug resistant (Feng *et al.*, 2018).

The *E.coli* strain with ESBL gene was isolated from cattle faeces in Abidjn district, Ivory Coast. A total of 420 faecal samples were collected, from which, 85 strains of *E.coli* were isolated. Among the isolates, 45 strains were confirmed as ESBL producers, identified by disc- diffusion method. When subjected to PCR test, 11 isolates showed positive results for *bla*$_{CTXM}$, 10 were *bla*$_{SHV}$ positive and 15 isolates were *bla*$_{TEM}$ positive (Yao *et al.*, 2018).

Na *et al.* (2019) reported six (4.1%) ESBL positive *E. coli*, carrying *bla*$_{CTX-M}$ genes from 146 *E. coli* isolates of duck faeces and carcass.

Yang *et al.* (2019) isolated ESBL producing *E. coli* from waterfowl birds. By double disc synergy test, 289 isolates were detected as ESBL producers out of 311 *E. coli* isolates and the *bla*$_{CTX-M}$ gene was found mostly (46.9%) followed by combination of *bla*$_{CTX-M}$ and *bla*$_{TEM}$ gene in 70 isolates.

ESBL type antimicrobial resistance (AMR) *E.coli* was detected from cattle farms and raw beef in North-West province, South Africa. A total of 151 samples consisting of 55 fecal swabs from cattle and 96 samples of raw beef were collected. A total of 114 samples were confirmed as*E.coli* by PCR technique. Among the *E.coli* isolates, 85.5%, 69.6% and 58% of the isolates were confirmed as *bla*$_{TEM}$, *bla*$_{SHV}$ and *bla*$_{CTXM}$, respectively, by PCR techniques. Fingerprinting study had also revealed that there was cross-contamination between the beef and fecal samples (Montso *et al.*, 2019).

A total of 120 *E.coli* isolates were recovered from the 206 samples (63 from the diseased cattle and 143 from swine). These isolates were found to be resistant against several classes of antibiotics, through disc-diffusion method. Resistant against streptomycin were found to be39.2%, against tetracycline were 32.5% and 30% against sulfamethoxazole. Three *E.coli* isolates were found to be positive for *bla*$_{TEM-52C}$ (Aasmae *et al.*, 2019).

One hundred and fourteen *E.coli* strains were isolated from 151 samples, comprising 55 faeces and 96 raw beef in North-West province, South Africa. PCR study showed that *bla*$_{TEM}$ wasthe most prevalent gene (85.5%), followed by *bla*$_{SHV}$ (69.6%) and *bla*$_{CTXM}$ (58%) (Montso *et al*, 2019).

ESBL producing *E.coli* was detected in bovine faeces and milk samples in North Gujarat,India. In this study, a total of 109 samples (42 faecal and 67 mastitic mik samples) were collected. Culturing the samples in selective media resulted in isolation of 71 *E.coli* strains. Antibiotic sensitivity test had shown that 30 isolates (42.25%) were ESBL positive, comprising 17 from milk samples and 13 from faeces. The most prevalent ESBl gene detected was *bla*$_{TEM}$, where 17 isolates out of 30 were positive (Prajapati *et al.*, 2019).

A total of 776 faecal samples were collected from beef cattle of 40 commercial farms in England, Wales and Scotland. Genotypic study had shown that ten of the farms tested positive. For ESBL producing *E.coli, bla*$_{CTXM}$ gene was the most prevalent gene, while 15 farms were positive for *ampC E.coli* (Velasova *et al.,* 2019).

ESBL producing carbapenem resistant *Enterobacteriaceae* were isolated from beef cattle in the North West province of South Africa. A total of 280 *Enterobacteriaceae* isolates were obtained from 233 faecal samples of cattle. The isolates were identified to be resistant against imipenem (42%), ertapenem (35%), doripenem (30%) and meropenem (28%). The resistant isolates were subjected to PCR for ESBL detection. The study revealed that 33.1% of the isolates were bla_{SHV} positive, 22.5% and 20.5% were bla_{TEM} and bla_{CTXM} positive, respectively (Tshitshi *et al.,* 2020).

A total of 34 *E.coli* strains were found to be ESBL producers, isolated from 151 faecal samples of cattle, in Brazil. PCR results had shown that $bla_{CTXM\text{-}8}$ was the most frequent gene (62.5%) amongst the ESBL producing *E.coli,* followed by $bla_{SHV\text{-}2a}$ (20%), $bla_{CTXM\text{-}2}$ (10%) and $bla_{CTXM\text{-}15}$ (7.5%) (Palmeira *et al.,* 2020).

Antibiotic resistant *Salmonella* were isolated from raw beef in Karachi, Pakistan. A total of 150 beef samples were collected, from which, 32 *Salmonella* isolates were recovered. PCR studies had revealed that bla_{TEM} was the most frequent ESBL type, followed by bla_{CTXM} and $bla_{SHV.}$ (Hussain *et al.,* 2020).

ESBL and *amp*C positive *E.coli* was harvested from grazing beef cattle in Florida, USA. A total of 1098 samples were collected including 840 fecal samples from cattle and 258 environmental samples from 17 commercial farms. Out of these samples, a total of 59 ESBL/ ampC producing *E.coli* were isolated and characterized. PCR study had revealed that 39 out of 59 samples were bla_{CTXM} positive (66.10%), 20 samples were bla_{CMY} positive (33.89%) and 32 samples were bla_{TEM} positive (54.23%) (Lee *et al.,* 2020).

A total of 339 cloacal swabs were collected from 34 broiler chicken farms located in six provinces of Korea, in 2019, from which, 332 *E.coli* strains were isolated. Antibiotic sensitivity test resulted in determination of more than 90% antibiotic resistant strains among the isolates. The study also determined that a total of 46 isolate (14%) were *ampC* positive (Song *et al.,* 2020).

Beta-lactamase producing *Enterobacteriacea* were isolated from domestic and farm animals in Pakistan. A total of 1273 faecal samples were collected from which 245 ESBL positive *Enterobacteriaceae* were isolated with 180 *E.coli* and 65 *Klebsiella pneumonia* strains. PCR studies had shown that 73.9% of the isolates were bla_{CXM} positive, 26.1% were positive for bla_{TEM} and 14.2% for bla_{SHV} (Ejaz *et al.,* 2021).

ESBL producing, multi-drug resistant *E.coli* strains were isolated from the faecal samplesof domestic animals and humans, and environmental samples, in North Eastern region of India. A total of 648 *E.coli* strains were isolated from faecal samples of calves, lambs, kids and humans, suffering from diarrhea, along with water samples. These isolates were found to be resistant against imipenem (71%), doripenem (70.47%), ertapenem (66%) and to amoxicillin, ampicillin, cefotaxime and gentamicin, all with greater than 80%. PCR techniques had found the presence of bla_{TEM}, bla_{CTXM} and bla_{SHV} genes amongst the isolates (Lalhruaipuii *et al.,* 2021).

A total of 222 *E.coli* isolates were recovered from 230 rectal swabs of healthy beef cattle in China. Of the *E.coli* isolates, 102 strains showed ESBL phenotype. A total of 21 isolates were found positive for bla_{CTXM} gene, confirmed by PCR, followed by 18 strains with bla_{SHV} gene (Zhang *et al.,* 2021).

Multidrug resistant ESBL producing *Salmonella* were isolated from beef cattle in Bangladesh. A total of 240 beef samples were collected from different butcher shops, out of which, 98 *Salmonella* strains were isolated through selective agar method. A total of 57 isolates were ESBL producers. All the ESBL producing Salmonella were found to be positive for bla_{TEM} (100%), and none were bla_{SHV} and bla_{CTXM} positive (Ali *et al.,* 2021).

ESBL producing ampC positive *E.coli* was isolated from dairy farms in New Zealand. Faecal samples were collected from the cattle of fifteen different dairy farms. A total of 184 *E.coli* isolates were recovered from them. PCR studies had found that 10 isolates were *ampC* positive. Besides, 03 isolates also possessed $bla_{CTXM\text{-}14}$ gene (Burgess, *et al.,* 2021).

Fecal samples were collected from 30 registered farms of broiler chicken in Alberta, Canada. A total of 120 isolates were confirmed as *E.coli* through molecular analysis. Antibiotic sensitivity tests had revealed that 37 *E.coli* isolates were multidrug resistant, out of which, 19 were phenotypically positive for ampicillin resistant. All the 19 isolates were positive for *ampC* (100%), confirmed by PCR (Tran *et al.,* 2021).

The prevalence of ESBL producing *E. coli* in raw chicken meat, pork and beef meat as 51% (109/213), 26.9% (58/216) and 7.3% (15/205) was reported by Guo *et al.* (2021). Among these ESBL isolates 76.4% carried $bla_{CTX\text{-}M}$, 45.3% carried bla_{TEM} and 23% carried bla_{SHV}. The most prevalent ESBL gene detected in this study were $bla_{CTX\text{-}M\text{-}55}$ and $bla_{CTX\text{-}M\text{-}65}$.

Fecal samples were collected from 30 registered farms of broiler chicken in Alberta, Canada. A total of 120 isolates were confirmed as *E. coli* through molecular analysis. Antibiotic sensitivity tests had revealed that 37 *E. coli* isolates were multi-drug resistant, out of which, 19 were phenotypically positive for ampicillin resistant. All the 19 isolates were positive for *AmpC* (100%), confirmed by PCR (Tran *et al.,* 2021).

A total of 242 *Salmonella* isolates were recovered from 9162 bovine faecal samples in California, USA. Out of those, 110 were found positive for $bla_{CMY\text{-}2}$ and bla_{SHV}, by 45% and 50%, respectively through PCR analysis (Basbas *et al.,* 2021).

Gazal *et al.* (2021) reported 66% (78/117) prevalence of ESBL producing *E. coli* in production pyramid in southern Bzazil. In this study, they collected samples from poultry litter, poultry (cloacae), feed, water and beetles in three different periods *i.e.* on the 1st day of the chick, between 20-25 day and 36-38 day of production pyramid. He reported increase in prevalence in poultry litter, poultry and beetles though out the pyramid and absence of ESBL genes in water.

Ninety three (6.8%) ESBL producing *E. coli* isolates were reported by Kim *et al.* (2021) in which 1376 samples were collected from poultry, meat, environmental samples and farm workers in Korea. Common ESBL types were *CTX-M-55* and *CTX-M-14*, followed by *CTX-M-1*, *CTX-M-15*, *CTX-M-65*, *CTX-M-27*, and *CTX-M-61*.

The *E. coli* strains harbouring bla_{CTXM} gene were isolated from the fecal samples of cattle in South West England. A total of 4581 samples were collected from the 53 dairy farms, out of which 4145 *E.coli* isolates were recovered, which were found to be resistant against amoxicillin (66%), streptomycin (36%), ciprofloxacin (6%) and tetracycline (69%). The bla_{CTXM} gene was detected in 224 isolates (5.4%) (Schubent *et al.,* 2021).

Antimicrobial resistant and pathogenic *E.coli* and *Salmonella* species were isolated from dairy cattle and poultry farms in Northeastern Ohio, USA. A total of 844 samples were collected,out of which, 15 were confirmed as *E.coli* O157 (1.8%) and 13 were confirmed as *Salmonella* (1.5%). The *E.coli* strains were found positive for bla_{TEM} while the *Salmonella* species were found as *ampC* positive (32.1%) (Hailu *et al.,*2021).

Faecal samples of cattle were found to be harbouring *amp*C positive bacteria of *Enterobactericeae* family in North West Province, South Africa. A total of 177 samples were collected including 61 cattle faecal sample, 104 environmental sample and 12 meat samples. A total of 150 *Enterobactericeae* strains were isolated and characterized, including 65 *E.coli*, 36 *Shigella* and 15 *Klebsiella*, respectively. Antibiotic susceptibility test showed that the resistance patterns amongst the isolates, where 55.4% of the *E.coli* was resistant against Ciprofloxacin, 33.8% against Ceftazidime, 100% against Amikacin. Again, 44.4% of the *Shigella* isolates were resistant to Ciprofloxacin, 30.6% against Cefepime, 27.8% against Aztreonam. The *Klebsiella pneumonae* isolates were also found to be resistant against Aztreonam (40%), Cefotaxime (33.3%) and Cefaroxime (26.7%). Further studies showed that 32.8% were *ampC* positive (Matloko *et al.,* 2021).

A total of 271 *Salmonella enterica* isolates were recovered from fecal samples of 146 poultry, 55 farm animal and 70 environmental samples in Uttar Pradesh, India. Antimicrobial resistance pattern were observed amongst the isolates, where they were found to be resistant against nalidixic acid (50.67%), followed by tetracycline (36.3%), ampicillin (30.82%) and streptomycin (29.45%). Molecular studies had revealed that 09 isolates were found to be bla_{TEM} positive and 02 isolates were *ampC* positive (Inbaraj *et al.,* 2022).

In Indonesia, Yanestria *et al.* (2022) reported 16 (9.14%) of the 175 environmental samples from poultry coon and waste water surrounding the farm were ESBL positive that suggested dissemination of MDR bacteria into the environment.

Fecal samples of human, poultry and cattle were found to be harboring ESBL positive *E. coli*, in north Indian region. A total of 139 *E. coli* isolates were recovered from the samples. PCR studies have shown that 07 isolates were $bla_{CTX\text{-}M}$ positive (5.03%), 10 were bla_{TEM} positive (7.19%) and 04 were bla_{SHV} positive (2.87%) (Tayyaba *et al.,* 2022).

AMR scenario in Livestock of Eastern India

β-lactamase producing *E. coli* was found in the fecal and milk samples of cattle and poultry, respectively in Odisha, India. A total of 305 samples were collected, 170 of poultry fecal samples and 135 of cattle milk samples. The number of *E. coli* strains isolated were 316, out of which, 18 isolates were confirmed as ESBL producers, by disc diffusion method. These isolates were further detected with ESBL genes by PCR where 17, 13, 09 and 02 isolates were found positive for bla_{SHV}, $bla_{CTX\text{-}M}$, bla_{TEM} and bla_{AmpC}, respectively (Kar *et al.,* 2015).

ESBL positive faecal coliforms were isolated from dairy cattle in Chhatisgarh, India. A total of 70 faecal swabs were collected from cattle in Durg, Chhatisgarh. A total of 120 bacterial isolates were recovered. Antimicrobial susceptibility testing showed that 75% of the coliform were found to be resistant against amoxicillin, cefixime, ceftaxidime, imipenem and neopenem. The PCR study had revealed that 31.6% and 20% of the isolates were positive for bla_{SHV} and bla_{TEM} genes, respectively, and bla_{SHV} and bla_{TEM} co-expressions were observed in 12.1% *E.coli* and 10% of *Klebsiella* isolates (Rawat *et al.,* 2018).

In the last decade (2012 onwards) several experiments were carried out in the Department of Veterinary Microbiology, WBUAFS on different food animals, viz. poultry birds, goat, pig, buffalo and cattle that are reared under various husbandry systems in different agro-climatic zones of West Bengal state. The objective of the study was to assess antimicrobial resistance (AMR) pattern besides the probable source of resistance, if any. The results and conclusive remarks drawn out of those studies were depicted in the following section to reveal the present scenario of local AMR menace that exists in livestock.

Samanta *et al.* (2014) isolated 272 (75.5%) *E. coli* from 360 samples collected from cloacal swabs of backyard poultry and its environment (feed, water and litter) from four agro-climatic zones of West Bengal, India. Among the 272 *E. coli* isolates, 78 strains (28.67%) were untypeable (UT) and the remaining isolates (194) were distributed among 47 different O-serogroups. The major serogroups isolated were UT, O84, O147, and O60. None of the isolates were positive for extended-spectrum beta-lactamases (bla_{TEM}, bla_{SHV}, and bla_{CTX-M}) or quinolone resistance (*qnrA*) genes.

To investigate the prevalence of ESBL/beta-lactamase producing *E. coli* in healthy pigs, 200 rectal swabs were collected from four organized and 10 backyard farms of W.B. Some *E. coli* isolates (n=12) were observed to possess ESBL/beta-lactamase genes studied. The presence of *blaCTX-M-9*, *blaSHV-12*, *blaTEM-1* was noticed upon molecular characterization of the isolates. Clonal relationship was detected in two pairs of isolates obtained from organized and backyard farms. The possibility of antibiotic gene transmission from organized to backyard farm was anticipated. Pigs of backyard farm were suspected to be major source of ESBL/beta-lactamase producing *E. coli* with typical pattern of antibiotic resistance (Samanta *et al.*, 2015).

Prevalence of beta-lactamase / AmpC-producing *Klebsiella* and *E. coli* in organized and backyard healthy pig of West Bengal was noted albeit the pigs had no history of antibiotic intake. Majority of beta-lactamase–producing isolates contained *blaCTX-M-9*. Further, 81% *Klebsiella* and all the *E. coli* isolates were having AmpC beta-lactamase ACBL producers. The possible role of contaminated environment as a source of beta-lactamase/ AmpC producing *Klebsiella* and *E. coli* in pigs was anticipated (Samanta *et al.*, 2018).

In another study, assessment was done on the presence of CTX-M-producing *Klebsiella* spp. in indigenous chicken, broiler, and kuroiler birds. The study was carried out in different districts of West Bengal during November 2014 through February, 2015. While assessing type of bacteria phenotypically, the isolates showed *Klebsiella* spp. in 10.7% cases with CTX-M producers. Polymerase chain reaction revealed the isolates had *blaCTX-M*, whereas 51.5% and 48.5% *Klebsiella* spp. isolates contained *blaSHV* and *blaTEM* along with *blaCTX-M*, respectively. This investigation revealed that the studied birds harbour CTXC-M-producing *Klebsiella* spp. which might be transmitted to the food chain either directly or indirectly (Mahanti *et al.*, 2018).

In an investigation, a total of 50% of the *E. coli* strains detected in the bovine milk samples were found to be positive for ESBL production. The isolates were resistant to the common antimicrobials revealing the gravity of the situation (Batabyal *et al.*, 2018).

Cloacal swabs (n=202) were collected from ducks of organized farms and backyard to study the prevalence of bacteria of *Enterobacteriaceae* group that produce betalactamase. It was observed that, 17.4%, 5.05% and 13.76% isolates contained *blaTEM*, *blaSHV* and *blaCTX-M* genes, respectively. Moreover, in the same study, 38.46% Salmonella was isolated. These were found to contain *blaCTX-M*. *Klebsiella pnemoniae* isolates possessed 33.33% *blaTEM*, 10.00% *blaSHV* and 13.33% *blaCTX-M*. Whereas, 79.82% *E. coli*, 46.15% *Salmonella* and 70% *K. pneumonia* isolates were found to contain *blaAmpC*. The backyard ducks, reared by marginal farmers in India, cannot afford to use antibiotics in feed or during therapy owing to high cost. This study provided a valuable proof that exposure to contaminated environment might be an additional source for generation of antimicrobial resistant bacteria in backyard ducks (Banerjee *et al.*, 2019).

Batabyal *et al.* (2020) recovered 89 (78.7%) *E. coli* isolates from 113 raw meat samples of chicken from different parts of West Bengal. Among 89 isolates 17(19.1%) were positive to ESBL gene whereas 78 strains (87.6%) were found to possess bla_{AmpC} gene.

Multi-drug resistant, β-lactamase producing, *ampC* positive *E.coli* was isolated from milksamples of cattle in West Bengal. A total of 450 milk samples were collected randomly from six agro-climatic zones of West Bengal. A total of 383 *E.coli* isolates were recovered, out of which, 231 were *ampC* positive, confirmed by PCR test. The isolates were found to be resistant against penicillin G (100%), cefoxitin (100%), cefotaxime (66.2%), ampicillin (42%), co-trimoxizole (13.5%) and levofloxoacin (5.2%), confirmed by disc assay (Mahanti *et al.*, 2020).

Out of 134, 107 (79.85%) *Escherichia coli* isolates and out of 33, 24 (72.73%) *Klebsiella pneumoniae* isolates were detected as phenotypically ESBL/ACBL producers based on double-disc synergy assays. During molecular detection of the resistance genes, a total of 36(26.86%) *E. coli* and 6 (18.18%) *K. pneumoniae* isolates were found to possess the $bla_{CTX\text{-}M}$ gene (540bp) along with other genes (bla_{TEM} and bla_{SHV}) (Mondal *et al.*, 2022).

A recent study was carried out with 550 samples comprising of rectal swabs from cattle (n=170), cloacal swabs from poultry birds (n=212) and milk samples from cattle (n=168). The samples were collected from five distinct agro-climatic zones of West Bengal viz. New Alluvial, Old Alluvial, Terrai, Coastal Saline and Red Laterite. PCR studies of the ESBL specific genes showed that 53 (16.26%), 38 (11.66%) and 34 (10.43%) number of isolates possessed bla_{CTXM}, bla_{TEM} and bla_{SHV} genes, respectively. In case of the *Salmonella* isolates, a total of 17 out of 172 total isolates were phenotypically ESBL positive (9.88%), confirmed by double-disc test. Further, it was found that 37 (21.52%), 23 (13.37%) and 08 (4.65%) number of *Salmonella* isolates possessed bla_{CTXM}, bla_{TEM} and bla_{SHV} genes, respectively. It was found that 210 *E. coli* isolates (64.42%) and 98 *Salmonella* isolates (57%) were ampicillin resistant, confirmed by the PCR of *ampC* genes. A total of 45 *Staphylococcus aureus* isolates out of 146 were methicillin resistant (30.82%) was confirmed by the PCR of *mecA* gene. Further, significant differences ($p<0.01$) were observed amongst the $bla_{CTX\text{-}M}$ isolates, when studied agro-climatic zone-wise. However, there were also differences ($P<0.05$) in data when the positive isolates from two different animal sources i.e. cattle and poultry were compared and between the $bla_{CTX\text{-}M}$ positive *E. coli* and *Salmonella* i.e. between the bacterial isolates. Similar kind of results were observed in cases of bla_{TEM} and bla_{SHV} isolates, when studied agro-climatic zone-wise ($p<0.01$). Also, there were differences in observations, when bla_{TEM} positive isolates from cattle and poultry, and bla_{SHV} positive *E. coli* and *Salmonella* were compared ($p<0.05$). Although, no such significant differences were observed amongst the data, when compared bacterial isolate wise for bla_{TEM}, and animal species wise for bla_{SHV}. Diversity in climate, topography, environmental condition may influence the frequency of occurrence of ESBL positive bacterial species, which might be the reason for the significant differences within the agro-climatic zones in all three cases of the ESBL specific genes viz. $bla_{CTX\text{-}M}$, bla_{TEM} and bla_{SHV}. The bla_{AmpC} gene was found to be the most prevalent ESBL genes in *E. coli* and *Salmonella* under present study. The observations differ significantly ($p<0.01$) when studied agro-climatic zone wise (Table-1) and also amongst the isolates of two different species (Bardhan, 2023).

Table 1: Zone wise occurrence of *bla*$_{AmpC}$ positive *E.coli* isolates

Zone	Number of *E.coli* isolates	
	Cattle	Poultry
New alluvial	33^{ap}	94^{bp}
Old alluvial	09^{aq}	17^{bq}
Terrai	-	07^{r}
Coastal saline	14^{ar}	03^{bs}
Red laterite	14^{ar}	19^{bq}
Total	**70**	**140**

Values bearing different superscript (depicted as a,b) in a row differ significantly (P<0.01). Values bearing different superscript (depicted as p,q,r,s) in a column differ significantly(P<0.01)

To explore the antimicrobial resistance patterns in ESBL producing Gram-negative *Enterobacteriaceae*, focusing on *Escherichia coli*, *Salmonella* spp., and *Klebsiella* spp. sourced from duck and their surrounding environments, recently a total of 462 samples, including cloacal and tracheal swabs, and environmental samples (soil, water and feed) were collected from some representative districts of West Bengal covering three agro-climatic zones. Among the isolates, 58.48% *E. coli*, 42.20% *Salmonella* spp., and 62.11% *Klebsiella* spp. were identified as ESBL producers. Among *E. coli* isolates, the prevalence of *bla*$_{CTX\text{-}M}$ (Fig.1) (Table 2), *bla*$_{TEM}$, *bla*$_{SHV}$ and *bla*$_{AmpC}$ genes was 22.38% (124/554), 39.71% (220/554), 37.55% (208/554), and 90.79% (503/554), respectively. In case of *Salmonella* spp. isolates, 36.47% (159/436) carried the *bla*$_{TEM}$ gene, 20.64% (90/436) had *bla*$_{CTX\text{-}M}$, 17.66% (77/436) harboured *bla*$_{SHV}$, and 32.57% (142/436) contained the *bla*$_{AmpC}$ gene. Among *Klebsiella* spp., the prevalence of these genes differed: 523 isolates (78.65%) harboured the *bla*$_{AmpC}$ gene, followed by 279 (41.95%) with *bla*$_{SHV}$, 252 (37.89%) with *bla*$_{TEM}$, and 195 (29.32%) with *bla*$_{CTX\text{-}M}$ gene-carrying isolates. In the entire dataset, the *bla*$_{AmpC}$ gene exhibited the highest prevalence, ranging from 32% to 90%, followed by the genes *bla*$_{TEM}$, *bla*$_{SHV}$, and *bla*$_{CTX\text{-}M}$. The antibiotic susceptibility testing revealed concerning resistance patterns, with Cefixime demonstrating complete resistance in *E. coli* isolates. Tetracycline and Cefixime displayed high resistance rates in *Salmonella* spp., while Enrofloxacin and Ticarcillin/Clavulanic acid resistance was prominent in *Klebsiella pneumonia* (Paul, 2023). The distribution of *bla*$_{CTX\text{-}M}$ positive isolates across different agro-climatic zones is shown in Table 3.

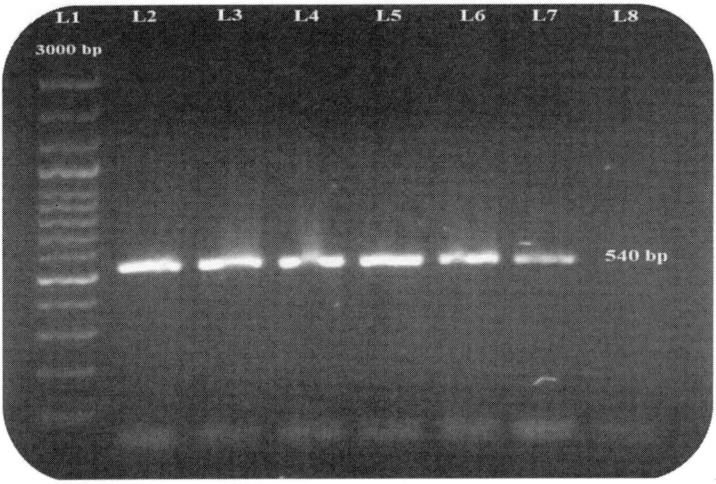

Fig. 1: Agarose gel electrophoresis showing amplified product of the $bla_{CTX\text{-}M}$ gene (540 bp) in bacterial isolates [L1: 100 bp DNA Ladder Plus, L2: Positive control, L3-L7: Test samples, L8: Negative control]

Table 2: Sample wise distribution of the $bla_{CTX\text{-}M}$ positive isolates

Bacterial Isolate	**Sample**	**No. of isolated bacteria**	**No. of $bla_{CTX\text{-}M}$ positive isolates**	**Percentage (%)**
Escherichia coli	Cloacal swab	244	60	24.59%
	Tracheal swab	224	46	20.54%
	Environmental	86	18	20.93%
Salmonella spp.	Cloacal swab	198	29	14.65%
	Tracheal swab	190	50	26.32%
	Environmental	48	11	22.92%
Klebsiella spp.	Cloacal swab	320	85	26.56%
	Tracheal swab	289	95	32.87%
	Environmental	56	15	26.79%

Table 3: Agro-climatic zone wise distribution of the $bla_{CTX\text{-}M}$ gene in different bacteria

Bacterial Isolate	**New Alluvial Zone**			**Coastal Saline Zone**			**Undulating Red & Laterite Zone**		
	No. of isolated bacteria	**$bla_{CTX\text{-}M}$ +ve**	**Percentage (%)**	**No. of isolated bacteria**	**$bla_{CTX\text{-}M}$ +ve**	**Percentage (%)**	**No. of isolated bacteria**	**$bla_{CTX\text{-}M}$ +ve**	**Percentage (%)**
Escherichia coli	346	77	22.25%	116	39	33.62%	92	08	8.7%
Salmonella spp.	232	62	26.72%	151	24	15.89%	53	04	7.55%
Klebsiella spp.	400	136	34%	159	37	23.27%	106	22	20.76%

Conclusions

The prevalence of ESBL genes in livestock-associated bacteria exhibits complex dynamics influenced by a myriad of factors, including antimicrobial usage, geographical location, and ecological interactions. Our laboratory studies contribute to the understanding of these variations, emphasizing the need for prudent antibiotic stewardship practices and continued surveillance to mitigate the potential risks associated with ESBL-producing organisms. Further research is warranted to elucidate the mechanisms driving these variations and to inform targeted interventions to curtail the spread of ESBL genes in livestock populations and the environment.

Good animal health and management practices having improved biosecurity measures should be encouraged to follow at the grass route, since animal environment is considered to be an important avenue of generating antimicrobial resistance in food animals. Better growth enhancers in form of natural products, enzymes, essential oils, antimicrobial peptides besides pro- pre- and syn-biotics should be propagated for replacing antibiotic growth promoters to avoid the chance of entering resistant bacteria in livestock. Moreover, monitoring and reporting antibiotic-use at the farmers' level should be executed meticulously for formulating fruitful strategies to address the menace of antimicrobial resistance in livestock population and in food chain.

Acknowledgements

Authors are thankful to the Vice Chancellor, WBUAFS for providing infrastructural facilities to carry out research in our laboratory. We acknowledge the funding agencies, viz. the Department of Biotechnology, Govt. of India (Grant no. BT/PR16149/NER/95/85/2015 dated19.01.2017) and the Department of Science & Technology and Biotechnology, Govt. of West Bengal (Grant no. 251 (Sanction.)-ST/P/S&T/17-G-2/2018, dated 25.2.2019) for their financial support. Thanks are also due to our Departmental colleagues, PG/PhD students and collaborators.

References

Aasmäe, B., Häkkinen, L., Kaart, T., and Kalmus, P. (2019). Antimicrobial resistance of Escherichia coli and Enterococcus spp. isolated from Estonian cattle and swine from 2010 to 2015. Acta Veterinaria Scandinavica 61(1): 1-8.

Abraham, S., Kirkwood, R. N., Laird, T., Saputra, S., Mitchell, T., Singh, M., Linn, B., Abraham, R,J., Pang, S., Gordon, D.M., Trott, D.J. and O'Dea, M. (2018). Dissemination and persistence of extended-spectrum cephalosporin-resistanceencoding IncI1-bla CTXM-1 plasmid among Escherichia coli in pigs. The ISME Journal 12(10): 2352-2362.

Abreu, R., Castro, B., Espigares, E., Rodríguez-Álvarez, C., Lecuona, M., Moreno, E., Espigares, M., and Arias, Á. (2014). Prevalence of CTX-M-Type Extended-Spectrum β-Lactamases in Escherichia coli Strains Isolated in Poultry Farms. Foodborne Pathogens and Disease, 11(11): 868-873. https://doi.org/10.1089/ fpd.2014.1796.

Ali, M.Y., Parvin, M.S., Talukder, S., Mandal, A.K., M.T. Rahman, M.T. and Islam, M.T. (2021). Multidrug resistant and extended spectrum -lactamase producing Salmonella spp. in red meat of cattle, Bangladesh. International Journal of Infectious Diseases 10.1016/j.ijid.2020.09.099

Aslam, M., Diarra, M. S., Service, C., and Rempel, H. (2009). Antimicrobial resistance genes in Escherichia coli isolates recovered from a commercial beef processing plant. Journal of Food Protection 72(5): 1089-1093.

Awosile, B. B., McClure, J. T., Sanchez, J., VanLeeuwen, J., Rodriguez-Lecompte, J. C., Keefe, G., and Heider, L. C. (2017). Extended-spectrum cephalosporin-resistant Escherichia coli in colostrum from New Brunswick, Canada, dairy cows harbor blaCMY-2 and blaTEM resistance genes. Journal of Dairy Science 100 (10): 7901-7905.

Azeredo, J., Azevedo, N.F., Briandet, R., Cerca, N., Coenye, T., Costa, A.R., Desvaux, M., Bonaventura, G.D., Hébraud, M., Jaglig, Z., Kačániová, M., Knøchel, S., Lourenço, A., Mergulhão, F., Meyer, R.L., Nychas, G., Simões, M., Tresse, O. & Sternberg, C., (2017). Critical review on biofilm methods. Critical Reviews in Microbiology 43(3): 313-351.

Banerjee, A., Bardhan, R., Chowdhury, M., Joardar, S. N., Isore, D. P., Batabyal, K., Dey, S., Sar, T. K., Bandyopadhyay, S. and Samanta, I. (2019). Characterization of beta-lactamase and biofilm producing Enterobacteriaceae isolated from organized and backyard farm ducks. Letters in Applied Microbiology 69(2): 110-115.

Bardhan, R. (2023). Molecular characteristics of biofilm producing, antibiotic resistant, prevalent pathogenic bacteria, isolated from cattle and poultry of differe nt agro- climatic zones of West Bengal. Ph.D. thesis submitted to West Bengal University of Animal and Fishery Sciences, pp.176.

Bardoň, J., Husičková, V., Chromá, M., and Kolář, M. (2013). Prevalence and characteristics of Escherichia coli strains producing extended-spectrum β-lactamases in slaughtered animals in the Czech Republic. Journal of Food Protection 76(10): 1773-1777.

Basbas, C., Byrne, B. A., Chigerwe, M., Escobar, E. D., Hodzic, E., Pires, A. F., and Pereira, R. V. (2021). Detection of Cephalosporin and Fluoroquinolone Resistance Genes via Novel Multiplex qPCR in Fecal Salmonella Isolates From Northern Californian Dairy Cattle, 2002–2016. Frontiers in Microbiology 12: 601924.

Batabyal, K., Banerjee, A, Pal, S., Dey, S., Joardar, S.N., Samanta, I., Isore ,D.P., Singh, A.D. (2018). Detection, characterization and anti-biogram of extended-spectrum beta-lactamase Escherichia coli isolated from bovine milk samples in West Bengal. Veterinary World 11: 1423- 1427.

Batabyal, K., Banerjee, A., Dey, S., Samanta, I., Isore, D.P. and Singh, A.D. (2020). Detection and Characterization of Multi Drug-resistant Extended-spectrum and pAmpC Beta-lactamases Producing Escherichia coli from Chicken Meat in West Bengal, India. International Journal of Current Microbiology and Applied Sciences 9(7): 80-89.

Blaak, H., Lynch, G., Italiaander, R., Hamidjaja, R. A., Schets, F. M., and de Roda Husman, A. M. (2015). Multidrug-resistant and extended spectrum beta-lactamase-producing Escherichia coli in Dutch surface water and wastewater. PLoS One 10(6): e0127752.

Borah, V. V., Bora, P., Roy, M., and Saikia, K. K. (2014). High prevalence of antibiotic resistance in Escherichia coli isolated from fecal sample of cows and assessment of antibacterial efficacy of indigenous medicinal plants from Assam, India. Austin Journal of Biotechnology and Bioengineering 1(1) :6.

Bradfor d, P. A. (2001). Extended-spectrum β-lactamases in the 21st century: characterization, epidemiology, and detection of this important resistance threat. Clinical Microbiology Reviews, 14(4): 933-951.

Braun, S.D., Ahmed, M.F.E., El-Adawy, H., Hotzel, H., Engelmann, I., Weiß, D., Monecke, S. and Ehricht, R. (2016). Surveillance of Extended-Spectrum Beta-Lactama[se]-Producing Escherichia coli in Dairy Cattle Farms in the Nile Delta, Egypt. Frontiers in Microbiology 7:1020. doi: 10.3389/fmicb.2016.01020

Burgess, S.A., Cookson, A.L., Brousse, L., Ortolani, E., Benschop, J., Akhter, R., Brightwell, G., McDougall, S. (2021). The epidemiology of AmpC-producing Escherichia coli isolated from dairy cattle faeces on pasture-fed farms. Journal of Medical Microbiology 70(10): 001447. doi: 10.1099/jmm.0.001447.

Carattoli, A. (2009). Resistance Plasmid Families in Enterobacteriaceae. Antimicrobial Agents and Chemotherapy 53(6). DOI: https://doi.org/10.1128/aac.01707-08.

Castellanos, L. R., Donado-Godoy, P., León, M., Clavijo, V., Arevalo, A., Bernal, J. F., Timmerman A.J., Mevius D.J., Wagenaar, D.J. and Hordijk, J. (2017). High heterogeneity of Escherichia coli sequence types harbouring ESBL/AmpC genes on IncI1 plasmids in the Colombian poultry chain. PloS one 12(1): e0170777.

Cizek, A. (2010). Antibiotic-resistant Escherichia coli bacteria, including strains with genes encoding the extended-spectrum beta-lactamase and QnrS, in waterbirds on the Baltic Sea Coast of Poland. Applied and Environmental Microbiology 76(24): 8126-8134.

Cottell, J. L., Kanwar, N., Castillo-Courtade, L., Chalmers, G., Scott, H. M., Norby, B. and Boerlin, P. (2013). $bla_{CTX-M-32}$ on an IncN plasmid in Escherichia coli from beef cattlein the United States. Antimicrobial Agents and Chemotherapy 57(2): 1096.

Dierikx, C., van der Goot, J., Fabri, T., van Essen-Zandbergen, A., Smith, H., and Mevius, D. (2 013). Extended spectrumβ lactamase and AmpC β-lactamase producing Escheric hia co li in Du tch broiler s an d broiler farmer s. Journal of Antimicrobial Chemotherapy 68(1): 60-67.

Dierikx, C. M., van Duijkeren, E., Schoormans, A. H. W., van Essen-Zandbergen, A., Veldman, K., Kant, A., Huijsdens, X.W., van der Zwaluw, K., Wagenaar, J.A. and Mevius, D. J. (2012). Occurrence and characteristics of extended-spectrum-β-lactamase-and AmpC-producing clinical isolates derived from companion animals and horses. Journal of Antimicrobial Chemotherapy 67(6): 1368-1374.

Ejaz, H., Younas, S., Abosalif, K. O., Junaid, K., Alzahrani, B., Alsrhani, A. and Hamam, S. S. (2021). Molecular analysis of blaSHV, blaTEM, and blaCTX-M in extended-spectrum β-lactamase producing Enterobacteriaceae recovered from fecal specimens of animals. PLoS One 16(1): e0245126.

Faruk, T, Hulya, T. Dilek, O. and Hakam, Y. (2016). Molecular characterization of ESBL-producing E. coli isolated from healthy cattle and sheep. Acta Veterinaria-Beograd 66 (4): 520-533. DOI: 10.1515/acve-2016-0045 0-533.

Feng, Y., Zhang, S., Shang, X., Wang, X., Wang, L., Yan, Z., Li-Hong, S. (2018). Prevalence and characteristics of extended spectrum β-lactamaseproducing Escherichia coli from bovine mastitis cases in China. Journal of Integrative Agriculture 17(6): 1246–1251.

Flemming, H. C., Wingender, J., Szewzyk, U., Steinberg, P., Rice, S. A. and Kjelleberg, S. (2016). Biofilms: an emergent form of bacterial life. Nature Reviews Microbiology 14(9): 563.

Gazal, L. E. D. S., Medeiros, L. P., Dibo, M., Nishio, E. K., Koga, V. L., Gonçalves, B. C., Kobayashi and R. K. T. (2021). Detection of ESBL/AmpC-producing and fosfomycin-resistant Escherichia coli from different sources in poultry production in Southern Brazil. Frontiers in Microbiology 11: 604544.

Geser, N., Stephan, R., Kuhnert, P., Zbinden, R., Kaeppeli, U., Cernela, N., & Haechler, H. (2011). Fecal carriage of extended-spectrum β-lactamase–producing Enterobacteriaceae in swine and cattle at slaughter in Switzerland. Journal of Food Protection 74(3): 446- 449.

Giedraitienė, A., Vitkauskienė, A., Naginienė, R. and Pavilonis, A. (2011). Antibiotic resistance mechanisms of clinically important bacteria. Medicina 47(3): 19. https://doi.org/10.3390/medicina47030019

Gonggrijp MA, Santman-Berends IMGA, Heuvelink AE, Buter GJ, van Schaik G, Hage JJ and Lam TJGM (2016). Prevalence and risk factors for extended-spectrum β-lactamase- and AmpC-producing Escherichia coli in dairy farms. Journal of Dairy Science 99(11): 9001-9013. doi: 10.3168/jds.2016-11134.

Guo, S., Aung, K. T., Leekitcharoenphon, P., Tay, M. Y. F., Seow, K. L. G., Zhong, Y., Ng, L. C., Aarestrup, F. M. and Schlundt, J. (2021). Prevalence and genomic analysis of ESBL-producing Escherichia coli in retail raw meats in Singapore. Journal of Antimicrobial Chemotherapy 76(3): 601-605. DOI: 10.1093/jac/dkaa461.

Haenni, M., Saras, E., Métayer, V., Doublet, B., Cloeckaert, A., and Madec, J. Y. (2012). Spread of the bla TEM-52 gene is mainly ensured by IncI1/ST36 plasmids in Escherichia coli isolated from cattle in France. Journal of Antimicrobial Chemotherapy 67(11): 2774-2776.

Hailu, W., Helmy, Y. A., Carney-Knisely, G., Kauffman, M., Fraga, D., and Rajashekara, G. (2021). Prevalence and antimicrobial resistance profiles of foodborne pathogens isolated from dairy cattle and poultry $_{manure}$ amended farms in northeastern Ohio, the United States. Antibiotics 10(12): 1450.

Hall, C. W., and Mah, T. F. (2017). Molecular mechanisms of biofilm-based antibiotic resistance and tolerance in pathogenic bacteria. FEMS Microbiology Reviews 41(3): 276-301.

Hasman, H., Mevius, D., Veldman, K., Olesen, I., Aarestrup, F. M. (2005). Beta-Lactamases among extended-spectrum beta-lactamase (ESBL)-resistant Salmonella from poultry, poultry products and human patients in The Netherlands. Journal of Antimicrobial Chemotherapy, 56(1): 115-21. DOI: 10.1093/jac/dki190.

Hiraki, A., Tsuchiya, Y., Fukuda, Y., Yamamoto, T., Kurniawan, A. and Morisaki, H. (2009). Analysis of how a biofilm forms on the surface of the aquatic macrophyte Phragmites australis. Microbes and Environments 24(3): 265-272.

Hiroi, M., Yamazaki, F, Harda, T., Takahashi, N., Iida, N., Noda, Y., Yagi, M., Nishio, T., Kanda, T., Kawamori, F., Sugiyama, K., Masuda, T., Hara-Kudo, Y., Ohashi, N. (2012). Prevalence of extended spectrum β lactamase- producing E. coli and Klebsiella pneumonia in food-producing animals. Journal of Veterinary Medical Science 74(2): 185-195. doi: 10.1292/jvms.11-0372

Hordijk J, Wagenaar JA, van de Giessen A, Dierikx C, van Essen-Zandbergen A, Veldman K, Kant A, Mevius D. (2013). Increasing prevalence and diversity of ESBL/AmpC-type β-lactamase genes in Escherichia coli isolated from veal calves from 1997 to 2010. Journal of Antimicrobial Chemotherapy 68(9):1970-1973. doi: 10.1093/jac/dkt132. Epub 2013 May 8. PMID: 23657803.

Horton, R.A, Randall, LP., Snary, E.L., Cockrem, H., Lotz, S., Wearing, H., Duncan, D., Rabie, A., McLaren, ., Watson, E., La Ragione, R.M. and Colddham, L.G. (2011). Fecal carriage and shedding density of CTX-M extended spectrum β- lactamase producing E. coli in cattle, chickens and pig: implications for environmental contamination and food production. Applied and Environmental Microbiology 77 (11): 3715-3719.

Hussain, A., Shaik, S., Ranjan, A., Nandanwar, N., Tiwari, S. K., Majid, M., Baddam, R., Qureshi, I. A., Semmler, T., Weiler, L. H., Islam, M. A., Chakravortty, D. and Ahmed, N.

(2017). Risk of transmission of antimicrobial resistant Escherichia coli from commercial broiler and free-range retail chicken in India. Frontiers in Microbiology 8: https://doi.org/10.3389/fmicb.2017.02120.

Hussain, M. A., Wang, W., Sun, C., Gu, L., Liu, Z., Yu, T., Ahmad Y, Jiang Z, and Hou, J. (2020). Molecular Characterization of pathogenic Salmonella spp from raw beef in Karachi, Pakistan. Antibiotics 9(2):73. doi: 10.3390/antibiotics9020073

Inbaraj, S., Agrawal, R. K., Thomas, P., Mohan, C., RK, S. A., Verma, M. R., and Chaudhuri, P. (2022). Antimicrobial resistance in Indian isolates of non typhoidal Salmonella of livestock, poultry and environmental origin from 1990 to 2017. Comparative Immunology, Microbiology and Infectious Diseases 80: 101719.

Ismael, G. K., and Nasser, H. H. (2017). Molecular determination of extended spectrum β-lactamases antibiotics resistance genes in E. coli isolated from diarrhea in cattle. Al-Qadisiyah Journal of Veterinary Medicine Sciences 16(1): 67-73.

Jacoby, G. A. and Munoz-Price, L. S. (2005). The new β-lactamases. New England Journal of Medicine 352(4): 380-391.

Kar, D., Bandyopadhyay, S., Bhattacharyya, D., Samanta, I., Mahanti, A., Nanda, P. K. and Singh, R. K. (2015). Molecular and phylogenetic characterization of multidrug resistant extended spectrum beta-lactamase producing Escherichia coli isolated from poultry and cattle in Odisha, India. Infection, Genetics and Evolution 29: 82-90.

Karim, A., Poirel, L., Nagarajan, S. and Nordmann, P. (2001). Plasmid-mediated extended-spectrum β-lactamase (CTX-M-3 like) from India and gene association with insertion sequence IS Ecp1. FEMS microbiology letters 201(2): 237-241.

Kim, H., Kim, Y. A., Seo, Y. H., Lee, H. and Lee, K. (2021). Prevalence and Molecular Epidemiology of Extended Spectrum-β-Lactamase (ESBL) Producing Escherichia coli from Multiple Sectors of Poultry Industry in Korea. Antibiotics 10: 1050.

Lalhruaipuii, K., Dutta, T. K., Roychoudhury, P., Chakraborty, S., Subudhi, P. K., Samanta, I., Bandyopadhay, S. and Singh, S.B. (2021). Multidrug-Resistant Extended-Spectrum β-Lactamase-Producing Escherichia coli Pathotypes in North Eastern R egi on of India : Backyard Smal l Ruminants–Human–Water Interface. Microbial Drug Resistance. DOI: 10.1089/mdr.2020.0365

Lee, .S, Teng, L., DiLorenzo, N., Weppelmann, T.A., Jeong, K.C. (2020). Prevalence and Molecular Characteristics of Extended-Spectrum and AmpC β-Lactamase Producing Escherichia coli in Grazing Beef Cattle. Frontiers in Microbioogy 10: 3076. doi: 10.3389/fmicb.2019.03076.

Li, L., Wang, B., Feng, S., Li, J., Wu, C., Wang, Y., Ruan, X., Zeng, M. (2014). Prevalence and Characteristics of Extended-Spectrum β-Lactamase and Plasmid-Mediated Fluoroquinolone Resistance Genes in Escherichia coli Isolated from Chickens in Anhui Province, China. PLoS ONE 9(8): e104356. DOI:10.1371/journal.pone.0104356.

Literak, I., Dolejska, M., Janoszowska, D., Hrusakova, J., Meissner, W., Rzyska, H., Bzoma, S. and

Livermore, D. M. (1995). Beta-Lactamases in laboratory and clinical resistance. Clinical Microbiology Reviews 8(4): 557-584.

Ma, J., Liu, J. H., Lv, L., Zong, Z., Sun, Y., Zheng, H., Chen, Z. L. and Zeng, Z. L. (2012). Characterization of extended-spectrum β-lactamase genes found among Escherichia coli isolates from duck and environmental samples obtained on a duck farm. Applied and Environmental Microbiology 78(10): 3668-3673.

Mahanti, A., Joardar, S. N., Bandyopadhyay, S., Ghosh, S., Batabyal, K., & Samanta, I. (2020). Milk from healthy or infected cattle as a source of multi-drug resistant, AmpC β-lactamase-producing Escherichia coli. Indian Journal of Dairy Science 73(4): 343-347.

Mahanti A, Ghosh P, Samanta I, Joardar SN, Bandyopadhyay S, Bhattacharyya D, Banerjee J, Batabyal S, Sar TK and T.K. Dutta (2018). Prevalence of CTX-M-producing Klebsiella spp. in broiler, kuroiler and indigenous poultry in West Bengal state, India. Microbial Drug Resistance 24: 299-306.

Matloko, K., Fri, J., Ateba, T. P., Molale-Tom, L. G., and Ateba, C. N. (2021). Evidence of potentially unrelated AmpC beta-lactamase producing Enterobacteriaceae from cattle, cattle products and hospital environments commonly harboring the blaACC resistance determinant. Plos one 16(7): e0253647.

McEwen SA and Fedorka-Cray, P J. Antimicrobial use and resistance in animals (2002). Clinical Infectious Diseases 34:S93-106.

Melo, L., Bott, T. R., Fletcher, M. and Capdeville, B. (Eds.). (2012). In: Biofilms-Scienc e and Technology. Vol. 223, Springer Science and Business Media. 13.

Mollenkopf, D. F., Weeman, M. F., Daniels, J. B., Abley, M. J., Mathews, J. L., Gebreyes, W. A., ad Wittum, T. E. (2012). Variable within-and between-herd diversity of CTX-M cephalosporinase-bearing Escherichia coli isolates from dairy cattle. Applied and Environmental Microbiology 78(13): 4552-4560.

Mondal, T., Batabyal, K., Dey, S., Joardar, S. N., Samanta, I., Isore, D. P., Samanta, S. and Paul, A. (2022). Detection and Characterization of β-lactamases and Biofilm producing Escherichia coli and Klebsiella pneumoniae from Ducks and Duck Environments in West Bengal. Indian Journal of Animal Research B-4915: 1-7.

Montso KP, Dlamini SB, Kumar A, Ateba CN (2019). Antimicrobial Resistance Factors of Extended-Spectrum Beta-Lactamases Producing Escherichia coli and Klebsiella pneumoniae Isolated from Cattle Farms and Raw Beef in North-West Province, South Africa. Biomed Res Int. 2019: 4318306. doi: 10.1155/2019/4318306. PMID: 31915693; PMCID: PMC6935440.

Na, S. H., Moon, D. C., Choi, M. J., Oh, S. J., Jung, D. Y., Sung, E. J., Kang, H. Y., Hyun, B. H. and Lim, S. K. (2019). Antimicrobial resistance and molecular characterization of extended-spectrum β-lactamase-producing Escherichia coli isolated from ducks in South Korea. Foodborne Pathogens and Disease 16(12): 799-806.

Pacholewicz, E., Liakopoulos, A., Swart, A., Gortemaker, B., Dierikx, C., Havelaar, A., and Schmitt, H. (2015). Reduction of extended-spectrum-β-lactamase-and AmpC-β-lactamase-producing Escherichia coli through processing in two broiler chicken slaughterhouses. International Journal of Food Microbiology 215: 57-63.

Palmeira, J.D., Haenni, M., Metayer, V., Madec, J-Y., Helena Maria Neto Ferreira, H.M. (2020). Epidemic spread of IncI1/pST113 plasmid carrying the Extended-Spectrum Beta-Lactamase (ESBL) blaCTX-M-8 gene in Escherichia coli o f Braz ilian cattle. Ve terinary Mi crobiology 243, 108629. doi.org/10.1016/j.vetmic.2020.108629.

Paul, A. (2023). Molecular characterization of biofilm producing antibiotic resistant bacteria from duck and associated environment in West Bengal. Ph.D. thesis submitted to West Bengal University of Animal and Fishery Sciences, pp.186.

Prajapati, B. I., Solanki, K. M., Devi, S., Katira, B. P., Patel, S. S., Raval, S. H., & Momin, R. R. (2020). Phenotypic and molecular characterization of ESBLs producing Escherichia coli in bovine faecal and milk samples of North Gujarat. Indian Journal of Animal Sciences 90(7): 987-992.

Rahman, S., Ahmad, S. and Khan, I. (2018). Incidence of ESBL Producing Escherichia coli in Poultry Farm Environment and Retail Poultry Meat. Pakistan Veterinary Journal, 39(1): 116-120. DOI: http://dx.doi.org/10.29261/pakvetj/2018.091.

Rawat, N., Singh, F., Hirpurkar, S. D., Sannat, C., and Gade, N. E. (2018). Detection and characterization of extended-spectrum beta-lactamase genes (blaTEM and blaSHV) among beta-lactam-resistant fecal coliforms of dairy cattle from Chhattisgarh, India. Turkish Journal of Veterinary & Animal Sciences 42(6): 503-511.

Reich, F., Atanassova, V., and Klein, G. (2013). Extended-spectrum β-lactamase–and AmpC-producing Enterobacteria in healthy broiler chickens, Germany. Emerging Infectious Diseases 19(8): 1253.

Rossi, F., Baquero, F., Hsueh, P. R., Paterson, D. L., Bochicchio, G. V., Snyder, T. A., Satishchandran, V., MacCarroll, K., DiNubile, M. J. and Chow, J. W. (2006). In vitro susceptibilities of aerobic and facultatively anaerobic Gram-negative bacilli isolated from patients with intra-abdominal infections worldwide: 2004 results from SMART (Study for Monitoring Antimicrobial Resistance Trends). Journal of Antimicrobial Chemotherapy 58(1): 205-210.

Ruiz, J. (2018). Etymologia: TEM. Emerging Infectious Diseases 24(4): 709. DOI:10.3201/eid2404.et2404.

Saliu, E-M., Vahjen, W. and Zentek, J. (2017). Types and prevalence of extended-spectrum beta-lactamase producing Enterobacteriaceae in poultry. Animal Health Research Reviews 18(1): 46-57. DOI: 10.1017/S1466252317000020.

Samaha-Kfoury, J. N. and Araj, G. F. (2003). Recent developments in β lactamases and extended spectrum β lactamases. British Medical Journal 327(7425): 1209-1213.

Samanta, I., Joardar, S. N., Das, P. K., Das, P., Sar, T. K., Dutta, T. K., and Isore, D. P. (2014). Virulence repertoire, characterization, and antibiotic resistance pattern analysis of Escherichia coli isolated from backyard layers and their environment in India. Avian diseases 58(1): 39-45.

Samanta A, Mahanti A, Chattaerjee S, Joardar SN, Bandyopadhyay S, Sar TK, Mandal GP, Dutta TK and Samanta I. (2018). Pig farm environment as a source of beta-lactamase or AmpC-producing Klebsiella pneumonia and Escherichia coli. Annals in Microbiology 68 : 781-791.

Samanta I, Joardar SN, Mahanti A, Bandyopadhyay S, Sar T K, and Dutta TK (2015). Approaches to characterize extended spectrum betalactamase/beta-lactamase producing Escherichia coli in healthy organized vis-à-vis backyard farmed pigs in India. Infection Genetics and Evolution 36: 224-230.

Sauer, K., Camper, A. K., Ehrlich, G. D., Costerton, J. W. and Davies, D. G. (2002). Pseudomonas aeruginosa displays multiple phenotypes during development as a biofilm. Journal of Bacteriology 184(4): 1140-1154.

Schubert, H., Morley, K., Puddy, E. F., Arbon, R., Findlay, J., Mounsey, O., Gould, V.C., Vass, L., Evans, M., Rees, G.M., Barrett, D.C., Turner, K.M., Cogan, T.A., Avison, M.B. and Reyher, K. K. (2021). Reduced antibacterial drug resistance and bla CTX-M β-lactamase gene carriage in cattle-associated Escherichia coli at low temperatures, at sites dominated by older animals, and on pastureland: implications for surveillance. Applied and Environmental Microbiology 87(6): e01468-20.

Seo, K. W., Kim, Y. B., Jeon, H. Y., Lim, S-K., Lee and Y. J. (2018). Comparative genetic characterization of third-generation cephalosporin-resistant Escherichia coli from chicken meat produced by integrated broiler operations in South Korea. Poultry Science 97(8): 2871–2879. DOI:10.3382/ps/pey127.

Sharif, N. M., Sreedevi, B., and Chaitanya, R. K. (2017). Occurrence of beta-lactam resistant Escherichia coli among clinical cases of livestock in Andhra Pradesh. International Journal of Science Environment andTechnology 6(2): 1608-1615.

Singh, S. B. (2021). Multidrug-Resistant Extended-Spectrum β-Lactamase-Producing Escherichia coli Pathotypes in North Eastern Region of India: Backyard Small Ruminants–Human–Water Interface. Microbial Drug Resistance 27(12): 1664-1671.

Song, H. J., Moon, D. C., Mechesso, A. F., Kang, H. Y., Kim, M. H., Choi, J. H., ... & Lim, S. K. (2020). Resistance profiling and molecular characterization of extended- spectrum/ plasmid-mediated Ampc β-lactamase-producing Escherichia coli isolated from healthy broiler chickens in South Korea. Microorganisms 8(9): 1434.

Steenackers, H., Hermans, K., Vanderleyden, J., & De Keersmaecker, S. C. (2012). Salmonella biofilms: an overview on occurrence, structure, regulation and eradication. Food Research International, 45(2): 502-531.

Sudarwanto, M. B., Lukman, D. W., Purnawarman, T., Latif, H., Pisestyani, H., & Sukmawinata, E. (2017). Multidrug resistance extended spectrum β-lactamase and AmpC producing Escherichia coli isolated from the environment of Bogor Slaughterhouse, Indonesia. Asian Pacific Journal of Tropical Biomedicine 7(8): 708-711.

Tamamura, Y., Uchida, I., Tanaka, K., Okazaki, H., Tezuka, S., Hanyu, H., Nakaoka, Y. and Akiba, M. (2011). Molecular epidemiology of Salmonella enterica serovar Typhimurium isolates from cattle in Hokkaido, Japan: evidence of clonal replacement and characterization of the disseminated clone. Applied and Environmental Microbiology 77(5): 1739-1750.

Tamang, M. D., Nam, H. M., Gurung, M., Jang, G. C., Kim, S. R., Jung, S. C., Park, Y.H. and Lim, S. K. (2013). Molecular characterization of CTX-M β-lactamase and associated addiction systems in Escherichia coli circulating among c attle, farm workers, and the farm environment. Applied and Environmental Microbiology 79(13): 3898-3905.

Tayyaba, U., Ahmed, S., Singh, A., and Shahid, M. (2022). Gut resistome with special reference to beta-lactamase-producers from human, poultry, and cattle from north-Indian region: A step towards "one health" approach. New Zealand Journal of Medical Laboratory Science 76(1): 18-25.

Tong, P., Sun, Y., Ji, X., Du, X., Guo, X., Liu, J., Zhu, L., Zhou, B., Zhou, W., Liu, G. and Feng, S. (2015). Characterization of Antimicrobial Resistance and Extended-Spectrum β -Lactamase Genes in Escherichia coli Isolated from Chickens. Foodborne Pathogens and Disease 12(4). DOI:10.1089/fpd.2014.1857.

Tran, T., Checkley, S., Caffrey, N., Mainali, C., Gow, S., Agunos, A., & Liljebjelke, K. (2021). Genetic Characterization of AmpC and Extended-Spectrum Beta-Lactamase Phenotypes in Escherichia coli and Salmonella from Alberta Broiler Chickens. Frontiers in Cellular and Infection Microbiology 11: 622195.

Tshitshi, L., Manganyi, M. C., Montso, P. K., Mbewe, M., & Ateba, C. N. (2020). Extended spectrum beta-lactamase-resistant determinants among carbapenem-resistant Enterobacteriaceae from beef cattle in the north West Province, South Africa: a critical assessment of their possible public health implications Antibiotics 9(11): 820.

Tzouvelekis, L. S., Tzelepi, E., Tassios, P. T. and Legakis, N. J. (2000). CTX-M-type β-lactamases: an emerging group of extended-spectrum enzymes. International Journal of Antimicrobial Agents, 14(2): 137-142.

Velasova, M., Smith, R.P., Lemma, F., Horton, R.A., Duggett, N.A., Evans, J., Tongue, S.C, Anjum, M.F., Randall, L.P. (2019). Detection of extended-spectrum β-lactam, AmpC and carbapenem resistance in Enterobacteriaceae in beef cattle in Great Britain in 2015. Journal of AppliedMicrobiology 126(4): 1081-1095.

Voets, G. M., Fluit, A. C., Scharringa, J., Schapendonk, C., van den Munckhof, T., Leverstein-van Hall, M. A., and Stuart, J. C. (2013). Identical plasmid AmpC beta-lactamase genes and plasmid types in E. coli isolates from patients and poultry meat in the Netherlands.

International Journal of Food Microbiology 167(3): 359-362.

Wickens, H. and Wade, P. (2005). Understanding antibiotic resistance. Pharmaceutical Journal 274(7346): 501-504.

Wieland, N., Boss, J., Lettmann, S., Fritz, B., Schwaiger, K., Bauer, J., and Hölzel, C. S. (2017). Susceptibility to disinfectants in antimicrobial resistant and susceptible isolates of Escherichia coli, Enterococcus faecalis and Enterococcus faecium from poultry– ESBL/ AmpC phenotype of E. coli is not associated with resistance to a quaternary ammonium compound, DDAC. Journal of Applied Microbiology 122(6): 1508-1517.

Yanestria, S. M., Dameanti, F. N. A. K. P., Musayannah, B. G., Pratama, J. W. A., Witaningrum, A. M., Effendi, M. H. and Ugbo, E. N. (2022). Antibiotic resistance pattern of Extended-Spectrum β-Lactamase (ESBL) producing Escherichia coliisolated from broiler farm environment in Pasuruan district, Indonesia. Biodiversitas 23(9): 4460-4465. DOI: 10.13057/biodiv/d230911.

Yang, H., Rehman, M. U., Zhang, S., Yang, J., Li, Y., Gao, J., Gu, L., Wang, M., Jia, R., Chen, S., Liu, M., Zhu, D., Zhao, X., Wu, Y., Yang, Q., Huan, J., Zhang, L., Liu, Y., Tian, B., Pan, L., Cheng, X. and Cheng, A. (2019). High prevalence of CTX-M belonging to ST410 and ST889 among ESBL producing E. coli isolates from waterfowl birds in China's tropical island, Hainan. Acta Tropica 194: 30-35.

Yao, R. K., Coulibaly, J. K., Tiekoura, B. K., Yapi, F. H., & Djaman, J. A. (2018). Molecular Characterization of Extended-Spectrum Beta-lactamase Producing Escherichia coli Isolated from Cattle Faeces in Abidjan District, Ivory Coast. Microbiology Research Journal International 25(5): 1-10.

Zhang, Y. L., Huang, F. Y., Gan, L. L., Yu, X., Cai, D. J., Fang, J., Zhong ZJ, Guo HR, Xie Y, Yi J, Wang ZS and Zuo, Z. C. (2021). High prevalence of bla_{CTX-M} and bla_{SHV} among ESBL producing E. coli isolates frombeef cattle in China's Sichuan-Chongqing Circle. Scientific Reports 11(1): 13725.

Zurfluh, K., Jakobi, G., Stephan, R., Hächler, H. and Nüesch-Inderbinen, M. (2014). Replicon typing of plasmids carrying $bla_{CTX-M-1}$ in Enterobacteriaceae of animal, environmental and human origin. Frontiers in Microbiology, 5: 555. DOI: 10.3389/fmicb.2014.00555.

7

Unusual Causes of Emergence of Antimicrobial Drug Resistance

Bhoj R. Singh, R. Karthikeyan and A. Yadav

Division of Epidemiology, Indian Veterinary Research Institute, Izatnagar Uttar Pradesh, India

Globally, antimicrobial resistance (AMR) is an important public health and development threat (WHO, 2020). Being one of the top 10 global public health threats, the ever-increasing rates in the occurrence of drug-resistant bacterial infections have become a grave public health concern for the governments (Laxminarayan *et al.*, 2013). Moreover, such infections would be difficult to treat and therefore can lead to worse clinical outcomes (Laxminarayan *et al.*, 2013). Worldwide, each year about 700,000 people die from antimicrobial-resistant infections and the mortality figures are projected to reach 10 million/ year by 2050 (O'Neill, 2016). The crude infectious disease mortality rate in India is more than 400 per 100,000 persons and at least 23,000 deaths in adults and 58,000 neonatal deaths per year are caused by AMR bacteria (Laxminarayan and Chaudhury, 2016). A 2017 estimate puts the cost of developing an antibiotic at around US$1.5 billion (Towse, *et al.* 2017). Meanwhile, industry analysts estimate that the average revenue generated from an antibiotic's sale is roughly $46 million per year. "That's tiny and nowhere near the amount needed to justify the investment," because the life of the antibiotic is not much. Globally about 35 billion doses of antibiotics (3500-5000 tons) are used for therapy and disease prevention in human medicine, and about 50000 tons for treatment and growth promotion in the livestock and agriculture sector. New Estimates are >100 000 tonnes of antibiotic use in livestock (OIE, 2019)

Causes of Emergence of AMR

There are some conventionally accepted main drivers of antimicrobial resistance (WHO, 2020) including,

- Exposure of bacteria to irrational/ inappropriate/ sub-therapeutic doses of antibiotics.

- Misuse and Overuse of antibiotics in human therapeutics.
- Routine use of antibiotics to grow faster the food animals.
- Lack or inefficient access to clean water, sanitation and hygiene (WASH).
- Poor infection and disease prevention and control in health-care facilities and farms.
- Poor access to quality, affordable medicines, vaccines, and diagnostics.
- Lack of awareness and knowledge and
- Lack of enforcement of legislation.

Wherefrom Antibiotic Exposure Come to Bacteria?

Over consumption of antibiotics (irrespective of proper or improper use) for therapeutic and preventive purposes by humans. It is claimed that doctors routinely receive compensation from pharmaceutical companies and pharmacists in exchange for antibiotic prescriptions. Overuse of antibiotics in the veterinary field for therapeutic and preventive purposes. Antimicrobial drug use in food production systems such as animals, birds, fish, agriculture. Waste generated in hospitals and laboratories containing antimicrobials.

New Dimensions in Emergence of AMR

Effect of Disinfectants, Antiseptics, and Biocides on AMR

Overuse/uncontrolled use of antimicrobials has long been believed to fuel antimicrobial resistance (AMR), but new research shows that simply lowering consumption is not enough. Poor sanitation, corruption, and low public health spending have a bigger role in pushing up drug-resistant infections in low and middle-income countries, including India. Use of non-antibiotic antimicrobials (NAAM) like biocides/ disinfectants and antiseptics are used in much larger quantities than antibiotics, resulting in high residual levels of NAAM chemicals in the wider environment. After the start of the covid-19 era, the sudden overuse of cleaning products and hand sanitizers could have lead to an increase in the number of antimicrobial-resistant bacteria; the impact may be felt afterward. Because these products contain ingredients like phenol and hydrogen peroxide which have the potential to extensively damage or alter the DNA of bacteria, leads to mutations (Morgan, 2020). Though most sanitizers claim 99.99% effective in killing germs, microbiologists in Ontario showed that just 46%-60% of bacteria were killed on the hands after the use of hand sanitizers (FDA, 2019). The antiseptics and disinfectants as 10% povidone-iodine, 4% chlorhexidine gluconate solution, 4.8% chloroxylenol Dettol, 2% Lysol, 2% glutaraldehyde, 1% sodium hypochlorite solution, 2% liquid phenol, chlorophenol can induce resistance gene in the microbes and AMR through mutation or horizontal gene transfer to be propagated to the hospital environment (Ghosh *et al.*, 2016; Lu and Guo, 2021). Studies have been reported the chlorhexidine induces the expression of VanA-type vancomycin resistance genes and genes associated with daptomycin nonsusceptibility (Bhardwaj *et al.*, 2016). Chlorinated phenols (chlorophenols) induced the *mex*AB-*opr*M-mediated antibiotic-resistant in *Pseudomonas aeruginosa* (Muller *et al.*, 2015). It is important to note that *mex*AB efflux pump activation is responsible for pan drug resistance in *Pseudomonas aeruginosa* even against herbal drugs (Vadhana *et al.*, 2017).

Consumption of liquid disinfectants in 2008 in India was 7339 (KiloLitres~ Tons) with a share of Dettol (4.8% Chloroxylenol, 84%), Savlon (4% chlorhexidine gluconate,13%), and Suthol (Cetrimide, Chlorhexidine Gluconate, Neem, Turmeric, Marigold and Aloe vera, 3%). (Karania, 2012; https://www.slideshare.net/DhirKarania/dettol-marketing). In COVID-19 era the sanitizers witnessed 400% jump in demand and use. The global surface disinfectant market to grow at a Compound Annual Growth Rate (CAGR) of 11.70% during the period 2017-2021 (https://ijpsr.com/bft-article/disinfectants-regulation-and-requirements-global-overview/?view=fulltext). The global surface disinfectants market is projected to reach USD 3.6 billion by 2025 from USD 3.1 billion in 2020, at a CAGR of 3.0% from 2020 to 2025. Some of the major factors driving the growth of this market are the increasing prevalence of hospital-acquired infections (HAIs) and the presence of stringent regulations for the use of surface disinfectants (https://www.marketsandmarkets.com/Market-Reports/surface-disinfectant-market-231286043.html). However, occurrence of COVID-19 has already modulated the disinfectant market and it will be known soon.

Biocides: Exposure to low concentrations of a variety of biocides especially antibacterial and dyes resulted in the appearance of resistant mutants. It leads to the adaptation of bacteria towards them in different ways including an increase in the number of efflux pumps in the bacteria. Because the efflux pumps can also rid the cell of some antibiotics, pathogenic bacteria with more pumps are a threat to patients as they could be more resistant to treatment. (Society for General Microbiology, 2008).

Health concerns on Triclosan (TCS): Triclosan can be found in many places today. It has been added to many consumer products—including clothing, kitchenware, furniture, and toys—to prevent bacterial contamination. Because of that, people's long-term exposure to triclosan is higher than previously thought, raising concerns about the potential risks associated with the use of this ingredient over a lifetime. It is used in over 2000 kinds of products such as toothpaste and hand washing liquids. In the US alone, 1.1 × 105 to 4.2 × 105 kg of TCS are discharged from wastewater treatment plants (WWTPs) every year (Dann and Hontela, 2011). There is evidence of triclosan-induced heritable multi-drug resistance in *E. coli*. The oxidative stress induced by TCS caused mutations in fabI, frdD, marR, acrR , and soxR. Mutations led to resistance by up-regulating beta-lactamase and multi-drug efflux pump (Lu *et al*., 2018).

Role of Government and Regulators in Emergence and Spread of AMR

Due to the transnational nature and multi-sector scope of AMR, there is an urgent need for specific, clear, and coherent guidance from the global level to enable countries to devise impactful national action plans in line with the global action plans. There are some flaws in the regulations designed at the national level for manufacturing antimicrobials which leads to the emergence and spread of AMR. Sub-therapeutic exposure of microbes to antimicrobials comes from the foul-play of administrators and pharmaceutical companies in India, as: Misuse of antibiotics as a preservative: Use of Enrofloxacin as preservative in FMD Vaccine in India (https://www.researchgate.net/publication/267705649_Testing_of_FMD_Vaccine_intended_to_be_used_under_FMD-CP_of_Govt_of_India_at_CCS_NIAH_Baghpat_UP_India). Flaws in the pharmaceutical waste disposal management cause the release of low doses of antimicrobials into the environment, which makes the microbes resistant by the action of selection pressure.

Emergence of AMR due to Pharma Companies

Antibiotic manufacturing processes can increase drug resistance in two main routes: by releasing antibacterial residue directly into the environment; and by manufacturing antibacterial with too little of the active ingredient. Both routes give microbes extra opportunities to develop resistance. Pharmaceutical waste from antibiotic-producing pharmaceuticals polluting water bodies and soil to make natural resources the breeding grounds for AMR bacteria (Alejandro, 2016). Indian and Chinese drug makers routinely release untreated waste fluid containing active ingredients into surrounding soil and waterways (Waxman and Corr, 2016) Reducing antibiotic-laden pollution from pharmaceutical manufacturing plants is a relatively easy, affordable part of the solution. However, in India releasing all noxious wastes into Ganges, its tributaries and other sacred rivers is much easier and cheaper using bribes.

Pharma Pollution

Large environmental contaminations, including those leading to resistant organisms, have repeatedly been identified around bulk drug manufacturing plants in India and China. "Particular bulk drug manufacturing plants in Hyderabad, South India, have been shown to dump waste into their surroundings or fail to treat manufacturing discharges appropriately, resulting in the contamination of rivers and lakes. In some cases, the pharmaceutical concentrations in the water samples they took were higher than those found in the blood of patients taking medicine. The concentration of ciprofloxacin, a broad-spectrum antibiotic, was approximately one million times greater than the levels that are regularly found in treated municipal sewage effluent (Larsson *et al.*, 2007). In a study conducted in Pakistan, the highest levels of both antibiotics and resistance genes were seen at rivers, canal, and near drug formulation facility, within an industrial estate with a low number of residents and no hospitals in the vicinity, which indicates that the levels of antibiotic resistance genes at this site were associated with the environmental levels of antibiotics (Khan *et al.*, 2013). Hyderabad is a global market for bulk drug purchasing with 50% of India's drug exports, pegged at over $3 billion, coming from the city. Researchers from Leipzig University Hospital, Germany, tested 28 water samples from different places in the city, including sewage from around pharma manufacturing units in Patancheru-Bollaram Industrial Development Area on the outskirts. They found "unprecedented antimicrobial drug contamination" in the samples collected from around the pharma units. The study claimed that Indian authorities have not done enough to ensure efficient treatment of wastewater discharged by the pharma industry (Rohit, 2017). Most major drug companies display a "shocking lack of concern" about pollution in their supply chains (Davis, 2015).

Indian Drug Companies Try to Gut Antibiotic Pollution Controls

In January 2020, the Indian government published a draft bill to introduce its first limits on the concentration of 121 common antibiotics that can be discharged into rivers and the surrounding environment. The bill came after several investigations by the Bureau and Changing Markets and campaigning by the Centre for Science and Environment in New Delhi and the Stockholm International Water Institute.

The Indian Drug Manufacturers Association (IDMA) has lobbied both the Ministry of Environment, Forests and Climate Change and the Central Pollution Control Board. In a letter to the ministry, the association claimed that if the proposed environmental measures go ahead, the industry would face "untold miseries from litigations and harassment by the activist and regulator alike". (https://www.thebureauinvestigates.com/stories/2020-03-31/indian-drug-companies-try-to-gut-antibiotic-pollution-controls). Being the most Pharma friendly Nation (https://azad-azadindia.blogspot.com/2021/01/india-worlds-most-corporate-pharma.html), the bill is dumped now.

Therapeutic use of Sub-Standard (NSQD) Antibiotics in Therapy

Recent surveys revealed that Asia is the single largest counterfeit drug-producing region. Within Asia, India is the leader followed by Egypt and China. About 75% of counterfeit drugs supplied in the world originate in India, followed by 7% in Egypt and 6% in China. Fake drugs and vaccines are responsible for more than a million deaths across the globe every year. Indian health ministry estimated that 5% of drugs in India are counterfeit, while 0.3% are spurious. In India 'Bhagirath Palace' Chandni Chowk, New Delhi is said to be the hub for counterfeit and spurious drugs. In the Indian Pharma market of 40,000 crore, 20% is of fake drugs. Multibillion-dollar business of Substandard and spurious Antibiotics for therapeutic use. (Singh, 2017). As per Central Drugs Standard Control Organization (CDSCO), India, about 6.3-10.64% of drugs were substandard (NSQD) and up to 0.47% were fake, in 2010 in India. (http://www.cdsco.nic.in/writereaddata/REPORT_BOOK_13-7-10.pdf). The estimated business of antibiotics in India in 2009 was Rs. 64.14 billion (Ganguly, 2011), in 2016, India consumed antibiotics worth more than Rs. 150 billion (Dutta PTJ, 2017).

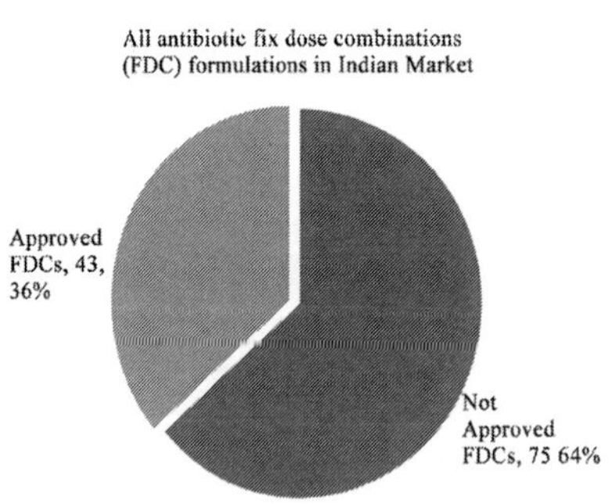

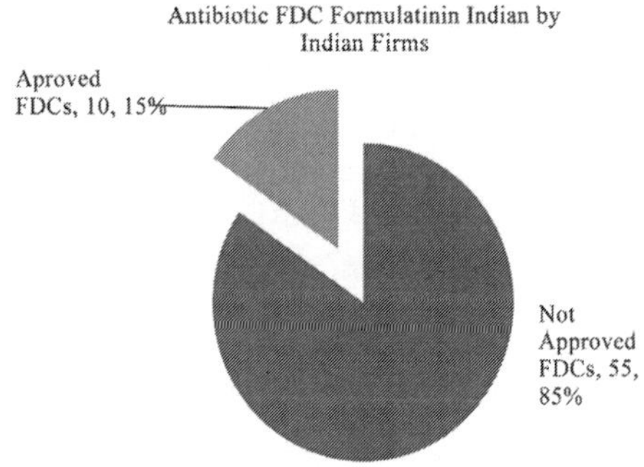

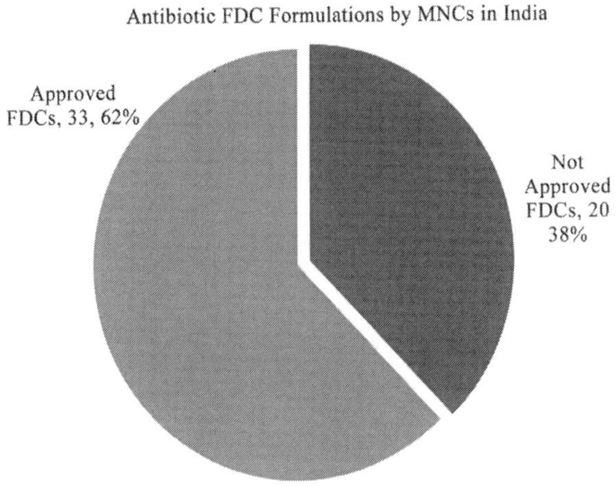
Antibiotic FDC Formulations by MNCs in India
Approved FDCs, 33, 62%
Not Approved FDCs, 20 38%

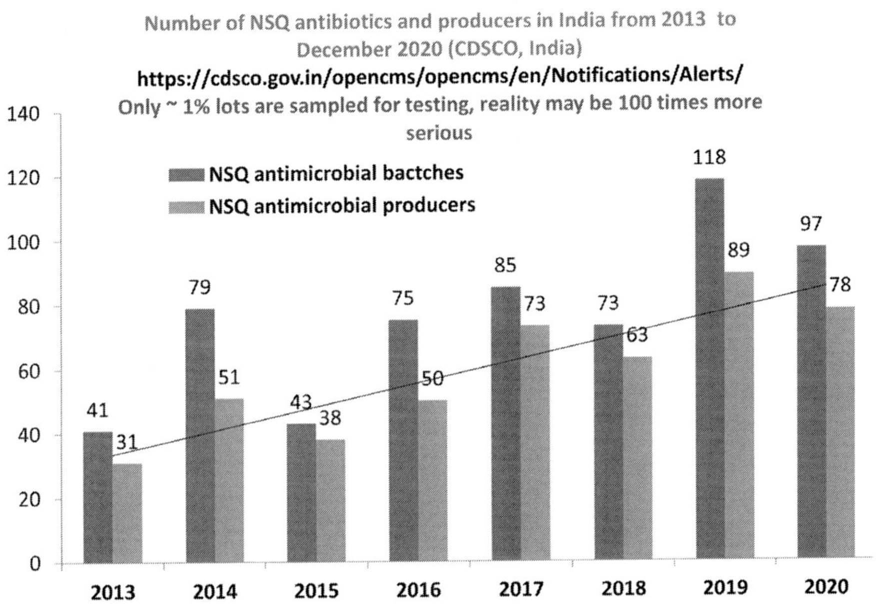
Number of NSQ antibiotics and producers in India from 2013 to December 2020 (CDSCO, India)
https://cdsco.gov.in/opencms/opencms/en/Notifications/Alerts/
Only ~ 1% lots are sampled for testing, reality may be 100 times more serious
NSQ antimicrobial bactches
NSQ antimicrobial producers
140
120
100
80
60
40
20
0
41
31
79
51
43
38
75
50
85
73
73
63
118
89
97
78
2013
2014
2015
2016
2017
2018
2019
2020

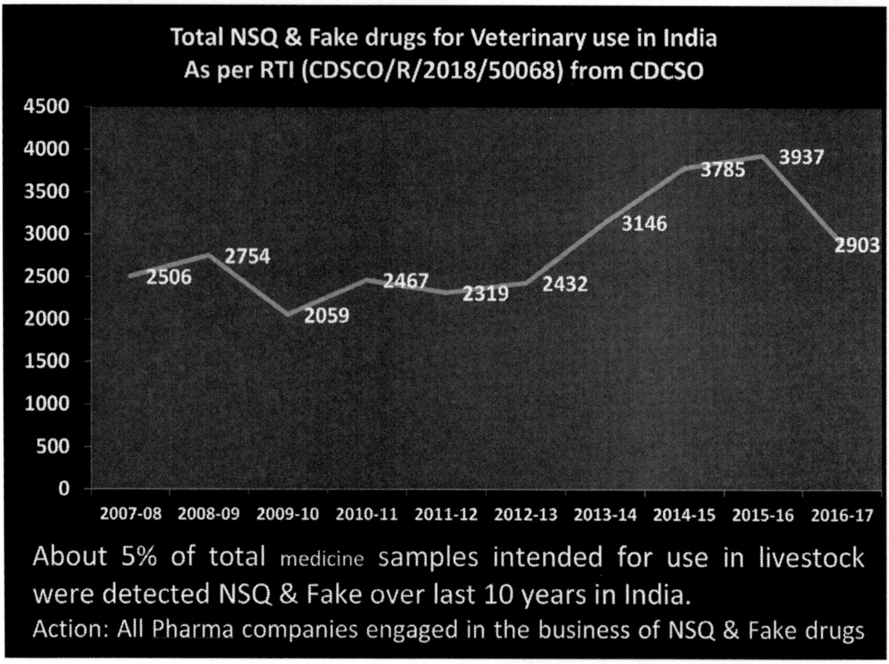

Conclusion

For identifying the risk of disinfectants and other antimicrobials on the emergence of AMR, there is a need for robust risk assessment to evaluate the environmental and public health risks of increased disinfection and its role in mediating the spread of AMR, particularly in the long term. The national health system should look into stamping out pollution in the antibiotics supply chain. They have to BLACKLIST pharmaceutical companies that are contributing to the spread of AMR through irresponsible manufacturing practices. There is high demand for transparency in the production and supply chain of the pharmaceutical industry. Along the major causes for the emergence of AMR, other factors like poor public health indicators, abolition of sub-standard (NSQD) antibiotics in therapy, and the availability of inexpensive antibiotics over the counter without a prescription need to be taken care of for the control of dissemination of antimicrobial resistance in World, particularly in India.

References

Bhardwaj, P., Ziegler, E. and Palmer, K.L. (2016). Chlorhexidine induces VanA-type vancomycin resistance genes in enterococci. Antimicrobial agents and chemotherapy. 60(4):2209-2221.

Dann, A.B. and Hontela, A. (2011). Triclosan: environmental exposure, toxicity and mechanisms of action. Journal of applied toxicology. 31(4):285-311.

Davies. (2015). How Big Pharma's industrial waste is fuelling the rise in superbugs worldwide? Available in: https://www.thebureauinvestigates.com/stories/2016-09-15/how-big-pharmas-industrial-waste-is-fuelling-the-rise-in-superbugs-worldwide).

FDA (2019). Antibacterial Soap? You Can Skip It, Use Plain Soap and Water. Available in https://www.fda.gov/consumers/consumer-updates/antibacterial-soap-you-can-skip-it-use-plain-soap-and-water

Ghosh et al., 2016; http://ijbamr.com/pdf/September%202016%20640-648.pdf.pdf

Khan, G.A., Berglund, B., Khan, K.M., Lindgren, P.E. and Fick, J. (2013). Occurrence and abundance of antibiotics and resistance genes in rivers, canal and near drug formulation facilities–a study in Pakistan. PloS one, 8(6):p.e62712.

Larsson, D.G.J., de Pedro, C., Paxeus, N. (2007). Efuent from drug manufactures contains extremely high levels of pharmaceuticals. J. Hazard. Mater. 148:751–755.

Laxminarayan, R. and Chaudhury, R.R. (2016) Antibiotic resistance in India: drivers and opportunities for action. PLoS Med . 13(3): e1001974.

Litovsky, A. (2016). Antibiotic waste is polluting India and China's rivers; big pharma must act. Available in: https://www.theguardian.com/sustainable-business/2016/oct/25/antibiotic-waste-pollution-india-china-rivers-big-pharma-superbugs-resistance

Lu, J., Wang, Y., Li, J., Mao, L., Nguyen, S.H., Duarte, T., Coin, L., Bond, P., Yuan, Z. and Guo, J. (2018). Triclosan at environmentally relevant concentrations promotes horizontal transfer of multidrug resistance genes within and across bacterial genera. Environment International. 121:1217-1226.

Lu, J. and Guo, J. (2021). Disinfection spreads antimicrobial resistance. Science. 371(6528):474-474.

Muller, J. F., Ghosh, S., Ikuma, K., Stevens, A. M. and Love, N. G. (2015). Chlorinated phenol-induced physiological antibiotic resistance in Pseudomonas aeruginosa. FEMS Microbiology Letters. 362 (21):fnv172, https://doi.org/10.1093/femsle/fnv172

O'Neill, J. (2016). Tackling drug-resistant infections globally: final report and recommendations.

Pesingi PV, Singh BR, Pesingi PK, Bhardwaj M, Singh SV, Kumawat M, Sinha DK, Gandham RK. MexAB-OprM Efflux Pump of Pseudomonas aeruginosa Offers Resistance to Carvacrol: A Herbal Antimicrobial Agent. Front Microbiol. 2019 Nov 19;10:2664. doi: 10.3389/fmicb.2019.02664. PMID: 31803171; PMCID: PMC6877666.

Rohit, 2017. Pharma effluents promoting drug resistance. Available in : https://www.thehindu.com/sci-tech/health/pharma-effluents-promoting-drug-resistance/article18516694.ece)

Singh BR, 2017. Why India Failed to Penalize those Responsible for the Circulation of Substandard Medicines and Vaccines while China Succeeded? DOI: 10.19080/GJPPS.2017.02.555599 https://www.researchgate.net/publication/317715214

Society for General Microbiology. "Disinfectants Can Make Bacteria Resistant To Treatment." ScienceDaily. ScienceDaily, 6 October 2008. Available in : www.sciencedaily.com/releases/2008/10/081005203059.htm>.

Towse, A., Hoyle, C.K., Goodall, J., Hirsch, M., Mestre-Ferrandiz, J. and Rex, J.H., 2017. Time for a change in how new antibiotics are reimbursed: Development of an insurance framework for funding new antibiotics based on a policy of risk mitigation. Health Policy, 121(10), pp.1025-1030.

Vadhana PA. Singh, B.R., Molecular studies on resistance against carvacrol in Escherichia coli / Pseudomonas aeruginosa. Ph.D. Thesis, ICARIndian Veterinary Research Institute, Izatnagar. 2017; Pp. 93.

Waxman, H. A. and Corr. B. (2016). Waste from pharmaceutical plants in India and China promotes antibiotic-resistant superbugs. Available in: https://www.statnews.com/2016/10/14/superbugs-antibiotic-resistance-india-china/

Winston Morgan, 2020. Heavy use of hand sanitizer boosts antimicrobial resistance. Available in https://phys.org/news/2020-04-heavy-sanitizer-boosts-antimicrobial-resistance.html

8

Common Mistakes Responsible for Therapeutic Failure Against AMR

Anu Rahal[1] and Amit Kumar[2]

[1]Division of Animal Health, ICAR-Central Institute for Research on Goats (CIRG), Makhdoom, Farah, Mathura, Uttar Pradesh, India
[2]Division of Animal Biotechnology, College of Biotechnology, Sardar Vallabhbhai Patel University of Agriculture and Technology (SVPUAT), Meerut, Uttar Pradesh, India

Abstract

Antimicrobial resistance (AMR) or resistance against drugs is currently a global challenge due to ever rising resistance in microorganisms including bacteria, fungi, and parasites leading to therapeutic failures. It is imposing the risk of more severe illnesses with more incidences of spreading such illnesses with increased morbidity and mortality. AMR is a natural adaptation process required for the survival of microbial population in adverse conditions like presence of antimicrobial agents. It involves the genetic changes in microbes; however multiple host factors can accelerate its transmission to other microbes leading to emergence and spread of new resistant strains or species. These factors mostly remain overlooked and continue to play crucial role in emergence as well as spread of AMR. The current chapter try to highlights such factors those can be a trigger point of AMR development and transmission.

Keywords: *Antimicrobial resistance, Quorum Sensing, Gut Microbiota, Pathophysiology, Host*

The response of any living cell to a xenobiotic (including antibacterial agent) is significantly affected by the prevailing local environmental conditions. In case of bacterial infection, it may include the presence of other microbes, no matter commensal or pathogenic, or biochemical alterations at that particular site of bacterial infection in host. All these host and bacterial factors play a critical role in the evolutionary responses of bacteria but usually go unconsidered while determining the microbial sensitivity to a particular antibiotic in a clinical setting. These also include the direct and indirect interspecies interactions that can affect the responses of individual bacterial species and surviving microbial communities to a particular antibiotic therapy. These interactions may significantly alter the qualitative and quantitative responses, potential phenotypic changes and the final trajectory of evolution of antimicrobial resistance. Due acknowledgement and plausible interpretation to these interactions may help to reduce the upsurge in AMR and its associated morbidity and fatality and pave path to more proficient clinical success.

The factors participating in drug- microbe interaction can be classified into two broad groups: host factors and microbial factors. The environmental milieu of the interaction is chiefly regulated by the gut microbiota with stressors causing deflections. The gastrointestinal bacteria amend host mental and physiological cadence via microbial metabolites such as butyrate, polyphenolic antioxidants, vitamins, and amines, affecting the overall ready perception and active rebuke to a stimulus. Lifestyle stressors such as fluctuating sleep and erratic eating patterns (western diet) disturb the host circadian system along with the gut microbiome. The overall impact is impaired detoxification (decreased conjugation of bile acids or increased production of hydrogen sulphide), substrate oxidation and energy regulation (reduced butyrate production) in the host affecting the overall health and productivity.

Gastrointestinal Microbiota

The first and foremost factor affecting the bacterial response to an antibiotic is gastrointestinal microbiota of host. A "Healthy Microbiota" in man means four dominant bacterial phyla (Firmicutes, Proteobacteria, Actinobacteria, and Bacteroidetes), with additional microbes (Chlamydia, Cyanobacteria, Deferribacteres, Deinococcus–Thermus, Fusobacteria, Spirochaetes, or Verrucomicrobia) in lower abundances. In totality, there are three known clusters of enterotypes, each specifically enriched in Bacteroides, Prevotella, and Ruminococcus alongwith a few minor genera like Parabacteroides, Desulfovibrio, and Akkermansia, respectively. Each enterotype has its own preferred routes for energy generation, and specialization to their ecological niches. Microbial richness and diversity are global parameters associated with health. Stability in bacterial configuration is considered as a vital feature of a healthy microbiota, and is considered to be related to resistance and resilience observed in a population (Dethlefsen *et al.*, 2007; Arumugam *et al.*, 2011; El Aidy *et al.*, 2015).

Changes in microbiota composition predisposes inflammation and, in turn, a higher incidence of infection. Western diet depletes the gut microbial diversity, and the change being characterized by an increase in Firmicutes and the family

Enterobacteriaceae and a decrease in the phylum Actinobacteria and the genus Prevotella. Bacterial species associated with anti-inflammatory status of the gut like *Akkermansia muciniphila, Faecalibacterium prausnitzii, Roseburia* spp., *Eubacterium hallii*, Clostridium clusters XIVa and IV, and Ruminococcus are reduced with an accompanied decrease in the capacity to produce beneficial metabolites. Furthermore, the circadian rhythm of microbiome also gets influenced by the changes in light–dark cycles, sunlight exposure, sleep, and dietary patterns. The consumption of food in a composed daily rhythm coinciding with the light phase of the light–dark cycle and the active phase of the day, imparts constructive regulation of the hosts' intestinal cell transcription, the rhythms of the circulating metabolites, and the gut microbiota composition and function (Stenvers *et al.*, 2012; Parkar *et al.*, 2019).

In ruminants, rumen is an anaerobic and methanogenic fermentation chamber thickly populated with diverse microbiome (bacteria, archaea, protozoa and fungi) that utilise and assimilate cellulolytic feeds. Bacteria are the most abundant microbes in rumen, with approximately 10^{10} – 10^{11} cells/ml and over 200 inhabiting species, with Prevotella, Butyrivibrio and Ruminococcus being the most dominant one. The gut microbiota is restricted at time of birth but undergoes dramatic changes before reaching the relative equilibrium at adulthood. The chartering of ruminal microbiota is governed by diverse factors including diet composition, energy requirements, and physiological demands or opposition to synthesis of toxic metabolic end-products (Castillo-Gonzalez *et al.*, 2014). It is mainly Gram negative in animals maintained on high forage diets. However, it has higher Gram positive bacteria fraction when the ruminal pH is low as observed after high grain diets (Oetzel, 2003; Scholtens *et al.*, 2012; Matamoros *et al.*, 2013; Sharon *et al.*, 2013)).

Rumen archaea are strictly anaerobic and are the only known microorganisms in the rumen capable of producing methane. Rumen methanogens mainly include Methanobrevibacter (63.2% of methanogen population), Methanomicrobium (7.7% of methanogen population), Methanosphaera (9.8%), Thermoplasma (7.4%), and Methanobacterium (1.2%). Out of these, only *Methanosphaera stadtmanae* produces methane through the reduction of methanol with H_2, thereby reducing hydrogen concentrations in the rumen, and allowing methanogens to promote the growth of other species, and enabling a more efficient fermentation. The type and ratio of gut microbiota mainly governed by the feed and feeding habit of the host. It directly affects the wellbeing and mental level of host through gut microbiota. These are included in host dietary effects. *Bacillus licheniformis* is a novel probiotic to reduce enteric methane emissions (Ishler *et al.*, 1996; Janssen and Kirs, 2008; Hook *et al.*, 2010; Patra *et al.*, 2017; Deng *et al.*, 2018).

Host Dietary Effect

Diet is a foreign matter to a living system. Any xenobiotic when introduced into the body, elicits an inflammatory response. Diet is most vital modulator of chronic inflammation and metabolic diseases and is responsible for more than 50% of the variability in the microbiota. The regular microbiota of any animal is synchronized over thousands of years of evolutionary and adaptive interaction between host physiological system, including the digestive mediators and metabolites, xenobiotics being added to the digestive lumen from time to time, and the luminal microbes. Substantial dietary alteration can shift the enterotype within 1–4 days but the effects get temporally diluted once the modified diet is withdrawn, and the microbiota tends to return to its original. It is also the most successful and appropriate way to reduce methane emissions and the related energy loss in the ruminants (Goodrich *et al.*, 2016; Oriach *et al.*, 2016; Statovci *et al.*, 2017; Rothschild *et al.*, 2018; Zinöcker and Lindseth, 2018).

While discussing dietary effects, highlighting the role of prebiotic, probiotics and synbiotics is inevitable. Prebiotics are natural feed additives, usually "an indigestible fermented diet substrate that selectively stimulate the composition, growth, and activity of microflora in gastrointestinal tract and thus confer a health benefit". Probiotics, on other hand, are "live micro-organisms which confer a health benefit on the host." These are likely to include species producing anti-inflammatory metabolites (*A. muciniphila, F. prausnitzii*) and butyrate. Synbiotic refers to the synergistic combination of prebiotic and probiotic, so that the prebiotic aid in the persistence of a probiotic in digestive system. Both prebiotics and probiotics can alleviate intestinal inflammation, promote immune regulation, or augment the intestinal barriers, thus producing a beneficial effect on the gut microbiota (Hill *et al.*, 2014; Rodríguez, 2015).

Prebiotics include galactooligosaccharides, fructooligosaccharides, and resistant starch. Fructose sugars promote Bifidobacterium, *F. Prausnitzii*, Lactobacillus, and the butyrate producers Ruminococcus, Faecalibacterium, and Oscillospira, along with reductions in the genera Phascolarctobacterium, Enterobacter, Turicibacter, Coprococcus, and Salmonella. Galactose sugars increase Bifidobacterium levels but decrease the population intensity of Ruminococcus, Dehalobacterium, Synergistes, and Holdemania. Galactose also improves butyrate production and the growth of butyrate producers, such as *Eubacterium rectale* (Walton *et al.*, 2012; Liu *et al.*, 2017; Tandon *et al.*, 2019).

Diet can be both a source of AMR and a solution to reduce AMR. The impact of local milieu on bacterial physiology is vast and certainly integrates into multiple life history traits, including health and longevity. Diversified diets high in fibre and low in animal protein lessen the prevalence of antibiotic resistance genes. Colostrum consumed by the newborn calves is a prone source of ARG these ARGs could then be suppressed by increasing fiber in the diet (Liu But *et al.*, 2019).

Oral administration of antibiotics for metaphylaxis (for animals suspected to be diseased), prophylaxis (to protect healthy animals when risk is established) or as antibiotic growth promoters in addition to treatment needs is a quite common practise in livestock rearing. Rather, as per the global data, consumption of antibiotics in the livestock sector as growth promoters is much higher than for treatment purpose. Adding the antibiotics directly to the feed as growth supplements has been one of the neglected causes for the global antimicrobial resistance (AMR) upsurge. Good feed and feeding habits decide gut microbiota. However, any pathophysiological change in host whether localized or general directly affect host microbiota.

Pathophysiological State of Host

The primary target of the physiological processes is to provide carbon and energy metabolism and in this process, it strongly restrict or promotes the evolutionary trajectories of antibiotic resistance. Once the antibiotic is administered to any animal, interplay between the natural microbiota, antibiotic and the physiological mediators becomes inevitable and directly as well as indirectly, through various physiological responses, compels the normal commensal biota to devise methods to counter it. The stress imposed on the host system due to any disease or any physiological alteration also affects the dynamics of resistance acquisition response of microbiota. Though mutation take place randomly, the environmental conditions play a decisive role in selection of condition-dependent compensatory mechanisms in antibiotic-resistant populations, including shifts in metabolic pathways, ultimately leading to establishment of a resistant mutant within the population (Zampieri *et al.*, 2017a).

The most efficient energy-producing metabolic pathway is aerobic cellular respiration, which includes glycolysis and the tricarboxylic acid (TCA) cycle. In case of fast energy demand or carbon source depletion, some bacterial pathogens such as *Pseudomonas aeruginosa*, switch towards less efficient anaerobic fermentative energy pathways, such as the nitrate respiratory chain, to maintain cellular homeostasis in oxygen-depleted environments. Switching to anaerobic energy metabolism is commonly used for evasion of host defence mechanisms and plays a vital role in increasing aminoglycoside tolerance. A shift from respiratory to fermentative metabolism is also observed along with over expression of efflux pumps, highlighting the role of metabolic adaptations in response to antibiotic selection pressure, perhaps an early bacterial response to antimicrobial compounds. It is also related to antibiotic adverse effects like unbalanced ammonia metabolism contributing to increased chloramphenicol toxicity, linking it to the generation of reactive oxygen species. Thus, the presence of any pathogen may directly or indirectly affect the evolution and transfer of resistance (Zampieri *et al.*, 2017a,b).

Site of Infections

A 5-day antibiotic cocktail regimen is a routine antibacterial regime, but what fails to get noticed by the clinician is the rapid upshoot of a new resistance phenotype in the bacterial population, which aims to capture a major share in the microbiota. The first bacteria to encounter the oral antibiotic is the gut microbiome and the latter depletes obligate anaerobes population, thereby reducing the production of short-chain fatty acids and favours bloom of inflammation-associated facultative anaerobes in colon. Antibiotics reduce gut clostridia count, which in turn disrupts peroxisome proliferator-activated receptor-γ (PPAR-γ) signalling and impairs colonocyte metabolism, releasing oxygen and other terminal electron acceptors into the gut, potentially expanding a niche for facultative anaerobes (Byndloss *et al.*, 2017; Litvak *et al.*, 2018).

One of the intriguing features of AMR is that the well controlled experimental results and the clinical findings usually do not complement each other. Actually, 'bacterial lifestyle' affects the phenotypic and genotypic expression of unique resistance strategies. For the bacteria grown in liquid culture, the most resistant lineage outcompetes the other bacterial lineages, allowing its offspring to rapidly take over the population. However, for the bacteria grown in biofilms or solid matrix, the movement is restricted and terms of interaction vary with the site in the alcove and multiple co-existing lineages may emerge.

Liquid-grown bacteria evolve low-level resistance mostly via efflux pump mutations or upregulation. These resistant cells then flourish and gain additional mutations. Biofilm-grown bacteria also evolve low-level resistance through pump protein production but do not accumulate additional mutations. In addition to this, biofilm-grown bacteria involve different efflux than their liquid-evolved counterparts. In absence of stimulus, the liquid evolved strains subside but the solid–evolved strains maintain themselves. The selective pressure imposed by the different lifestyles of the bacteria limits the evolutionary pathways, and thus the outcomes available to each lifestyle.

Coadministered Drugs

Resistance of bacteria to antibiotics or drugs in general, is mediated by three primary molecular mechanisms-decrease the intracellular levels of the drugs, modify the drug target through mutation or post-translational modification or inactivate the antimicrobial agent by enzymatic modification. The resistance to an antimicrobial agent can be mono (caused by a unique mechanism) or multifactorial (caused by more than one mechanism simultaneously). For example, some strain of carbapenems-resistant *P. aeruginosa* commonly have different mechanisms, including the production of carbapenemase, decreased expression or mutation of the outer membrane porin and overexpression of efflux-pumps.

Resistance to certain antibiotics frequently ensure rise in susceptibility or resistance to some other drugs. In an evolutionary trade-off known as collateral sensitivity, the resistance mechanism to a particular drug regulates the hypersensitivity to other drugs. Antibiotics belonging to a single class share common cellular target, and show cross-resistance, though the level of cross-resistance may differ amongst the members. Carbapenems are more effective than penicillin and cephalosporins owing to intrinsic resistance to β-lactamases.

Co-resistance occurs between antibiotics of different classes, owing to accumulation of different mechanisms encoded by mutated or acquired genes. For example, MRSA accumulates resistance to β-lactams, macrolides, tetracycline, aminoglycosides, and fluoroquinolones. Coresistance to non-β-lactams antibiotics (tetracycline, fluoroquinolones, and aminoglycosides) amongst ESBL-producing Gram-negative bacteria is mediated by integrons and plasmids. In addition to these, collateral sensitivity frequently arises between two agents with different microbial inhibitory mechanisms as a pleiotropic evolution due to mutation and, or acquisition of resistance genes. Therefore, antibiotic combination therapy might promote coresistance and coselection procedures that enhance the chance of developing persistent isolates (Cantón and Ruiz-Garbajosa, 2011; Tacão *et al.*, 2014; Malik *et al.*, 2017; Roemhild *et al.*, 2020).

Bacterial Quorum Sensing

Adaptation is the hallmark of life. Microbes have a remarkable aptitude to spread, interact, and adapt to the environment. Bacteria sense environmental changes (eg. nutrient availability, osmotic pressure, pH, redox state, signalling mediators, antibiotics or membrane stress), and respond to them using quorum sensing or a two-component regulatory system (TCS) comprising a pair of at least two proteins, namely the sensor kinase (SK) and the response regulator (RR). While SK senses any alteration in the external conditions, RR optimises survival and adaptation of bacteria through modulation of bacterial genes expression. The resulting regulatory action often involves activation of antibiotic defences and changes to cell physiology that increase antibiotic resistance. The response to the stimulus is chaotically dynamic because the environmental conditions for the microbial may be constantly shifting. Even without antibiotics and contagious threats, the nutrient abundance is sure to change with temporal alterations of the animal habitat, creating a selection pressure and leading to a shift in phenotypic expression from the same genotype.

The rate of environmental change affects both demographic and genetic aspects of evolutionary survival instinct, especially in the context of unprecedented anthropogenic shifts. A drastic change in environment limits mutational opportunities, by reducing viable population size and eliminating specific sets of possible evolutionary options. To further add to this, bacterial populations evolved under sturdy selection pressure show amplified cross-resistance against multiple antibiotics in comparison to those evolving under milder selection, indicating that strongly selected populations hold superior genetic mutations specific to the target pathways of the drugs used for selection [Lindsey *et al.*, 2013; Oz *et al.*, 2014).

The phenotypic expression usually lags behind genetic AMR; the phenotypic delay being attributed to either effective polyploidy, dilution of antibiotic-sensitive molecules or accumulation of resistance-enhancing molecules. For each possible target for mutation, sensitive and resistant variants coexist. The effective polyploidy does not influence genetic population ratio, but the dilution of sensitive molecules threatens the survival of mutant in case of therapy as well as underrates the recessive mutation. Accumulation of antibiotic resistance gene (ARG) mutations enhance the expression of drug efflux pumps, antibiotic degrading enzymes (β-lactamase), or ribosomal mutations affecting translational modifications.

Resilience is the property of any dynamic system to return to its normal stable state following a perturbation. Resilience genes are "markers" of the typical microbiota, and variation in their content indicates evolutionary adaptation in the community. Exposure to altered concentrations of xenobiotics (eg. diversification in nutrients, mediators, threats, or antibiotic) leads to altered phenotypic expression of the microbiota. Intrinsic resistance is steadily preserved over several generations, and provides adaptive capacity to recover from deep antibiotic perturbations. Persistent xenobiotic exposure may alter the efficiency of resilience genes. Distinguishing resilience genes within the overall resistance genes is crucial for real time assessment of the AMR risk in a microbiota.

Role of Microbiota in Pathogenic AMR

For young ruminants, most of the early colonized microbiome derives from their dams' teats, faeces, and milk. Though the gut microbiota is mainly commensal, it act as a reservoir for ARGs, which can be transferred between livestock and humans. In physiological conditions, the gut microbiome is stable, but when perturbative events occur (e.g., dietary changes, infections, stress, antibiotic administration, environmental changes), the population of the commensal microbiome alongwith the pathogenic bacteria changes. The gut resistome is complex and dynamic with ARGs present in all the bacteria, viruses, archaea, and eukaryotes lining the gut (Hu *et al.*, 2013; Shreiner *et al.*, 2015; Hu *et al.*, 2017; Wang *et al.*, 2019).

The response of pathogenic bacteria to antibiotics is significantly affected by the presence of other interacting microbes. Commensal tries to escape killing by suitable genotyping or phenotypic modifications like secretary metabolites, β-lactamase, biofilm, etc. In this process, they support the pathogenic bacteria against the antibiotic and facilitate therapeutic failure, even though the antibiotic kinetic profile meet the therapeutic standards. These changes may involve ensuring permanency to newly emerged resistant bacterial strain or transferring resistance to the commensals. These interactions are not typically accounted for when determining pathogen sensitivity to antibiotics *in vitro*. Therefore, AMR evolutionary responses to antibiotic, co-administered supportive treatment or coinfections should not be considered only a trait of an individual bacteria species but also an emergent property of the microbial community in which pathogens are embedded (Perry *et al.*, 2014; Card *et al.*, 2017; Gargiullo *et al.*, 2019; Wallace *et al.*, 2020).

Interspecies interactions are not typically accounted for when assessing antibiotic sensitivity and resistance evolution in the context of antibiotic treatments but they lead to horizontal gene transfer (HGT) of AMR, and ultimately, predicted clinical susceptibility of polymicrobial infections may not be achieved, especially when the pathogens are entrenched in complex multispecies microbial communities. In addition, the sub-MIC antibiotic concentrations can positively select for resistance mutations, increase HGT of antimicrobial resistance genes (ARGs), and elevate mutation rates (Aminov, 2011; Cooper *et al.*, 2017).

Bacterial Resistance or Tolerance

Bacterial resistance is a heritable ability of a bacterial cell to grow at high concentrations of an antibiotic, irrespective of the duration of exposure. In contrast, tolerance describes the ability of a bacterial population to survive transient exposure to a high concentration of an antibiotic without a change in their MIC mostly due to their environmental context. It involves slowing down essential cellular processes following a lack of resources, interactions with a host's immune system or interactions with other bacterial species, resulting in a reduced death rate in the presence of antibiotic. Alternatively, tolerance can be a heritable trait or acquired in the process of evolution through the optimisation of survival during intermittent antibiotic exposure (Biswas *et al.*, 2009; Nguyen *et al.*, 2011; Fridman *et al.*, 2014; Arnoldini *et al.*, 2014).

Bacteria secrete various compounds ranging from signalling molecules involved in quorum sensing to exotoxins involved in virulence and competition. Secreted products within communities directly alter gene expression, metabolic processes and the growth dynamics of co-residing bacterial species, altering their ability to survive antibiotic exposure. For example, indole secreted by *E. coli* activates the expression of an indole-dependent multi-drug efflux pump in *Pseudomonas putida*. In addition, bacterial exotoxins can also persuade the transition of competing bacterial species into an antibiotic-tolerant physiological state. For example, *P. aeruginosa* induces highly tolerant minor variants of *S. aureus* through the secretion of 4-hydroxy-2-heptylquinoline-*N*-oxide, which inhibits the electron transport chain, dramatically slowing down the growth rate of *S. aureus*. These community interactions are mutualistic, and provide protection to the sensitive microbial community members. These interactions in the community may either be collective resistance (generalised increase in the MIC of the community), collective tolerance (altered metabolic cell state during brief antibiotic exposure without an increase in MIC) or exposure protection, (reducing the effective concentration of antibiotic). These interactions are mutually non-exclusive and density-dependent (Molina and Santiago *et al.*, 2014; Vega and Gore, 2014; Meredith *et al.*, 2015).

In case of coinfection, prolonged use of supportive drugs like acid suppressing medications is a regular feature. These supportive medications alter the typical tissue characteristics and allow bacterial colonization. Gastric acid suppression also impairs neutrophil and natural killer cell function, which are a critical component of host immunity. The effect of co-infection largely depends upon the species involved in the infection. The environmental conditions customized by metabolites released one species also affect the response from the other microbial populations. *Pseudomonas quinolone* signal significantly disrupts biofilm and quorum sensing in *S. aureus* along with lesser tissue damage as compared to mono-infections. The most common resistance transmission is associated with co-infection and presence of one resistant bacteria is likely to produce more transmission. The type of antibiotic used and its duration and dose are key influential factors (Kedika *et al.*, 2009).

Conclusion

AMR continues to persist as a multifactorial global challenge with host and bacterial factors playing a crucial role. Microbial factors of AMR are mainly responsible for the acquisition and transmission of resistance genes horizontally as well as vertically. They also quite frequently give rise to collateral sensitivity, co-resistance, or cross-resistance amongst clinical drugs. The diversity and assortment of gut microbiota is directly related to feed and feeding habits of the host. Thus, feed is considered as second most critical factor that determines the gut microbial population and affects indirectly the evolution and spread of resistance among gut microbes. AMR against a primary drug may lead to a dual outcome, inducing either heightened or reduced susceptibility to other drugs concurrently.

References

Aminov RI. Horizontal gene exchange in environmental microbiota. Front Microbiol. 2011;2:158.

Arnoldini M, Vizcarra IA, Peña-Miller R, Stocker N, Diard M, Vogel V, et al. Bistable expression of virulence genes in salmonella leads to the formation of an antibiotic-tolerant subpopulation. PLOS Biol. 2014;12:e1001928.

Arumugam, M., Raes, J., Pelletier, E., Le Paslier, D., Yamada, T., Mende, D.R., Fernandes, G.D.R., Tap, J., Bruls, T., Batto, J.M., et al. Enterotypes of the human gut microbiome. Nature 2011, 473, 174–180.

Biswas L, Biswas R, Schlag M, Bertram R, Götz F. Small-colony variant selection as a survival strategy for staphylococcus aureus in the presence of *Pseudomonas aeruginosa*. Appl Environ Microbiol. 2009;75:6910–2.

Byndloss MX, Olsan EE, Rivera-Chávez F, Tiffany CR, Cevallos SA, Lokken KL, Torres TP, Byndloss AJ, Faber F, Gao Y, Litvak Y, Lopez CA, Xu G, Napoli E, Giulivi C, Tsolis RM, Revzin A, Lebrilla CB, Bäumler AJ. 2017. Microbiota activated PPAR-g signaling inhibits dysbiotic Enterobacteriaceae expansion. Science 357:570–575.

Cantón R, Ruiz-Garbajosa P. Co-resistance: an opportunity for the bacteria and resistance genes. Curr Opin Pharmacol. 2011; 11: 477-485.

Card RM, Cawthraw SA, Nunez-Garcia J, Ellis RJ, Kay G, Pallen MJ, et al. An in vitro chicken gut model demonstrates transfer of a multidrug resistance plasmid from Salmonella to Commensal Escherichia coli. mBio 2017;8:e00777–17.

Castillo-Gonzalez AR, Burrola-Barraza ME, Dominguez-Viveros J, Chavez-Martinez A. Rumen microorganisms and fermentation Microorganismos y fermentación ruminal. Arch Med Vet. 2014;46:349–361.

Cooper RM, Tsimring L, Hasty J. Inter-species population dynamics enhance microbial horizontal gene transfer and spread of antibiotic resistance. eLife Sci. 2017;6:e25950.

Deng KD, Xiao Y, Ma T, Tu Y, Diao QY, Chen YH, Jiang JJ. Ruminal fermentation, nutrient metabolism, and methane emissions of sheep in response to dietary supplementation with *Bacillus licheniformis*. Anim Feed Sci Technol. 2018; 241(November 2017):38–44.

Dethlefsen, L., McFall-Ngai, M., Relman, D.A. An ecological and evolutionary perspective on humang-microbe mutualism and disease. Nature 2007; 449: 811–818.

Edwards, C.A., Parrett, A.M. Intestinal flora during the first months of life: New perspectives. Br. J. Nutr. 2002; 88 (Suppl. S1): s11.

El Aidy, S., Dinan, T.G., Cryan, J.F. Gut Microbiota: The Conductor in the Orchestra of Immune-Neuroendocrine Communication. Clin. Ther. 2015; 37: 954–967.

Fridman O, Goldberg A, Ronin I, Shoresh N, Balaban NQ. Optimization of lag time underlies antibiotic tolerance in evolved bacterial populations. Nature. 2014;513:418–21.

Gargiullo L, Del Chierico F, D'Argenio P, Putignani L. Gut microbiota modulation for multidrug-resistant organism decolonization: present and future perspectives. Front Microbiol. 2019;10:1704.

Goodrich, J.K., Davenport, E., Beaumont, M., Jackson, M., Knight, R., Ober, C., Spector, T.D., Bell, J.T., Clark, A.G., Ley, R.E. Genetic Determinants of the Gut Microbiome in UK Twins. Cell Host Microbe 2016; 19:731–743.

Hill, C., Guarner, F., Reid, G., Gibson, G.R., Merenstein, D.J., Pot, B., Morelli, L., Canani, R.B., Flint, H.J., Salminen, S., et al. The International Scientific Association for Probiotics and Prebiotics consensus statement on the scope and appropriate use of the term probiotic. Nat. Rev. Gastroenterol. Hepatol. 2014; 11: 506–514.

Hook SE, Wright A-DG, McBride BW. Methanogens: methane producers of the rumen and mitigation strategies. Archaea [Internet]. 2010; 2010:1–11.

Hu Y, Gao GF, Zhu B. The antibiotic resistome: gene flow in environments, animals and human beings. Front Med. 2017; 11:161–8.

Hu Y, Yang X, Qin J, Lu N, Cheng G, Wu N, et al. Metagenome-wide analysis of antibiotic resistance genes in a large cohort of human gut microbiota. Nat Commun. 2013,4:1–7.

Ishler V, Heinrichs J, Varga G. From feed to milk: understanding rumen function. 1996.

Janssen PH, Kirs M. Structure of the Archaeal Community of the Rumen. Appl Environ Microbiol. 2008, 74(12):3619–3625.

Kedika, R. R., Souza, R. F., Spechler, S. J. (2009). Potential anti-inflammatory effects of proton pump inhibitors: a review and discussion of the clinical implications. Dig Dis. Sci. 54 (11), 2312–2317. doi: 10.1007/s10620-009-0951-9.

Lindsey, H.A., Gallie, J., Taylor, S., Kerr, B. Evolutionary Rescue from Extinction Is Contingent on a Lower Rate of Environmental Change. Nature 2013, 494, 463–467.

Litvak Y, Byndloss MX, Bäumler AJ. 2018. Colonocyte metabolism shapes the gut microbiota. Science. 362:eaat9076.

Liu, F., Li, P., Chen, M., Luo, Y., Prabhakar, M., Zheng, H., He, Y., Qi, Q., Long, H., Zhang, Y., et al. Fructooligosaccharide (FOS) and Galactooligosaccharide (GOS) Increase Bifidobacterium but Reduce Butyrate Producing Bacteria with Adverse Glycemic Metabolism in healthy young population. Sci. Rep. 2017, 7, 1–12.

Liu J, Taft DH, Maldonado-Gomez MX, Johnson D, Treiber ML, Lemay DG, DePeters EJ, Mills DA. 2019. The fecal resistome of dairy cattle is associated with diet during nursing. Nat Commun 10:4406.

Malik SZ, Linkevicius M, Göransson U, Andersson DI. Resistance to the cyclotide cycloviolacin O2 in salmonella enterica caused by different mutations that often confer cross-resistance or collateral sensitivity to other antimicrobial peptides. Antimicrob Agents Chemother. 2017; 61:e00684-17.

Matamoros, S., Gras-Leguen, C., Le Vacon, F., Potel, G., De La Cochetiere, M.F. Development of intestinal microbiota in infants and its impact on health. Trends Microbiol. 2013, 21, 167–173.

Meredith HR, Srimani JK, Lee AJ, Lopatkin AJ, You L. Collective antibiotic tolerance: mechanisms, dynamics and intervention. Nat Chem Biol. 2015,11:182–8.

Molina-Santiago C, Daddaoua A, Fillet S, Duque E, Ramos J-L. Interspecies signalling: Pseudomonas putida efflux pump TtgGHI is activated by indole to increase antibiotic resistance. Environ Microbiol. 2014,16:1267–81.

Nguyen D, Joshi-Datar A, Lepine F, Bauerle E, Olakanmi O, Beer K, et al. Active starvation responses mediate antibiotic tolerance in biofilms and nutrient-limited bacteria. Science. 2011,334:982–6.

Oetzel GR. Introduction to Ruminal Acidosis in DairyCattle. Technology. 2003,15:307–317.

Oriach, C.S., Robertson, R.C., Stanton, C., Cryan, J.F., Dinan, T.G. Food for thought: The role of nutrition in the microbiota-gut-brain axis. Clin. Nutr. Exp. 2016, 6, 25–38.

Oz, T., Guvenek, A., Yildiz, S., Karaboga, E., Tamer, Y.T., Mumcuyan, N., Ozan, V.B., Senturk, G.H., Cokol, M., Yeh, P., et al. Strength of Selection Pressure Is an Important Parameter Contributing to the Complexity of Antibiotic Resistance Evolution. Mol. Biol. Evol. 2014, 31, 2387–2401.

Parkar, S.G., Kalsbeek, A., Cheeseman, J.F. Potential Role for the Gut Microbiota in Modulating Host Circadian Rhythms and Metabolic Health. Microorganisms 2019; 7: 41.

Patra A, Park T, Kim M, Yu Z. Rumen methanogens and mitigation of methane emission by anti-methanogenic compounds and substances. J Anim Sci Biotechnol [Internet]. 2017,8(1):13.

Perry JA, Westman EL, Wright GD. The antibiotic resistome: what's new? Curr Opin Microbiol. 2014; 21:45–50.

Rodríguez, J.M. Probióticos: Del laboratorio al consumidor. Nutr. Hosp. 2015; 31: 33–47.

Roemhild R, Linkevicius M, Andersson DI. Molecular mechanisms of collateral sensitivity to the antibiotic nitrofurantoin. PLoS Biol. 2020; 18:e3000612.

Rothschild, D., Weissbrod, O., Barkan, E., Kurilshikov, A., Korem, T., Zeevi, D., Costea, P.I., Godneva, A., Kalka, I.N., Bar, N., et al. Environment dominates over host genetics in shaping human gut microbiota. Nature, 2018; 555: 210–215.

Scholtens, P.A.M.J., Oozeer, R., Martín, R., Ben Amor, K., Knol, J. The Early Settlers: Intestinal Microbiology in Early Life. Annu. Rev. Food Sci. Technol. 2012; 3: 425–447.

Sharon, I., Morowitz, M.J., Thomas, B.C., Costello, E.K., Relman, D.A., Banfield, J.F. Time series community genomics analysis reveals rapid shifts in bacterial species, strains, and phage during infant gut colonization. Genome Res. 2013; 23; 111–120.

Shreiner AB, Kao JY, Young VB. The gut microbiome in health and in disease. Curr Opin Gastroenterol. 2015; 31:69–75.

Statovci, D., Aguilera, M., MacSharry, J., Melgar, S. The impact of western diet and nutrients on the microbiota and immune response at mucosal interfaces. Front. Immunol. 2017, 8, 838.

Stenvers, D.J., Jonkers, C.F., Fliers, E., Bisschop, P.H., Kalsbeek, A. Nutrition and the circadian timing system. Prog. Brain Res. 2012; 199: 359–376.

Tacão M, Moura A, Correia A, Henriques I. Co-resistance to different classes of antibiotics among ESBL-producers from aquatic systems. Water Res. 2014; 48: 100-107.

Tandon, D., Haque, M.M., Gote, M., Jain, M., Bhaduri, A., Dubey, A.K., Mande, S.S. A prospective randomized, doubleblind, placebo-controlled, doseresponse relationship study to investigate efficacy of fructooligosaccharides (FOS) on human gut microfora. Sci. Rep. 2019; 9; 5473.

Vega NM, Gore J. Collective antibiotic resistance: mechanisms and implications. Curr Opin Microbiol. 2014; 21:28–34.

Wallace MJ, Fishbein SRS, Dantas G. Antimicrobial resistance in enteric bacteria: current state and next-generation solutions. Gut Microbes. 2020; 12:1799654.

Walton, G., Heuvel, E.V.D., Kosters, M.H.W., Rastall, R.A., Tuohy, K., Gibson, G.R. A Randomised Crossover Study Investigating the E_ects of Galacto-Oligosaccharides on the Faecal Microbiota in Men and Women Over 50 Years of Age. Br. J. Nutr. 2012; 107: 1466-1475.

Wang Y, Hu Y, Cao J, Bi Y, Lv N, Liu F, et al. Antibiotic resistance gene reservoir in live poultry markets. J Infect. 2019; 78:445–53.

Zampieri, M., Enke, T., Chubukov, V., Ricci, V., Piddock, L., Sauer, U. Metabolic Constraints on the Evolution of Antibiotic Resistance. Mol. Syst. Biol. 2017a, 13, 917.

Zampieri, M., Zimmermann, M., Claassen, M., Sauer, U. Nontargeted Metabolomics Reveals the Multilevel Response to Antibiotic Perturbations. Cell Rep. 2017b; 19:1214–1228.

Zinöcker, M.K., Lindseth, I.A. The Western Diet-Microbiome-Host Interaction and Its Role in Metabolic Disease. Nutrients, 2018; 10: 365.

9

Understanding Antimicrobial Resistance: Basics and Beyond

Surendra Upadhyay[1], Amit Kumar[1] and Anu Rahal[2]

[1]Division of Animal Biotechnology, College of Biotechnology, SVPUAT Meerut, Uttar Pradesh, India
[2]Division of Animal Health, ICAR-CIRG, Mukhdoom, Mathura Uttar Pradesh, India

Abstract

The discovery of antimicrobial agents and antibiotics had raised a hope of infection free era. However, microbes have proven that it is beginning of an ongoing saga of emergence of anti microbial resistance along with side-by-side development of new anti microbial drugs particularly antibiotics. The golden age of antibiotic development lost its glittering effect due to continuous up scaling of AMR. To understand the process of AMR development, it is always censorious to understand the timeline of AMR development and its correlation with introduction of new antibiotics. This chapter brings an insight of this with glimpses of mechanism of AMR development in microbes and transmission of AMR from resistant to sensitive microbes.

Keywords: AMR, Mechanism, Transmission, Alternate mechanism

Antibiotics, often referred to as "magic bullets" in the battle against bacteria, stand out as one of the most remarkable medical breakthroughs of the 20th century. Their advent revolutionized the therapeutic landscape, consistently saving millions of lives from bacterial infections (WHO, 2020). Undoubtedly, antibiotics are a blessing to humanity, not merely for their medicinal applications but also for their diverse uses. They have long been employed in various contexts, including animal husbandry and production, serving as preventive measures in numerous underdeveloped and developing nations for decades (Majumder *et al.*, 2020). A range of antimicrobial agents, including antibiotics, antifungals, antivirals, disinfectants, and food preservatives, function to either inhibit microbial growth or eradicate them altogether.

Among these, antibiotics, specifically tailored to combat bacterial infections, are the most widely used class of antimicrobials. With their increasing and often improper use, microorganisms have developed antimicrobial resistance (AMR) (Murray *et al.*, 2022).

Antimicrobial resistance is an inevitable evolutionary process observed in all microorganisms, and is driven by genetic mutations aimed at resisting the lethal pressures of selection. Bacteria, adapt to environmental selection pressures by developing resistance to antibacterial drugs, thereby diminishing the efficacy of these treatments (Murray *et al.*, 2022). The widespread use of antibiotics, particularly in developing nations, further flares up the process, leading to significant repercussions such as increased rates of morbidity and mortality (WHO, 2020). The incidence and prevalence of antimicrobial-resistant bacterial infections have reached alarming levels in the 21st century, posing a substantial threat to global public health akin to a silent pandemic. Antibiotic resistance knows no borders and can impact individuals of any age or gender, regardless of their location. In its present state, antimicrobial resistance (AMR) stands as one of the foremost threats, not only to global health but also to food security (Murray *et al.*, 2022).

The evolution and dissemination of AMR are concurrently affected by a multitude of interdependent factors related to healthcare and agriculture, including pharmaceuticals, inappropriate waste management, trade, and finance, making AMR one of the most complex public health concerns worldwide (World Health Organization, 2020). The rapid global spread of "superbugs," has elevated the issue of drug-resistant pathogens to a tangible and alarming level. Recognized as one of the top three major public health threats by the World Health Organization (WHO), antimicrobial resistance (AMR) rank third among the leading causes of death, following cardiovascular diseases (CDC, 2019). According to a significant study published 2023, an estimated 1.27 million deaths were linked to antimicrobial-resistant infections in 2019 alone, while nearly 5 million deaths were associated with drug-resistant infections in some way (Salam *et al.*, 2023). This figure is projected to escalate to 10 million per year by 2050, surpassing deaths from cancer by a significant margin (Murray *et al*, 2022).

In this series, Methicillin-resistant *Staphylococcus aureus* (MRSA) stands as a prominent example of the first "superbug," linked to a significant death toll from antimicrobial-resistant infections worldwide. Currently, 3.5% of active tuberculosis (TB) cases and 18% of previously treated TB cases worldwide are classified as MDR-TB (multidrug-resistant tuberculosis) (WHO, 2020). There is growing concern regarding XDR-TB (extensively drug-resistant tuberculosis) among a significant portion of MDR-TB cases. Beyond human healthcare, the indiscriminate use of antimicrobials in livestock feed in many developing nations has also been a major contributing factor. This underscores the need for heightened surveillance to assess the impact of excessive and unregulated antibiotic use in animal feeds, aiming to mitigate the incidence of drug-resistant bacteria. Pharmaceutical companies have largely withdrawn their focus from antibiotic discovery, citing various reasons, and have ceased significant expansion of their antibiotic portfolios since the 1980s. Fluoroquinolones marked the last addition to the group of broad-spectrum antibiotics discovered in the 1980s and were introduced to the market in 1987. Since then, there has been a paucity of new antibiotic development, with only a few new antibiotic classes in the pipeline (Centers for Disease Control and Prevention, 2020). Considering that antimicrobials are indispensable for treating and preventing infectious diseases, it has become imperative to safeguard the effectiveness of existing antimicrobials, especially given the lack of significant discoveries of new molecules in recent decades (The Lancet, 2022).

Timeline of AMR

The dawn of the modern antibiotic era can be traced back to Paul Ehrlich's discovery of salvarsan and neosalvarsan in 1910, synthetic prodrugs used to treat syphilis caused by *Treponema pallidum*. Subsequently, bacteriologist Gerhard Domagk's discovery of prontosil, a sulfonamide prodrug, gradually replaced salvarsan. In the 1930s, Selman Waksman, an American microbiologist and biochemist, conducted the first systematic assessment of soil microbes and their ability to produce compounds with antimicrobial properties. He uncovered numerous antibiotics from filamentous actinomycetes dwelling in the soil, including streptomycin, a widely used antibiotic against tuberculosis. Waksman defined an antibiotic as "a compound made by a microbe to destroy other microbes." Meanwhile, Sir Alexander Fleming, a Scottish physician and microbiologist, discovered penicillin from a mold called *Penicillium rubens* in 1928, igniting the golden era of antibiotic discovery, which peaked until the mid-1950s. The period from the 1940s to the 1960s is often termed the "Golden Age" of antibiotic discovery, as most of the antibiotics still in use today were discovered. However, since then, there has been a gradual decline in antibiotic discovery, accompanied by the evolution of drug-resistant pathogens (Hutchings *et al*, 2019).

Bacterial resistance to antibiotics has been acknowledged almost since the inception of the antibiotic era. Several years prior to the therapeutic introduction of penicillin in 1940, the first penicillin-resistant Staphylococcus strain was documented. Methicillin was introduced in 1959 as the first semisynthetic penicillinase-resistant penicillin. Surprisingly, a methicillin-resistant Staphylococcus strain was reported in 1960, merely a year after its introduction (Uddin *et al*, 2021) In 1958, vancomycin, a glycopeptide, was introduced as a last-resort treatment for infections caused by methicillin-resistant *Staphylococci*. In 1979, strains of coagulase-negative Staphylococci (CoNS) exhibiting resistance to vancomycin were identified, followed by the discovery of vancomycin-resistant Enterococcus (VRE) a decade later. Over time, vancomycin's effectiveness against *Staphylococcus aureus* diminished, leading to the identification of vancomycin-intermediate *Staphylococcus aureus* (VISA) in 1997 and vancomycin-resistant *Staphylococcus aureus* (VRSA) in 2002 (Parmar *et al*., 2018).

On similar lines, cephalosporin, a β-lactam antibiotic discovered in 1945, was introduced into clinical practice in 1964 to combat penicillin-resistant infections. Since then, several generations of cephalosporin have been introduced, with the fifth generation currently being available for clinical use. Though they were initially highly effective, particularly against extended-spectrum beta-lactamases (ESBLs) producing gram-negative bacteria, all the generations of cephalosporins have faced increasing resistance over time. Tetracycline, another important antibiotic discovered in 1950, was successfully employed for treating numerous common infections, including gastrointestinal diseases. However, within a decade of its discovery, tetracycline was reported to be ineffective against certain Shigella strains in 1959. Levofloxacin, a member of the third-generation fluoroquinolone class, was added to the antibiotic arsenal in 1996. Yet, levofloxacin-resistant Pneumococcus strains were reported in the same year, highlighting the ongoing challenge of antimicrobial resistance (Zaman *et al*, 2017). Carbapenem, a type of β-lactam antibiotic, was introduced in 1980 and reserved as a last-resort drug for treating infections caused by members of *Enterobacterales*, particularly in cases resistant to cephalosporins. However, with its heightened usage from the 1990s to the 2000s, carbapenem-resistant *Enterobacterales* (CRE) have repeatedly been reported in various countries since 2006 (Suay-García & Pérez-Gracia, 2019). The timeline of antibiotic discovery indeed reveals a concentrated period of new class production by pharmaceutical industries spanning approximately two decades, from 1960 to 1980. Subsequently, there was a notable decline in the pace of discovery until recent years.

Different Mechanisms Involved in Drug Resistance

Antimicrobial resistance is not a new phenomenon. In nature, microbes are constantly evolving in order to optimise their survival in the environment. The development of antimicrobial drugs and their widespread clinical use has simply provided another selective pressure that promotes further evolution. Several important factors can accelerate the evolution of drug resistance, including the overuse and misuse of antimicrobials, inappropriate prescribing, subtherapeutic dosing, and patient noncompliance with the recommended course of treatment. These factors contribute to the emergence of AMR through various mechanisms, as illustrated in Figure 1.

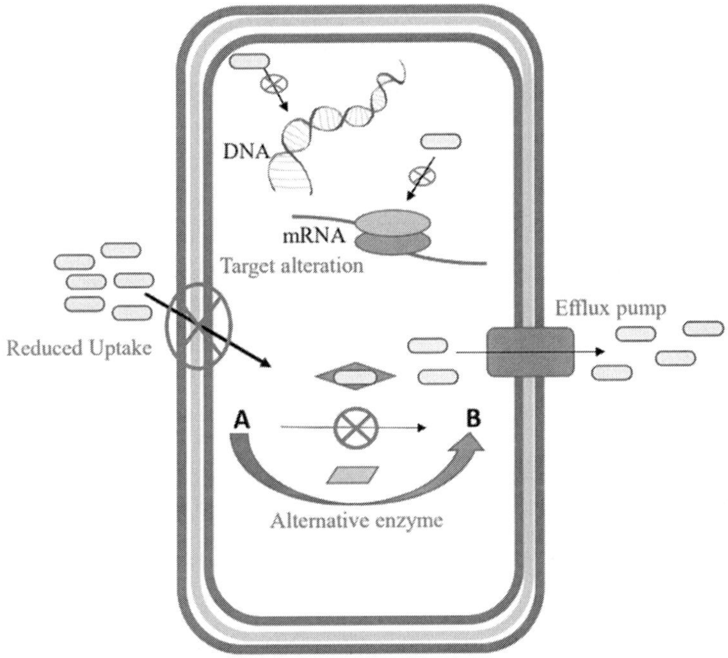

Fig 1: Schematic representation of various mechanism that leads to development of AMR

Drug Modification or Inactivation

Resistance genes may code for enzymes that chemically modify an antimicrobial, thereby inactivating it, or destroy an antimicrobial through hydrolysis. Resistance to many types of antimicrobials occurs through this mechanism.

Prevention of Cellular Uptake or Efflux

Microbes may inhibit the accumulation of an antimicrobial drug at the site of action, which then prevents the drug from reaching its threshold at the cellular target. This strategy is common among gram-negative pathogens and can involve changes in outer membrane lipid composition, porin channel selectivity, and/or porin channel concentrations.

Target Modification

Antimicrobial drugs have very specific targets. Any structural changes to those targets can prevent drug binding, rendering the drug ineffective. Through spontaneous mutations in the genes encoding antibacterial drug targets, bacteria have an evolutionary advantage that allows them to develop resistance to drugs. This mechanism of resistance development is quite common.

Target Overproduction or Enzymatic Bypass

Antimicrobial drug can function as an antimetabolite, and target a specific metabolic enzyme to inhibit its activity. in such case, microbial resistance may occur via two ways. First, the microbe may overproduce the target enzyme such that there is a sufficient amount of antimicrobial-free enzyme to carry out the proper enzymatic reaction. Second, the bacterial cell may develop a bypass that circumvents the need for the functional target enzyme. Both of these strategies have been found as mechanisms of sulfonamide resistance.

Target Mimicry

Target mimicry is a fascinating resistance mechanism developed by certain bacteria . In this context, bacteria produce proteins that mimic the natural targets of antibiotics. These mimic proteins bind to the antibiotics, thereby preventing them from interacting with their actual targets, such as ribosomal RNA or enzymes involved in cell wall synthesis. (Gualerzi *et al*, 2013)

Various Mechanism Involved in Target Mimicry

Decoy Targets: Bacteria synthesize proteins or RNA molecules that resemble the antibiotic's original target, effectively acting as decoys. When an antibiotic bind to this mimic, it is sequestered away from the true target, ultimately the effective antibiotic concentration at the site of acion is below threshold, and renders the antibiotic ineffective.

Protection of Vital Structures: Some mimicry proteins protect essential bacterial structures (like the ribosome) by binding to antibiotics in a competitive manner, reducing the antibiotic's ability to reach its intended target.

Evolutionary Adaptation: Target mimicry is believed to have evolved as a defence mechanism in response to the selective pressure exerted by antibiotics. This mechanism is often encoded by genes that bacteria acquire through horizontal gene transfer, making it a potent tool in the spread of antimicrobial resistance (AMR).

AMR Transmission

Evolutionary Mechanisms

Genetic Mutation: Bacteria can develop resistance through spontaneous mutations in their genetic material. These mutations can alter the target sites of antibiotics, reduce drug uptake, or increase drug efflux, rendering the antibiotic ineffective (Blair *et al.*, 2015).

Horizontal Gene Transfer (HGT): AMR genes can be transferred between bacteria through mechanisms such as conjugation, transformation, and transduction. This allows for rapid dissemination of resistance traits across bacterial populations, even across different species (Martínez, 2018).

Selective Pressure

Overuse and Misuse of Antibiotics: The over-prescription of antibiotics in human medicine, agriculture, and aquaculture creates selective pressure that favours the survival of resistant strains. Inappropriate use, such as not completing a prescribed course, further exacerbates this issue by allowing partially resistant bacteria to survive and proliferate (Ventola, 2015).

Environmental Factors: Antibiotics released into the environment through waste from hospitals, farms, and pharmaceutical factories can create hotspots of resistance. Environmental bacteria exposed to these drugs can develop resistance and transfer these genes to pathogenic bacteria (Kümmerer, 2009).

Global Spread

Travel and Trade: The globalization of trade and travel facilitates the rapid spread of resistant bacteria across borders. For instance, resistant strains can be transmitted through food, animals, and human travel, making AMR a global concern (Laxminarayan *et al.*, 2013).

Healthcare-Associated Infections: Hospitals and other healthcare settings are hotspots for the development and spread of AMR. Resistant bacteria, such as Methicillin-resistant Staphylococcus aureus (MRSA), can spread rapidly in these environments due to the high usage of antibiotics and the presence of vulnerable patients (Weiner-Lastinger *et al.*, 2020).

Antimicrobial Resistance (AMR) Detection

Detecting antimicrobial resistance (AMR) is critical for guiding appropriate treatment and mitigating the spread of resistant strains. Presence of a AMR gene does not certify the appearance of resistant phenotype. It only suggests the likelihood of appearance of a resistant strain under certain conditions. Various methods are employed in clinical and research settings to identify and characterize AMR, ranging from traditional culture-based techniques to advanced molecular diagnostics.

Phenotypic Methods

Phenotypic methods are used to evaluate the growth of microorganisms in the presence of antimicrobial agents to determine their susceptibility or resistance. These methods typically measure two key parameters:

a. Minimum Inhibitory Concentration (MIC): This is the lowest concentration of an antimicrobial agent that inhibits visible growth of a microorganism. Determining the MIC helps to understand the effectiveness of an antimicrobial and the concentration needed to inhibit the growth of the pathogen.

b. Minimum Bactericidal Concentration (MBC): This is the lowest concentration of an antimicrobial agent required to kill a particular bacterium. The MBC provides insight into the potency of an antimicrobial to eliminate the pathogen, rather than just inhibiting its growth.

By assessing MIC and MBC, phenotypic methods can provide a comprehensive understanding of the antimicrobial resistance profile of microorganisms.

Disk Diffusion Method: Also known as the Kirby-Bauer test, this method involves placing antibiotic-impregnated disks on an agar plate inoculated with the test organism. After incubation, the inhibition zones around the disks are measured to determine susceptibility. This method is widely used due to its simplicity and cost-effectiveness (Bauer *et al.*, 1966).

Broth Microdilution and Agar Dilution: These methods involve exposing bacteria to serial dilutions of antibiotics in a liquid (broth) or solid (agar plates) medium to determine the minimum inhibitory concentration (MIC), the lowest concentration that inhibits visible growth. These tests are considered the gold standard for antibiotic susceptibility testing (Jorgensen & Ferraro, 2009).

Automated Systems: Automated systems like VITEK and BD Phoenix use optical or fluorometric methods to measure bacterial growth in the presence of antibiotics, providing rapid and standardized results (Hindler & Stelling, 2007).

Molecular Methods

Molecular methods target specific genetic determinants of resistance, allowing for rapid and precise identification.

Polymerase Chain Reaction (PCR): PCR is used to amplify and detect specific resistance genes, such as mecA in methicillin-resistant Staphylococcus aureus (MRSA) or blaKPC in carbapenem-resistant Enterobacteriaceae (CRE). This method is highly sensitive and specific, making it suitable for detecting known resistance genes (Alekshun & Levy, 2007).

Multiplex PCR and DNA Microarrays: These techniques allow for the simultaneous detection of multiple resistance genes in a single test. DNA microarrays can analyse the expression of a wide array of genes, providing a comprehensive resistance profile (Cantón & Morosini, 2011).

Whole Genome Sequencing (WGS): WGS provides a complete genetic blueprint of an organism, enabling the identification of all known resistance genes and potential novel mechanisms of resistance. It is increasingly used in epidemiological studies and outbreak investigations to trace the spread of resistant strains (Zankari *et al.*, 2012).

Rapid Diagnostic Tests

Rapid diagnostics are crucial for timely treatment decisions.

Lateral Flow Assays: These are point-of-care tests that detect specific resistance proteins or genes in clinical samples. They are easy to use and provide results in minutes, making them suitable for use in resource-limited settings (Cohen *et al.*, 2019).

Matrix-Assisted Laser Desorption Ionization-Time of Flight (MALDI-TOF) Mass Spectrometry:

MALDI-TOF is a rapid technique that identifies bacteria based on protein profiles. Recent advancements have allowed for the detection of resistance mechanisms, such as β-lactamase production, directly from bacterial cultures (Sparbier *et al.*, 2012).

Conclusions

Antibiotic resistance has significant impacts on human and animal health, manifesting in both therapeutic and preventive realms. Therapeutically, its implications are direct, evident in treatment failures and complications. Preventively, antibiotic resistance compromises treatment options in immunosuppressive scenarios like cancer chemotherapy, advanced surgical procedures such as transplantation, and invasive procedures like intubation or catheterization. Urgent interventions are imperative to address this escalating crisis.

The timeline of AMR development clearly indicate the ability of microbes to develop resistance against almost all the antibiotics in very short span. The indiscriminate use of antibiotics is considered as main cause of these emerging resistances. Thus, it is imperative to save critically important antibiotics for the prevention and cure of critical illnesses. Further, the understanding of mechanism involved in emergence of resistance and its transmission from resistant to non-resistant microbes is also crucial to find out the path to overcome resistance. The ongoing interaction and history of resistance development reveals that the battle against AMR is far from over. The knowledge and strategies discussed may serve as essential tools in our ongoing efforts to combat this global health threat, emphasizing the need for continued vigilance, innovation, and international cooperation to preserve the efficacy of antimicrobial treatments for future generations.

References

Alekshun, M. N., & Levy, S. B. (2007). Molecular mechanisms of antibacterial multidrug resistance. Cell, 128(6), 1037-1050. https://doi.org/10.1016/j.cell.2007.03.004

Bauer, A. W., Kirby, W. M., Sherris, J. C., &Turck, M. (1966). Antibiotic susceptibility testing by a standardized single disk method. American Journal of Clinical Pathology, 45(4), 493-496. https://doi.org/10.1093/ajcp/45.4_ts.493

Blair, J. M. A., Webber, M. A., Baylay, A. J., Ogbolu, D. O., &Piddock, L. J. V. (2015). Molecular mechanisms of antibiotic resistance. Nature Reviews Microbiology, 13(1), 42-51. https://doi.org/10.1038/nrmicro3380

Cantón, R., &Morosini, M. I. (2011). Emergence and spread of antibiotic resistance following exposure to antibiotics. FEMS Microbiology Reviews, 35(5), 977-991. https://doi.org/10.1111/j.1574-6976.2011.00296.x

Cohen, R., Levy, C., Thollot, F., &Wollner, A. (2019). Rapid diagnostic tests for respiratory tract infections: clinical relevance and guidelines. Archives de Pédiatrie, 26(4), 214-219. https://doi.org/10.1016/j.arcped.2019.03.011

Gualerzi, C. O., Brandi, L., Fabbretti, A., &Pon, C. L. (Eds.). (2013). Antibiotics: targets, mechanisms and resistance. John Wiley & Sons.

Hindler, J. A., &Stelling, J. (2007). Analysis and presentation of cumulative antibiograms: a new consensus guideline from the Clinical and Laboratory Standards Institute. Clinical Infectious Diseases, 44(6), 867-873. https://doi.org/10.1086/511864

Hutchings M.I., Truman A.W., Wilkinson B. Antibiotics: Past, present and future. Curr. Opin. Microbiol. 2019;51:72–80. doi: 10.1016/j.mib.2019.10.008.

Jorgensen, J. H., & Ferraro, M. J. (2009). Antimicrobial susceptibility testing: a review of general principles and contemporary practices. Clinical Infectious Diseases, 49(11), 1749-1755. https://doi.org/10.1086/647952

Kümmerer, K. (2009). Antibiotics in the aquatic environment – A review – Part I. Chemosphere, 75(4), 417-434. https://doi.org/10.1016/j.chemosphere.2008.11.086

Laxminarayan, R., Duse, A., Wattal, C., Zaidi, A. K. M., Wertheim, H. F. L., Sumpradit, N., .& Cars, O. (2013). Antibiotic resistance—the need for global solutions. The Lancet Infectious Diseases, 13(12), 1057-1098. https://doi.org/10.1016/S1473-3099(13)70318-9

Majumder, M. A. A., Rahman, S., Cohall, D., Bharatha, A., Singh, K., Haque, M., &Gittens-St Hilaire, M. (2020). Antimicrobial stewardship: fighting antimicrobial resistance and protecting global public health. Infection and drug resistance, 4713-4738. Available at: https://www.cdc.gov/drugresistance/index.html

Martínez, J. L. (2018). General principles of antibiotic resistance in bacteria. Drug Resistance Updates, 33-35, 1-2. https://doi.org/10.1016/j.drup.2018.09.005

Murray, C. J., Ikuta, K. S., Sharara, F., Swetschinski, L., Aguilar, G. R., Gray, A., ... &Tasak, N. (2022). Global burden of bacterial antimicrobial resistance in 2019: a systematic analysis. The lancet, 399(10325), 629-655.

Parmar A., Lakshminarayanan R., Iyer A., Mayandi V., Leng Goh E.T., Lloyd D.G., Chalasani M.L.S., Verma N.K., Prior S.H., Beuerman R.W., et al. Design and Syntheses of Highly Potent Teixobactin Analogues against Staphylococcus aureus, Methicillin-Resistant Staphylococcus aureus (MRSA), and Vancomycin-Resistant Enterococci (VRE) in Vitro and in Vivo. J. Med. Chem. 2018;61:2009–2017. doi: 10.1021/acs.jmedchem.7b01634.

Salam, M. A., Al-Amin, M. Y., Salam, M. T., Pawar, J. S., Akhter, N., Rabaan, A. A., &Alqumber, M. A. A. (2023). Antimicrobial Resistance: A Growing Serious Threat for Global Public Health. Healthcare (Basel, Switzerland), 11(13), 1946.

Sparbier, K., Schubert, S., Weller, U., Boogen, C., &Kostrzewa, M. (2012). Matrix-assisted laser desorption ionization–time of flight mass spectrometry-based functional assay for rapid detection of resistance against β-lactam antibiotics. Journal of Clinical Microbiology, 50(3), 927-937. https://doi.org/10.1128/JCM.05737-11

Suay-García B., Pérez-Gracia M.T. Present and Future of Carbapenem-resistant Enterobacteriaceae (CRE) Infections. Antibiotics. 2019;8:122. doi: 10.3390/antibiotics8030122.

Uddin T.M., Chakraborty A.J., Khusro A., Zidan B.R.M., Mitra S., Emran T.B., Dhama K., Ripon M.K.H., Gajdács M., Sahibzada M.U.K., et al. Antibiotic resistance in microbes: History, mechanisms, therapeutic strategies and future prospects. J. Infect. Public Health. 2021;14:1750–1766. doi: 10.1016/j.jiph.2021.10.020.

Ventola, C. L. (2015). The antibiotic resistance crisis: Part 1: Causes and threats. P & T: A Peer-Reviewed Journal for Formulary Management, 40(4), 277-283. https://www.ncbi.nlm.nih.gov/pmc/articles/PMC4378521/

Weiner-Lastinger, L. M., Abner, S., Edwards, J. R., Kallen, A. J., Karlsson, M., Magill, S. S., ... &Dudeck, M. A. (2020). The impact of coronavirus disease 2019 (COVID-19) on healthcare-associated infections in 2020: A summary of data reported to the National Healthcare Safety Network. Infection Control & Hospital Epidemiology, 1-14. https://doi.org/10.1017/ice.2020.1413

World Health Organization (WHO). (2020). Antimicrobial resistance. Available at: https://www.who.int/news-room/fact-sheets/detail/antimicrobial-resistance

Zaman S.B., Hussain M.A., Nye R., Mehta V., Mamun K.T., Hossain N. A Review on Antibiotic Resistance: Alarm Bells are Ringing. Cureus. 2017;9:e1403. doi: 10.7759/cureus.1403.

Zankari, E., Hasman, H., Kaas, R. S., Seyfarth, A. M., Agersø, Y., Lund, O., ... &Aarestrup, F. M. (2012). Genotyping using whole-genome sequencing is a realistic alternative to surveillance based on phenotypic antimicrobial susceptibility testing. Journal of Antimicrobial Chemotherapy, 68(4), 771-777. https://doi.org/10.1093/jac/dks496

10

Understanding Quorum Sensing to Mitigate Transfer of Drug Resistance Genes

Mrinal Srivastava, Malyaj R Prajapati, Anamika Bhordia Anu Rahal and Amit Kumar

College of Biotechnology, Sardar Vallabhbhai Patel University of Agriculture and Technology, Meerut, Uttar Pradesh, India

Abstract

In the current scenario of AMR, transmission of drug resistance among microbes is a major threat and it is mainly through quorum sensing. Quorum Sensing is interconnected with cell density, a cell-to-cell communication process that greatly lives in our microbiome. In bacteria, chemical communication mean production, release, detection and responses to a small hormone like molecules 'Autoinducers'. Increases in the density can produce ample amount of small molecular signals to activate a verity of downstream cellular process including resistance mechanism, virulence and tolerate antibiotics. Due to quorum sensing bacteria enables them to act as multicellular organism because maximum quorum sensing controlled processes are ineffective when under taken by separate bacterium acting alone but becomes favourable when carried out by large number of cell i.e. multicellularly. This review contains general introduction to resistance mechanism like drug efflux pump and microbial biofilm formation regulation and we have also discussed about two component quorum sensing in gram positive and LUXI\LUXR quorum sensing in gram negative bacteria.

Keywords: *Quorum sensing, Autoinducers, AMR, Biofilm, LUXI\LUXR*

Microbial Resistance Mechanism

Huge use of antibiotics in nosocomical environment has lead to the occurrence of multidrug resistance mechanism by microorganism against particular antibiotics (Munita *et al.*, 2016; Zhao *et al.*, 2020). Main operation includes chemical modification, efflux pump through passivation, modification of drug targeting gene and systemic elimination of antibiotics as many of them can form biofilm (Rajput *et al.*, 2018) which can show extreme resistance. Chemical and enzymatic mechanism can include inactivation, activity loss, degradation and derivatizaton of antibiotics chemical group (Liu *et al.*, 2019). Best idea may include production of enzymes or they can also expel antibiotic to efflux pump. Antibiotics drug efflux resistance can be accomplished by drug efflux pump playing an important role in microbial resistance. A different type of efflux pump system has been identified that include lipophilic and hydrophilic efflux system targeting the drug at different chemical properties (Wasaznik *et al.*, 2009; Kumar *et al.*, 2012). Another strategy adopting in resistance mechanism is modification of drug targeting gene. This mechanism makes the changes in drug to lose its target through drug targeting gene modification. Another important resistance mechanism is effectiveness of antibiotics by interfering with the target site. Therefore, bacteria has evolved different mechanism that include target site protection. A bactericidal role played by beta lactum antibiotics in inhibition of mucopeptide synthase and bacterial penicillin binding protein (PBP) in cell wall transpeptidation reaction that prevents the formation of complete call wall and hence dies (Sauvage *et al.*, 2016). Bacteria also developed its own strategies to cope up with the environmental stress that can also include human body. In course of gaining the advantage bacteria needs to compete for nutrients and to keep away from the molecules produced by other competing organism (Zhao *et al.*, 2019). Recently researchers have found the importance of biofilm resistance in bacteria. Bacterial biofilm resistance produce by complex and systematic drug resistance mechanism.

Principle of drug resistance can be concluded in 3 points (Stewart *et al.*, 2002; Balcazar *et al.*, 2015; Hathroubi *et al.*, 2017).

1. Biofilm itself can reduce its antibiotics permeability through an effective drug barrier. Bacteria especially connected through extracellular polysaccharide protein and DNA forming an insuperable barrier, which can improve survival rate in biofilm and reduction in permeability of antibiotics drugs.

2. Bacterial membrane produce heterogenicity to regulate antibiotics resistance so that they can create a special microenvironment.

3. Changes in the environmental factors outside the biofilm includes changes in pH, concentration of certain chemicals, change in temperature may affect in bacterial biofilm regulates its biochemical and physiological function and decrease its growth efficiency for antibiotics resistance (Zhong *et al.*, 2019).

In contract to conventional design, quorum sensing encourages the coincident expression of target gene across the population of bacteria. Currently quorum sensing processes continuous time ON mode of sub population of cell in quorum sensing where as remaining population mode will be OFF for quorum sensing (Anetzberger *et al.*, 2009; Pérez *et al.*, 2010; Pradhan *et al.*, 2014; Cárcamo-Oyarce *et al.*, 2015; Plener *et al.*, 2015; Grote *et al.*, 2015).

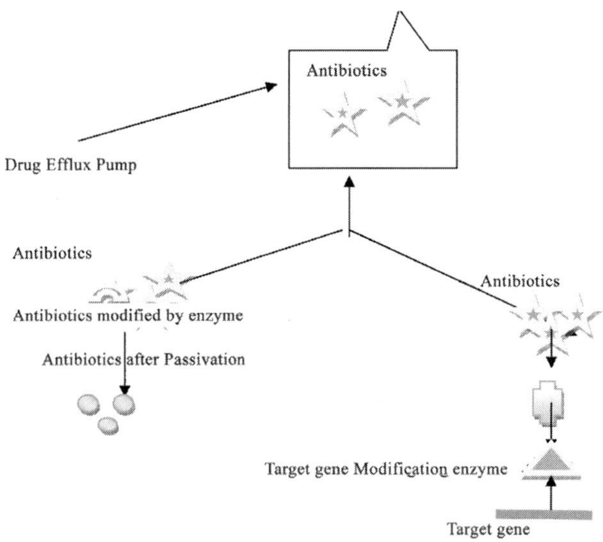

Fig. 1: Common mechanism of microbial resistance (Zhao *et al.*, 2020).

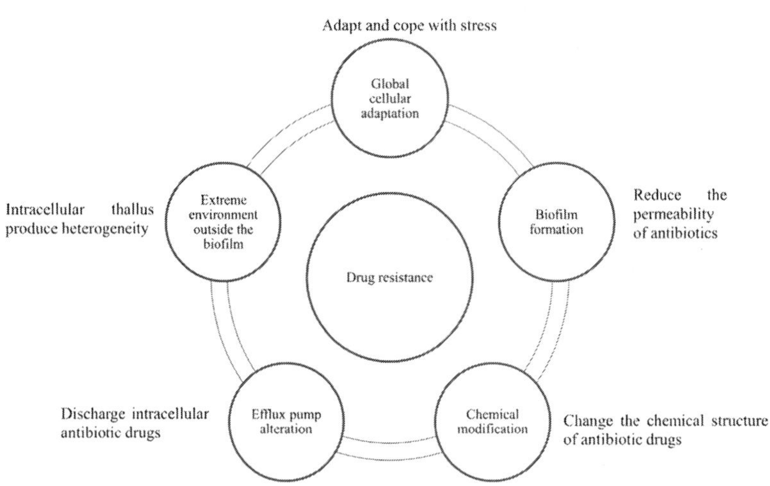

Various resistance mechanisms of bacteria and their action involved

Quorum Sensing

In bacteria, changes in the cell density in response to regulation of gene expression is called as 'Quorum Sensing'. Quorum sensing bacteria produce, release and respond to a Chemical Signalling Molecule termed as Autoinducers (AIs) that accumulates in the environment as the cell density increases. When the required stimulatory concentration of Autoinducer is attained, a signal transduction cascade is inaugurated that eventually is translated into a behaviour change of organism (Engebrecht *et al.*, 1983; Bainton *et al.*, 1992; Passador *et al.*, 1993; Piper *et al.*, 1993). Many classes of AIs have been reported till date. Originally, quorum sensing was described in *Vibrio fischeri* and *Vibrio hareyi* where it functions as control apparatus for light creation and many more traits (Eberhard *et al.*, 1981; Engebrecht *et al.*, 1983 & 1984; Ruby *et al.*, 2007). *V harveyi* owns two quorum sensing system that controls the expression of bioluminescence (Lux) parallelly in density dependent manner. Density sensing system of *V. hareyi* i.e. signalling system 1 and signalling system 2 sensor and a cognate autoinducer. Therefore, autoinducer1 (AI1) respond to sensor 1 of signalling system 1 and Autoinducer 2 (AI2) detects sensor 2 of signalling system 2 (Bassler *et al.*, 1995). AI2 is a species non-specific signal uses by both gram positive and gram negative bacteria (Surette *et al.*, 1999) and has been found in at least 55 strain produced by LuxS gene (Bassler *et al.*, 1997). Most intensely studied AIs in Gram-negative bacteria are N-acyl homoserine lacton (AHLs) and in gram positive AIs are peptide type, a class of AI2 whose structure is unknown (Antunes and Ferreira, 2009). AHLs are usually detected and activated through binding to cytoplasmic receptor proteins. It detects signal and dimerize upon promoter region to bind on target gene activation or transcriptional repression (Fuqua *et al.*, 1994). For years it was considered that this was happening to only some of the marine organism but quorum sensing, now widely acknowledged by many bacterial species as a part of their regulatory machinery (Lyon *et al.*, 2004; Bassler and Losick, 2006; Smith *et al.*, 2006).

Two component Quorum Sensing in Gram Positive Bacteria

In Gram positive bacteria's AIs are detected via membrane bound tow component transduction system i.e. oligo- autoinducing peptides as signalling molecules (Otto *et al.*, 1998; Ji *et al.*, 1995; Solomon *et al.*, 1996). AIPs has diversified sequence and structure that are encoded as 'precusors' (Magnuson *et al.*, 1994; Lazazzera, 2001; Nakayama *et al.*, 2001; Kalkum *et al.*, 2003; Okada *et al.*, 2005; Thoendel *et al.*, 2011). As cell membrane is impermeable to peptide so a specialized transporters are required for transport of peptide secrete AIPs. Therefore, precursors i.e. pro-AIPs get modified by post-translational modification in between the size range of 5 to 17 amino acid and that can either in the cyclised or linear form (Ruby, 1996; Okada *et al.*, 2005; Bouillaut *et al.*, 2008). At extracellular site AIPs are detected by two component membrane bound sensor kinases. When by AIPs, sensor kinases autophosphorylates themselves at conserved histidines. Now phosphoryl group is passed to conserved aspartate from histidine at cognate cytoplasmic respond regulator that controls quorum sensing gene expression. An operon has been meant for histidine kinase receptor and response regulator quorum sensing circuits.

LUXI\LUXR Quorum Sensing in Gram-negative Bacteria

Gram negative has similar quorum sensing system as in *Vibrio fischeri* (a marine bioluminescent bacteria) (Engebrecht and Silverman, 1984; Hastings and Greenberg, 1999). AI synthase catalyses the reaction between SAM and an acyl carrier protein (ACP), an homolog of LUXI system that can produce a freely diffusible acyl homoserine lacton (AHL) AI (Engebrecht *et al.*, 1983; More *et al.*, 1996; Schaefer *et al.*, 1996; Ng and Bassler, 2009). At increased concentration of AHL. AI binds to LUXR type transcription factor at cytoplasmic site. When AI is free i.e. not in bound form the LUXR type proteins are quickly degraded, so that they can avoid short-circuiting of quorum sensing system. AI binding stabilizes the LUXR type protein, allowing them to bind to DNA, activate target gene transcription factor (Engebrecht and Silverman, 1984; Stevens *et al.*, 1994; Zhu and Winans; 1999, Case *et al.*, 2008). LUXI protein expression can also be activated by LUXR forming feed forward autoinducer loop that increase the level with AI. In more than 100 species of gram negative bacteria' LUXI\LUXR has been identified (Cárcamo-Oyarce *et al.*, 2015). Different bacteria possess different length side chain and side chain decorations produced by AHLs. C4 and C18 in acyl chain has been identified with modification at C3 position at hydroxy and carboxyl moieties this chemical diversity encourage intra-species cell-cell communication with LUXR partner are commonly highly specific.

In contract to conventional design, quorum sensing encourages the coincident expression of target gene across the population of bacteria. Currently quorum sensing processes continuous time ON mode of sub population of cell in quorum sensing where as remaining population mode will be OFF for quorum sensing (Anetzberger *et al.*, 2009; Pérez *et al.*, 2010; Pradhan *et al.*, 2014; Cárcamo-Oyarce *et al.*, 2015; Plener *et al.*, 2015; Grote *et al.*, 2015).

Conclusion

Quorum sensing is an important decisive system used by many bacterial species to command collaborative traits that can provide bacteria to utilize particular nich. Bacterial population use quorum sensing to control the antibiotic resistance mechanism which provide member of population, higher level of resistance .So as we discussed in the above example bacteria that makes their living by accomplishing eukaryotic hosts have coupled the production of resistance mechanism necessary for antibiotics resistance by detecting changes in cell population density. it is also understandable that QS gene regulation is the outcome of regulatory networks mounted onto the primary AI detection and production mechanism. Although with constant improvement in molecular biology and synthetic biology subsequent research on QS will certainly undertake a new stage and this will definitely make a new contribution in antibiotic resistance mechanism.

References

Anetzberger, C., Pirch, T. and Jung, K. (2009). Heterogeneity in quorum sensing-regulated bioluminescence of Vibrio harveyi. Mol. Microbiol. 73, 267–277.

Antunes, L. C. and Ferreira, R. B. (2009). Intercellular communicationin bacteria. Crit Rev Microbiol 35, 69–80.

Bainton, N. J., Bycroft, B. W., Chhabra, S., Stead, P., Gledhill, L.,Hill, P. J., Rees, C. E. D., Winson, M. K., Salmond, G. P. C.,Stewart, G. S. A. B. & Williams, P. (1992). A general role for the lux autoinducer in bacterial cell signalling: control of antibiotic biosynthesis in Erwinia. Gene 116, 87–91.

Balcazar J.L., Subirats J., Borrego C.M. (2015). The role of biofilms as environmental reservoirs of antibiotic resistance. Front. Microbiol. 6 doi: 10.3389/fmicb.2015.01216.

Bassler, B. L., E. P. Greenberg, and A. M. Stevens. (1997). Cross-speciesinduction of luminescence in the quorum-sensing bacterium Vibrio harveyi. J.Bacteriol. 179:4043–4045.

Bassler, B. L. and Losick, R. (2006). Bacterially speaking. Cell 125, 237–246.

Bassler, B. L. and Silverman, M. R. (1995) in Two-ComponentSignal Transduction, eds. Hoch, J. A. and Silhavy, T. J. (Am. Soc.Microbiol., Washington, DC), pp. 431–445.

Bouillaut L, Perchat S, Arold S, Zorrilla S, Slamti L, Henry C, Gohar M, Declerck N, Lereclus D. (2008). Molecular basis for group-specific activation of the virulence regulator PlcR by PapR heptapeptides. Nucleic Acids Res 36: 3791–3801.

Case R.J., (2008). Labbate M, Kjelleberg S. AHL-driven quorum-sensing circuits: their frequency and function among the Proteobacteria. Isme J 2: 345–349.

Cárcamo-Oyarce, G., Lumjiaktase, P., Kümmerli, R. & Eberl, L. (2015). Quorum sensing triggers the stochastic escape of individual cells from Pseudomonas putida biofilms. Nat. Commun. 6, 5945.

Eberhard, A., Burlingame, A. L., Eberhard, C., Kenyon, G. L.,Nealson, K. H. and Oppenheimer, N. J. (1981). Structural identificationof autoinducer of Photobacterium fischeri luciferase. Biochemistry 20, 2444–2449.

Engebrecht, J., Nealson, K. and Silverman, M. (1983) Bacterial bioluminescence: isolation and genetic analysis of functions from Vibrio fischeri. Cell 32,773–781.

Engebrecht J, and Silverman M. (1984). Identification of genes and gene products necessary for bacterial bioluminescence. Proc Natl Acad Sci 81: 4154–4158.

Engebrecht J, Nealson K, and Silverman M. (1983). Bacterial bioluminescence: Isolation and genetic analysis of functions from Vibrio fischeri. Cell 32: 773–781.

Fuqua, W. C., Winans, S. C. and Greenberg, E. P. (1994). Quorumsensing in bacteria: the LuxR–LuxI family of cell density-responsivetranscriptional regulators. J Bacteriol. 176, 269–275.

Grote, J., Krysciak, D. and Streit, W. R. (2015). Phenotypic heterogeneity, a phenomenon that may explain why quorum sensing does not always result in truly homogenous cell behavior. Appl. Environ. Microbiol. 81, 5280–5289.

Hastings JW, and Greenberg EP. (1999). Quorum sensing: The explanation of a curious phenomenon reveals a common characteristic of bacteria. J Bacteriol 181: 2667–2668.

Hathroubi S., Mekni M.A., Domenico P., Dao N., and Jacques M. (2017). Biofilms: Microbial Shelters Against Antibiotics. Microb. Drug Resist. 23:147–156.

Ji G., Beavis R.C., and Novick R.P. (1995). Cell density control of staphylococcal virulence mediated by an octapeptide pheromone. Proc Natl Acad Sci 92: 12055–12059.

Kalkum M, Lyon GJ, and Chait BT. (2003). Detection of secreted peptides by using hypothesis-driven multistage mass spectrometry. Proc Natl Acad Sci 100: 2795–2800.

Kumar S. and Varela M.F. (2012). Biochemistry of Bacterial Multidrug Efflux Pumps. Int. J. Mol. Sci. 13:4484–4495.

Lazazzera, B.A. (2001). The intracellular function of extracellular signaling peptides. Peptides 22: 1519–1527.

Liu L.Y., Ye C.X., Soteyome T., Zhao X.H., Xia J., Xu W.Y., Mao Y.Z., Peng R.X., Chen J.X., Xu Z.B., et al. (2019). Inhibitory effects of two types of food additives on biofilm formation by foodborne pathogens. Microbiology Open. 8:9.

Lyon, G. J. and Novick, R. P. (2004). Peptide signaling in Staphylococcusaureus and other Gram-positive bacteria. Peptides 25, 1389–1403.

Magnuson R., Solomon J., and Grossman A.D. (1994). Biochemical and genetic characterization of a competence pheromone from B. subtilis. Cell 77: 207–216.

More MI, Finger LD, Stryker JL, Fuqua C, Eberhard A, and Winans SC. (1996). Enzymatic synthesis of a quorum-sensing autoinducer through use of defined substrates. Science 272: 1655–1658.

Munita J.M. and Arias C.A. (2016). Mechanisms of Antibiotic Resistance. Microbiol. Spectr. 4:24.

Nakayama J, Cao Y, Horii T, Sakuda S, Akkermans AD, de Vos WM, and Nagasawa H. (2001). Gelatinase biosynthesis-activating pheromone: A peptide lactone that mediates a quorum sensing in Enterococcus faecalis. Mol Microbiol 41: 145–154.

Ng WL and Bassler BL. (2009). Bacterial quorum-sensing network architectures. Annu Rev Genet., 43: 197–222.

Okada M., Sato I., Cho S.J., Iwata H., Nishio T., Dubnau D., and Sakagami Y. (2005). Structure of the Bacillus subtilis quorum-sensing peptide pheromone ComX. Nat Chem Biol 1: 23–24.

Otto M, Sussmuth R, Jung G, and Gotz F. (1998). Structure of the pheromone peptide of the Staphylococcus epidermidis agr system. FEBS Lett 424: 89–94.

Passador, L., Cook, J. M., Gambello, M. J., Rust, L. and Iglewski, B. H. (1993). Expression of Pseudomonas aeruginosa virulence genes requires cell-to-cell communication. Science 260, 1127–1130.

Piper, K. R., Beck von Bodman, S. and Farrand, S. K. (1993). Conjugation factor of Agrobacterium tumefaciens regulates Ti plasmid transfer by autoinduction. Nature(London) 362, 448–450.

Plener, L. et al. (2015). The phosphorylation flow of the Vibrio harveyi quorum-sensing cascade determines levels of phenotypic heterogeneity in the population. J. Bacteriol. 197, 1747–1756.

Pradhan, B. B. and Chatterjee, S. (2014). Reversible non-genetic phenotypic heterogeneity in bacterial quorum sensing. Mol. Microbiol. 92, 557–569.

Pérez, P. D. and Hagen, S. J. (2010). Heterogeneous response to a quorum-sensing signal in the luminescence of individual Vibrio fischeri. PLOS ONE 5, e15473.

Rajput A., Thakur A., Sharma S., and Kumar M. (2018). A Biofilm: A resource of anti-biofilm agents and their potential implications in targeting antibiotic drug resistance. Nucleic Acids Res. 46: D894–D900.

Ruby, E. G. and Greenberg, E. P. (2007). Transcriptome analysis of the Vibrio fischeri LuxR–LuxI regulon. J Bacteriol 189, 8387–8391.

Ruby E.G. (1996). Lessons from a cooperative, bacterial-animal association: The Vibrio fischeri-Euprymna scolopes light organ symbiosis. Annu Rev Microbiol. 50: 591–624.

Sauvage E., and Terrak M. G. (2016). lycosyltransferases and Transpeptidases/Penicillin-Binding Proteins: Valuable Targets for New Antibacterials. Antibiotics.2016;5:12.

Schaefer A.L., Val D.L., Hanzelka B.L, Cronan J.E Jr, Greenberg E.P. (1996). Generation of cell-to-cell signals in quorum sensing: Acyl homoserine lactone synthase activity of a purified Vibrio fischeri LuxI protein. Proc Natl Acad Sci. 93: 9505–9509.

Smith, D., Wang, J. H., Swatton, J. E., Davenport, P., Price, B., Mikkelsen, H., Stickland, H., Nishikawa, K., Gardiol, N. and other authors (2006). Variations on a theme: diverse N-acyl homoserinelactone-mediated quorum sensing mechanisms in Gram-negative bacteria. Sci Prog. 89, 167–211.

Solomon J.M., Lazazzera B.A. and Grossman A.D. (1996). Purification and characterization of an extracellular peptide factor that affects two different developmental pathways in Bacillus subtilis. Genes Dev. 10: 2014–2024.

Stevens A.M., Dolan K.M. and Greenberg E.P. (1994). Synergistic binding of the Vibrio fischeri LuxR transcriptional activator domain and RNA polymerase to the lux promoter region. Proc Natl Acad Sci. 91: 12619–12623.

Stewart P.S. (2002). Mechanisms of antibiotic resistance in bacterial biofilms. Int. J. Med. Microbiol. 292:107–113.

Surette, M. G., M. B. Miller, and B. L. Bassler. (1999). Quorum sensing in Escherichia coli, Salmonella typhimurium, and Vibrio harveyi: a new family of genes responsible for autoinducer production. Proc. Natl. Acad. Sci. USA. 96:1639–1644.

Thoendel M., Kavanaugh J.S., Flack C.E., and Horswill AR. (2011). Peptide signaling in the staphylococci. Chem Rev 111: 117–151.

Wasaznik A., Grinholc M., and Bielawski K.P. (2009). Active efflux as the multidrug resistance mechanism. Postepy Hig. I Med. Dosw. 63:123–133.

Zhao, X., Yu, Z., and Ding, T. (2020). Quorum-Sensing Regulation of Antimicrobial Resistance in Bacteria. Microorganisms, 8(3), 425.

Zhao X.H., Xia J. and Liu Y. (2019). Contrast of Real-Time Fluorescent PCR Methods for Detection of Escherichia coli O157:H7 and of introducing an Internal Amplification Control. Microorganisms.7:14. doi: 10.3390/microorganisms7080230.

Zhao X.H., Zhao F.H., and Zhong N.J. (2020). Production of diacylglycerols through glycerolysis with SBA-15 supported Thermomyces lanuginosus lipase as catalyst. J. Sci. Food Agric. 100:1426–1435.

Zhong J. and Zhao X. (2019). Transcriptomic Analysis of viable but non-culturable Escherichia coli O157:H7 formation induced by low temperature. Microorganisms. 7:634.

Zhu J. and Winans S.C. (1999). Autoinducer binding by the quorum-sensing regulator TraR increases affinity for target promoters in vitro and decreases TraR turnover rates in whole cells. Proc Natl Acad Sci., 96: 4832–4837.

11

Transfer of Antimicrobial Resistance Through Mobile Genetic Elements

Joycee Jogi, Daljeet Chhabra, Rakesh Sharda, Rakh Gangil, Ravi Sikrodia and Neetu Rajput

College of Veterinary Science & A.H., Mhow, NDVSU, Jabalpur, Madhya Pradesh, India

Abstract

Strains of bacteria resistant to antibiotics, particularly those that are multiresistant, are an increasing major health care problem around the world. It is now abundantly clear that both Gram-negative and Gram-positive bacteria are able to meet the evolutionary challenge of combating antimicrobial chemotherapy, often by acquiring preexisting resistance determinants from the bacterial gene pool. This is achieved through the concerted activities of mobile genetic elements able to move within or between DNA molecules, which include insertion sequences, transposons, and gene cassettes/ integrons, and those that are able to transfer between bacterial cells, such as plasmids and integrative conjugative elements. Together these elements play a central role in facilitating horizontal genetic exchange and therefore promote the acquisition and spread of resistance genes. This article aims to outline the characteristics of the major types of mobile genetic elements involved in acquisition and spread of antibiotic resistance in both Gram-negative and Gram positive bacteria, focusing on the so-called ESKAPEE group of organisms (Enterococcus faecium, Staphylococcus aureus, Klebsiella pneumoniae, Acinetobacter baumannii, Pseudomonas aeruginosa, Enterobacter spp., and Escherichia coli), which have become the most problematic hospital pathogens.

Introduction

Antibiotic-resistant bacteria are a major cause of health care-associated infections around the world, and resistance has also emerged in infections in the wider community. Infections caused by multi resistant organisms significantly increase morbidity, mortality, and health care costs. Molecular analyses have revealed that widespread multi resistance has commonly been achieved by the acquisition of preexisting determinants followed by amplification in response to selection. The capture, accumulation, and dissemination of resistance genes are largely due to the actions of mobile genetic elements (MGE), a term used to refer to elements that promote intracellular DNA mobility (e.g., from the chromosome to a plasmid or between plasmids) as well as those that enable intercellular DNA mobility.

Insertion sequences (IS) and transposons (Tn) are discrete DNA segments that areable to move themselves (and associated resistance genes) almost randomly to newlocations in the same or different DNA molecules within a single cell. Other elements, such as integrons (In), use site-specific recombination to move resistance genes between defined sites. As these types of MGE are often present in multiple copies indifferent locations in a genome, they can also facilitate homologous recombination(exchange of sequences between identical or related segments). Intercellular mechanisms of genetic exchange include conjugation/mobilization (mediated by plasmidsand integrative conjugative elements [ICE]), transduction (mediated by bacteriophages), and transformation (uptake of extracellular DNA). Interactions between thevarious types of MGE underpin the rapid evolution of diverse multi resistant pathogens in the face of antimicrobial chemotherapy. Primarily the most important and/ or topical elements in Gram-negative and Gram-positive bacterial species of particular concern clinically, namely, Enterococcus faecium, Staphylococcus aureus, *Klebsiella pneumoniae*, *Acinetobacter baumannii*, *Pseudomonas aeruginosa*, and *Enterobacter* spp. (the so-called ESKAPE group) (Rice LB., 2008) as well as Escherichia coli (giving the ESKAPEE group) (Llaca-Díaz J.M. *et al.*,2012); nonetheless, many of the MGE types described are of course broadly relevant to many other bacterial taxa.

Insertion Sequence (Is)and Composite Transposons

IS are generally small mobile elements that typically carry little more than one (sometimes two) transposase (tnp) gene.They can be divided into groups based partly on active site motifs in Tnp, designated by key amino acids that come together in the active site, most commonly DDE (Asp, Asp, and Glu) but also DEDD and HUH (two His residues separated by a large hydrophobic amino acid) (Hickman and Dyda, 2015) and/or based on whether transposition is a conservative, cut-and-paste mechanism, where the IS is simply excised from the donor and inserted into the recipient, or replicative (Hallet and Sherratt,1997). Replicative transposition can occur by a copy-and-paste mechanism (the IS is replicated to join the donor and recipient in a cointegrate, which is then resolved to give the original donor plus the recipient with the IS or a copy-out-paste-in mechanism (the IS is replicated into a double-stranded circular intermediate that then integrates into the recipient).Traditionally IS were not thought of as carrying "passenger" genes, but they can move resistance genes as part of a composite (also called compound) transposon, a region bounded by two copies of the same or related IS that can move as a single unit.

Gene Cassettes and Integrons

A gene cassette is a small mobile element (0.5 to 1 kb) consisting of a single gene(occasionally two), typically lacking a promoter, and an attC recombination site. Gene cassettes can exist in a free circular form but are nonreplicative and are usually found inserted into an integron, characterized by an intI gene, an attI recombinationsite, and a promoter (Pc). intI encodes an atypical site-specific tyrosine recombinase, which has an extra domain compared to other members of this family (Escudero*et al.*, 2015.), that catalyzes recombination between the attI site of the integron and the attC site of acassette. This inserts the cassette into the integron in the orientation that allows expression of the cassette-borne gene from the Pc promoter. Multiple cassettes may be inserted into the same integron to create a cassette array (often incorrectly referred toas a "cassette") that may confer multiresistance. Different classes of integrin have been defined based on the sequence of IntI (called IntI1, IntI2, IntI3, etc., withcognate attI1, attI2, and attI3 sites), with class 1 being the first reported and most common in antibiotic-resistant clinical isolates.

Cassette Integration and Expression

attC sites associated with different cassettes differ in sequence, but all include twopairs of conserved 7 or 8bp core sites at their outer ends (Partridge *et al.*, 2009.). These are separated by a region of variable length that usually shows inverted repeatedness. Although the sequence similarity between different attC sites islow, single-stranded versions each form a conserved secondary structure, with two orthree unpaired, protruding extrahelical bases. These are recognized by the IntI recombinase and are important in directing recombination to the bottom strand, ensuring that insertion occurs in one orientation only.

Gene Cassettes and Antibiotic Resistance

A wide variety of gene cassettes containing resistance genes (named after the gene carried) have been identified. The most clinically relevant are those carrying genes encoding B-lactamases oraminoglycoside-modifying enzymes. The former include metallo-B-lactamases (MBL; classB), with the VIM and IMP types being the most common. Cassette-borne genes also encodeclass A GES enzymes, which are either ESBL or carbapenemases (with a mutation at aminoacid 170), and class D OXA-10-like (which include ESBL variants) and OXA-1-likeenzymes.

Gene Cassettes and Integrons in Gram-Positive Bacteria

Gene cassettes and/or integrons have been reported for a few Gram-positive bacterial species, including *Corynebacteriumglutamicum* (on a plasmid transferable to*E. coli*) (Nesvera *et al.*, 1998.), Staphylococcus (Nandi *et al.*, 2004), and Enterococcus (e.g., on a transferable plasmid) (Clark*et al.*,1999.). However, many studies report only detection of intI1 by PCR, with sequencing of fragments in some cases. Searches with the class 1 integron5'-CS or 3'-CS against sequences from Staphylococcus and Enterococcus species inGenBank (including the whole-genome shotgun contigs [WGS] database [accessed May2018]) identified very few examples, most of which were fragments and none of which provided evidence of linkage to the chromosome or plasmids. Thus, there is presently no conclusive evidence demonstrating the existence of integrons in these genera.

MITEs AND TIMEs

MITEs are nonautonomous (i.e., incapable of self-transposition) derivatives of bacterial IS or transposons that retain the inverted repeats but which have lost central parts, including thet ransposase gene(s) (Delihas, 2011). Pairs of MITEs, including Tn3-derived inverted-repeat miniature elements (TIMEs) (Zuplewska *et al.*, 2014), appear to have been involved in mobilization of resistance genes.

Resistance Plasmids

Plasmids are important vehicles for the carriage of other MGE and acquired antimicrobial resistance genes associated with these elements in both Gram-negative and Gram-positive genera, and they vary in size from less than a kilobase to several megabases (Shintani *et al.*, 2015). Their extra chromosomal existence stems from their ability to replicate and hence be inherited in a growing population of host cells, which often requiresa cadre of gene systems dedicated to their efficient vertical inheritance. Conjugation or mobilization functions may also be present, allowing plasmids to spread horizontally. Together the genes encoding these functions form a "backbone" (Thomas, 2000) that represents a core of plasmid housekeeping functions to which can be added "accessory" niche adaptive activities that might benefit the host cell (and hence the plasmid itself) in a particular environment. In resistance plasmids, these accessory regions are typicallymade up of one or more resistance genes and associated mobile elements of the typesdescribed above (IS, Tn, and/or

In). Closely related backbones may have different insertions and/or resistance regions, and conversely, different backbones may housethe same resistance genes and associated mobile elements.

Replication Initiation and Copy Number Control

Plasmid replication initiates at a defined region, the origin (ori), triggered either byan RNA transcript or, more commonly, by the binding of an initiation protein (Rep),encoded by a rep gene on the plasmid, to proximal iterated DNA repeat sequences termed iterons. The ori and the (typically colocated) initiator gene form the basic component of all plasmids, the minimal replicon. Thus, plasmids encode their own replication initiation but usually exploit the host's chromosomally encoded replication machinery (helicase, primase, polymerase, etc.) for DNA synthesis itself. Interactions with and dependence on host-encoded DNA replication proteins are among the factors that limit the host range of plasmids. Some plasmids are efficiently maintained only inclosely related bacterial taxa and are hence termed narrow-host-range plasmids, whereas others are referred to as broad-host-range plasmids because they have been found or shown to replicate in quite diverse genera. Factors other than replication,particularly whether it is transmissible by conjugation or mobilization, can also influence a plasmid's host range. Conjugation can be an extraordinarily promiscuous process, capable of even transkingdom genetic exchange (Lacroix and Citovsky, 2016). Transfer of resistance plasmids into hosts in which they cannot replicate is therefore likely to be common place, with other MGE (e.g., IS, Tn, and In) providing intracellular mobilitymechanisms that give resistance genes an opportunity to "escape" to other functional replicons (the chromosome or other resident plasmids). Thus, even narrow-host-rangeplasmids can act as suicide vectors for the horizontal spread of resistance genes into divergent hosts.

Plasmid Maintenance

Once replicated, plasmids must be distributed between daughter cells when division takes place. For small plasmids maintained at a high copy number, efficientinheritance by both daughter cells can be achieved by random segregation. However,larger plasmids usually exist at a low copy number to minimize the burden on theirhosts, which risk being outcompeted by plasmid-free counterparts in the environment.Large low-copy-number plasmids thus usually possess functional modules that contribute to plasmid maintenance.

Conjugation

Plasmid propagation is facilitated not only through vertical transmission via celldivision but also via horizontal transmission to other bacterial cells. Conjugative(self-transmissible) plasmids possess genetically complex systems for horizontal plasmid transfer, which significantly increase the size of their conserved backbone.

Genomic Islands

A genomic island (GI) is a distinct region of a bacterial chromosome that has beenacquired via horizontal transfer; in many cases, GIs are flanked by direct repeats. GIs vary in size (they may be composed of several hundred genes) and can be classified based on the phenotype(s) that they encode. For example, GIs that contain multiple resistance determinants are referred to as resistance islands, whereas those that contain virulence factors are often called pathogenicity islands. A broad definition of GIs (Delavat*et al.*, 2017) encompasses elements with mobility functions, such as ICE, integrative mobilizable elements(IME), which require helper functions to conjugate, and elements that are excised fromthe chromosome and may be transferred horizontally via phage-mediated mechanisms(Novick*et al.*, 2010), such as staphylococcal cassette chromosome elements (SCCmec) and *S. aureus* pathogenicity islands (SaPI).

Integrative Conjugative Elements (ICE)

ICE (Burrus*et al.,* 2002) constitute a diverse group of mobile elements found in both Gram-negative and Gram-positive bacteria and have been reviewed recently. Likeplasmids, ICE are self-transmissible by conjugation, but they integrate into the host chromo some and are replicated as part of it, although replication of excised ICE hasnow been demonstrated (Carraro and Burrus, 2015.). ICE typically consist of a backbone (containing phage like integration/ excision functions, plasmid-like conjugation/maintenance components,and a regulation module) into which accessory genes are inserted.

Staphylococcal Cassette Chromosome

SCCmec is a type of resistance island carried on the chromosome of MRSA isolates that confers resistance to methicillin, penicillin, and other B-lactam antibiotics. This element contains the mecA gene or the more recently identified mec C gene, both of which encode related low-affinity penicillin-binding proteins called PBP2a, and the divergently transcribed regulatory genes, mecR1 (for the signal transducer proteinMecR1) and mecI (for the repressor protein MecI) (Ito *et al.*, 2004).

Staphylococcal Pathogenicity Islands

SaPIs are genomic islands that integrate at specific sites, are flanked by direct repeats, and utilize the capsids ofhelper phages for their movement. They encode phage-like proteins that facilitate this process, including a master repressor (Stl) that controls SaPIexcision via interaction with helper phage antirepressor proteins; these interactions are SaPI and phage specific (Novickand Ram, 2016.). In most cases, SaPIs also encode one or more virulence factors, such as superantigens, but they rarely carry resistance determinants. However,some exceptions are SaPIj50, which encodes resistance to penicillin (bla) (Iwao*et al*., 2012.), and SaRIfusB, which encodes resistance to fusidic acid (fusB). Note that while SaRIfusBis related to classical SaPIs, it does not encode any known virulence factors and is therefore referred to as a resistance island (O'Neill *et al*., 2007).

Using Wgs to Better Understand Mobile Antibiotic Resistance

The increasing availability of next-generation DNA sequencing methods, including their use for tracking outbreaks of resistant organisms, has led to an explosion in the number of bacterial whole-genome sequences. Analysis of these data has underscoredthe significance of MGE, and the increasing use of this technology to characterize bacterial pathogens presents opportunities for understanding the evolution of resistance but also creates challenges. It is increasingly apparent that the boundaries between types of elements historically viewed as distinct are becoming blurred (e.g., IS with passenger genes resembling unit transposons, excised ICE replicating as plasmidsdo, etc.), and this needs to be borne in mind when naming new elements. Using existing resources to obtain names/numbers for novel IS (ISfinder [https://www-is.biotoul.fr]) (Siguier*et al*., 2006.), transposons (Transposon Registry [http://transposon.lstmed.ac.uk])(Roberts *et al*., 2008), gene cassettes (INTEGRALL [http://integrall.bio.ua.pt] (Moura *et al*., 2009) and RAC [http://app.spokade.com/rac/feature/list]) (Tsafnat*et al*., 2011.), and SCCmec elements (http://www.sccmec.org)(International Working Group on the Classification of Staphylococcal Cassette Chromosome Elements, 2009) and submitting elements to these sites help to reduce confusion.

While use of long-read sequencing methods is becoming more common, many plasmid sequences in International Nucleotide Sequence Database Collaboration (INSDC) databases (GenBank, EMBL-EBI, and DDBJ) were derived from short-read methods, as these were more widely available and are more economical. However, complex resistance regions in plasmids or genomic islands present challenges for assembly from short-read data, as multiple copies of the same mobile element in different locations constitute repeats that are generally significantly longer than read lengths. Mostassembly programs will collapse reads covering these repeats down to a single contig,while regions between repeats are usually found as separate contigs, potentially with fragments of repeats on each end. Methods such as plasmidSPAdes (Antipov*et al.*, 2016) may help toidentify contigs derived from plasmids, and those such as PLACNET (Lanza *et al.*, 2014) may help to group contigs from a particular plasmid, but it can still be difficult to correctly assign resistance regions to particular plasmids (Orlek*et al.*, 2017).

Classification of plasmids also needs to move on from typing based on experimentally defined incompatibility, which may not be reflected adequately in sequence identity, and expanded to consider the whole backbone rather than just the replicon and/or relaxase region. At present, different types of schemes exist for different plasmid types, based on analyses by different groups of researchers, and some plasmid typeshave been neglected. Developing a more universal system will require cooperation between experts in pertinent fields, including plasmid biology and bioinformatics, aswell as consultation and broad acceptance from the relevant research community.

Conclusions

Horizontal gene transfer plays an important role in the acquisition of new properties,such as pathogenicity and antibiotic resistance, underpinning the formidable adaptive potential of bacteria. This helps us to understands the diverse toolkit of MGE that the species of interest exploit to access an extended gene pool in order to overcome the evolutionary challenge that antimicrobial chemotherapy represents. It also helps us to know that how various mobile element types interact with each other, since it is largely the synergistic amalgamation of their differing properties that underpins the adaptive capacity of these bacteria. Although there aresome notable differences between the elements important in Gram-negative andGram-positive bacteria, such as the significant roles of integrons/gene cassettes in theformer and of small RC plasmids in the latter, there are many more similarities. Transposable and integrative elements mediate the insertion of resistance genes into chromosomes and plasmids, with the latter serving as key vehicles of intercellulartransmission. Nonetheless, recent findings remind us that there is still a lot to learn about MGE.

Improved analysis methods for the annotation and classification of MGE will also be needed to obtain full value from the vast quantities of sequence data that are being generated, but the increasing diversity of sequenced elements means that there arerarely obvious approaches, and effective changes to nomenclature require broad consultation to ensure that these changes are taken up. Likewise, continued research into the basic biology of mobile elements will be needed for meaningful understanding of the properties of known and yet-to-be-discovered elements. Finally, it needs to berecognized that the current knowledge is based largely on analysis of clinical strains, representing a very limited snapshot of relevant bacterial ecology. It is becoming increasingly feasible to investigate intra- and interspecies linkages between organisms within health care settings, and to other niches in the broader environment, which should provide a more comprehensive understanding of the ecological pathways that ultimately lead to resistance in bacterial pathogens.

References

Antipov, D., Hartwick, N., Shen, M., Raiko, M., Lapidus, A. and Pevzner, P.A. (2016). plasmidSPAdes: assembling plasmids from whole genome sequencing data. Bioinformatics, 32(22):3380-3387, doi: 10.1093/bioinformatics/btw493

Burrus, V., Pavlovic, G., Decaris, B. and Guedon, G.(2002). Conjugative transposons: the tip of the iceberg. Molecular Microbiology, 46(3):601-10, doi: 10.1046/j.1365-2958.2002.03191.x.

Carraro, N. and Burrus, V. (2015).The dualistic nature of integrative and conjugative elements. Mobile Genetic Elements, 5(6):98-102, doi: 10.1080/2159256X.2015.1102796

Clark,R., Anderson, N.B., Clark, V.R. and Williams, D.R.(1999). Racism as a stressor for African Americans. A biopsychosocial model. American Psychologist, 54(10):805-16. doi: 10.1037//0003-066x.54.10.805.

Delavat, F., Miyazaki, R., Carraro, N., Pradervand, N. and Meer, J.R.V.D.(2017). The hidden life of integrative and conjugative elements. FEMS Microbiology Reviews, 41(4):512-537, doi: 10.1093/femsre/fux008

Delihas, N.(2011). Impact of small repeat sequences on bacterial genome evolution. Genome Biology and Evolution, 3:959-73, doi: 10.1093/gbe/evr077

Escudero, J.A., Loot, C., Nivina, A. and Mazel, D.(2015). The Integron: Adaptation On Demand. Microbiology Spectrum, 3(2):MDNA3-0019-2014

Hallet, B. and Sherratt, D.J. (1997). Transposition and site-specific recombination: adapting DNA cut-and-paste mechanisms to a variety of genetic rearrangements. FEMS Microbiology Reviews, 21(2):157-78

Hickman, A.B. and Dyda, F. (2015). Mechanisms of DNA Transposition. Microbiology Spectrum,3(2):MDNA3-0034-2014

Ito, T., Ma, X.X., Takeuchi, F., Okuma, K., Yuzawa, H. and Hiramatsu K. (2004). Novel type V staphylococcal cassette chromosome mec driven by a novel cassette chromosome recombinase, ccrC. Antimicrobial Agents Chemotherapy, 48: 2637–2651.

Lacroix, B. and Citovsky, V. (2016). Transfer of DNA from Bacteria to Eukaryotes. mBio, 7(4):e00863-16, doi: 10.1128/mBio.00863-16

Lanza,V.F., Baquero, F., Martínez, J.L., Ramos-Ruiz, R., González-Zorn, B., Andremont, A., Valenzuela, A.S., Ehrlich, S.D., Kennedy, S., Ruppe, E., Schaik, W.V., Willems, R.J., Cruz, F.D.L. and Coque, T.M.(2014). In-depth resistome analysis by targeted metagenomics. Microbiome, 6:11 doi:10.1186/s40168-017-0387-y

Llaca-Díaz, J.M., Soraya, M.O., Camacho-Ortiz, A.,,Flores, S. and Garza-González, E., (2013). One-Year Surveillance of ESKAPE Pathogens in an Intensive Care Unit of Monterrey, Mexico. Chemotherapy, 58(6):475-481

Moura A., Soares M., Pereira C., Leitao N., Henriques I., Correia A. (2009). INTEGRALL: a database and search engine for integrons, integrases and gene cassettes. Bioinformatics, 25:1096–1098. 10.1093/bioinformatics/btp105.

Nandi, S., Maurer, J.J., Hofacre, C. and Summers, A.O. (2004). Gram-positive bacteria are a major reservoir of Class 1 antibiotic resistance integrons in poultry litter. Proceedings of the National Academy of Sciences of the United States of America, 101(18):7118-22, doi:10.1073/pnas.0306466101

Nesvera, J.,Hochmannová, J. and Pátek, M.(1998.). An integron of class 1 is present on the plasmid pCG4 from Gram-positive bacterium Corynebacterium glutamicum. FEMS Microbiology Letters, 169(2): 391–395, https://doi.org/10.1111/j.1574-6968.1998.tb13345.x

Novick, R.P., and Ram, G. (2016). The Floating (Pathogenicity) Island: A Genomic Dessert. Trends in Genetics, 32 (2), 114–126. doi:10.1016/j.tig.2015.11.005

Novick, R. P., Christie, G. E., and Penades, J. R. (2010). The phage-related chromosomal islands of gram-positive bacteria. Nature Reviews Microbiology, 8:541–551. doi: 10.1038/nrmicro2393

Orlek, A., Phan,H., Sheppard, A.E., Doumith, M., Ellington, M., Peto, T., Crook, D., Walker, A.S., Woodford, N., Anjum, M.F. and Stoesser, N. (2017) A curated dataset of complete Enterobacteriaceae plasmids compiled from the NCBI nucleotide database. Data in Brief ,12: 423-426.

O'Neill, A. J., Larsen, A.R., Skov, R., Henriksen, A.S. and Chopra, I. (2007). Characterization of the Epidemic European Fusidic Acid-Resistant Impetigo Clone of Staphylococcus aureus. Journal of Clinical Microbiology, 45(5): 15-30. doi: https://doi.org/10.1128/jcm.01984-06

Partridge, S.R., Tsafnat, G., Coiera, E. and Iredell, J.R.(2009.). Gene cassettes and cassette arrays in mobile resistance integrons. FEMS Microbiology Reviews, 33(4):757-84. doi: 10.1111/j.1574-6976.2009.00175.x.

Rice, L.B. (2008). Federal funding for the study of antimicrobial resistance in nosocomial pathogens: no ESKAPE. Journal of Infectious Diseases, 197(8):1079-81

Roberts, A.P., Chandler, M. and Couvalin, P. (2008). Revised nomenclature for transposable genetic elements. Plasmid, 60: 167-173

Shintani, M., Sanchez, Z.K. and Kimbara, K. (2015). Genomics of microbial plasmids: classification and identification based on replication and transfer systems and host taxonomy. Frontiers in Microbiology, 6:242, doi: 10.3389/fmicb.2015.00242

Siguier,P., Perochon, J., Lestrade, L., Mahillon, J. and Chandler, M. (2006.). ISfinder: the reference centre for bacterial insertion sequences. Nucleic Acid Research, 34:D32-6, doi: 10.1093/nar/gkj014.

Thomas C. M. (2000). Paradigms of plasmid organization. Molecular Microbiology, 37:485–491 10.1046/j.1365-2958.2000.02006.x

Tsafnat, G., Copty, J. and Partridge, S. R. (2011). RAC: Repository of Antibiotic resistance Cassettes. Database, bar054, https://doi.org/10.1093/database/bar054

12

Resistomes-Informed Combating of Antibiotic Resistance in the Frame of One Health

Ajit Singh

Scientist Emeritus, Department of Veterinary Microbiology, LUVAS Hisar, Haryana, India

Abstract

A strategic joint initiative has been taken to combat the current pandemic of antibiotic resistance (AR). It includes interventions in the holistic 'One Health' framework, which takes into account the interconnected human-animal-plant-environment health. AR is an ancient biological phenomenon of the bacterial world. It is determined by ubiquitous, evolving, and a diverse array of AR genes (ARGs). AR emerges due to intricate mechanisms involving intrinsic and mobile genetic elements-encoded factors and restrictive growth conditions. Anthropogenic activities and climate change events are fueling the pace of emergence and spread of AR pathogens over the past 80 years or so. Functional and sequence-based metagenomics, in combination with computational biology and bioinformatics tools, have led to identification, annotation, and cataloguing of the entire sets of ARGs, called the 'antibiotic resistomes', of bacterial communities in diverse environments. These studies have clearly established that ARGs have bidirectional flow capabilities to interconnect ecosystems in the micro-biosphere. They are exchanged among pathogens, commensals, and environmental bacteria in diverse habitats. The contaminated habitats are the 'hotspots' of ARG exchange. Only a few studies have been conducted on the antibiotic resistomes of different habitats in India. Overall, resistomes provide more valuable information than the current practices for AR surveillance. They help in spotting the hotspots of ARG emergence and exchange, identification of critical control points, evaluation of the waste treatment methods, and the antibiotic stewardship in hospitals. In addition, resistomes can improve the diagnostics for AR pathogens and serve as screens in the discovery of new antimicrobials. This text provides an overview of the next-generation approaches to sourcing information about AR phenomenon in diverse habitats. It also highlights the implications of this information for combating AR in the frame of One Health.

Keywords: *Antibiotic resistomes; next generation methodologies; One Health; combating antibiotics resistance*

Introduction

Resistance to antibiotics in the bacterial world is a genetically determined phenomenon that was first observed within a few years after the introduction of antibiotics for therapeutic purposes. In Nature, ARGs are believed to have originated about three billion years ago as an intrinsic defense mechanism in antibiotic-producing bacteria (Perry *et al.*, 2016; Iskandar *et al.*, 2022), and subsequently, evolved by complex and quantum jump trajectories to mobilize, diversify and interconnect all ecosystems in the micro-biosphere. Bacterial genomes exhibit plasticity and continue to evolve under the selection pressure of antibiotics and other stressors (Patel, 2016). The ARGs in circulation at present are thus a mixture of ancient and modern counterparts. Recently, the interplay between bacterial metabolism and antibiotic resistance has also been revealed (Zampieri, 2021).

The use of antimicrobials in health management, livestock, and food industry is driving the emergence of resistant microbes at a rapid pace (Wall *et al.*, 2016; Adegoke *et al.*, 2016; Hu *et al.*, 2017). As a result, AR pathogens have spread globally to cause loss of lives, production, productivity, and negatively impact economic growth. Recently, AR pathogens in a large study have been found directly responsible for millions of deaths, and the figures are likely to increase in the coming decades (Murray *et al.*, 2022). The pace of the emergence of AR can however be slowed down by improving human interventions. The global and local AR combat plans implemented during the past few years have enhanced the mass awareness of the pandemic problem (WHO, 2015; FAO, 2016; NAP, GOI, 2017; WHO, 2022; WOAH, 2022). These Action Plans on AR containment encourage avoiding of indiscriminate use of antibiotics for the treatment of sick humans and animals, recommend the ban on the use of antibiotics as growth promoters in food animals, promote AR surveillance and monitoring, and support the 'One-Health' strategy and application of the biosecurity principles for containment of the resistant microbes.

AR or susceptibility is traditionally tested in axenic cultures, with the aim of either selecting the most appropriate antibiotic for clinical use or profiling the AR of pathogenic bacteria (Clinical and Laboratory Standards Institute, 2006). In addition, standard methods in microbial genetics available for decades have been used for the discovery of the ARGs. However, these methods are inadequate for AR profiling of the non-cultivable bacteria from different niches. These limitations were overcome when the tools that enabled the study of metagenomes of entire bacterial communities in an ecosystem became available. Demonstration of AR in the commensals in the human and animal guts, and other niches, and their exchange with the pathogens stimulated further investigations on the metagenomes of various habitats (Schmieder & Edwards, 2012; Forsberg *et al.*, 2012).

Whole genome sequencing (WGS) could accurately identify AR genes in the metagenomic libraries, with subsequent functional/phenotypic validation by the functional metagenomics, and the annotation by bioinformatics tools and computational analysis (Schmieder & Edwards, 2012; Mullany, 2014; Beatson & Walker, 2014; Gibson *et al.* 2014; Bengtsson-Palme *et al.* 2017; Crofts *et al.* 2017; Alcock *et al.*, 2020). Whole sets of the ARGs in an ecosystem could then be determined. Although thousands of ARGs have been identified, annotated, and catalogued, the total number of ARGs probably remains unknown. Technologies are being further refined and updated. Antibiotic resistome may be defined as a full complement of the ARGs, including the proto-resistance genes and the cryptic/silent genes' (Canton, 2009; Martínez & Baquero, 2014; Crofts *et al*, 2017; Inda-Díaz *et al.* 2023). These data on the antibiotic resistomes of various ecosystems have been made available in various public databases (Papp and Solymosi, 2022). The antibiotic resistome data are more useful than the clinically- relevant- but- limited AR data for devising strategies to combat AR.

Natural habitats of the microbial communities and the associated antibiotic resistome have increasingly been affected by anthropogenic activities, including modern agricultural practices, livestock agriculture, industrial operations, transportation, etc. (Zhu Y-G. *et al.*, 2017; Czatzkowska *et al.*, 2022). Humans and animals are the hosts to microbiomes of commensals and the associated antibiotic resistomes in the oral cavity, gut, respiratory tract, urogenital system, skin, etc., and shed these via excretion into wastewater and sewage treatment systems, farmlands, water-bodies, environment, etc. Bacterial pathogens of humans and animals, about 60% of which are zoonotic, and 75% are the causal agents of emerging and re-emerging infectious diseases, closely interact with the microbiomes of commensals, opportunists and saprophytes in various habitats, where they exchange ARGs by HGT (Martínez, 2008; Walsh, 2013; Nesme *et al.*, 2014; Pal *et al.*, 2016; Parnanen *et al.* 2016).

Environmental resistome is a vast resource of the ARGs with the potential to be mobilized into a relatively limited number of pathogens (Canton, 2009; Parnanen *et al.*, 2016; Bengtsson-Palme *et al.*, 2017). No habitat can escape from the exchange of the ARGs and the hotspots of HGT exist in the terrestrial and aquatic environments. Multiple clinical and ecological factors contribute to multiple routes of dissemination of the ARGs and the AR bacteria, ultimately entering humans and animals to be shed again into the environment (Nesme *et al.*, 2014; Parnanen *et al.*, 2016).

The use and abuse of antibiotics in agriculture, animals, humans, and food industry heighten the selective pressure for the emergence of the AR bacteria (Walsh, 2013; Nesme *et al.*, 2014; Wall *et al.*, 2016; Adegoke *et al.*, 2016; Thanner *et al.*, 2016; Singh, 2017; Millan, 2018; Singh, 2020). Often the ARGs are co-located and hence co-selected with genes for resistance to metals and antimicrobials/biocides in the wastewater, sewage, sludge, hospital biomedical waste, and industrial effluents in rivers (Amarasekara *et al.*, 2023). These environments are thus a serious threat to allow emergence and spread of AR pathogens, more particularly in developing countries, which have suboptimal waste treatment methods. Resistance develops against all classes of antibiotics. The plasmid-mediated ARGs emerge and disseminate quicker than the chromosomally-located ones. Moreover, concentrations below the minimum inhibitory concentration (MIC) of antibiotics in polluted and chemically complex environments can create selective pressure for the ARGs to emerge in bacteria (Canton, 2009; Nesme *et al.*, 2014; Khan *et al.*, 2017; Karkman *et al.*, 2018; Manaia *et al.*, 2018).

One Health concept recognizes the interconnection and interdependence of the health of humans, animals, and the ecosystems/environment, and provides a frame to achieve optimal health outcomes by a collaborative, multi-sectoral, and trans-disciplinary approach (Evans & Leighton, 2014; Lebov *et al.*, 2017; Xie *et al.*, 2017; Destoumieux-Garzon *et al.*, 2018; Kim & Cha, 2021). Humans and animals are closely connected by zoonosis and the food supply chain. The inclining trend of the animal protein demand-driven shift towards larger and more complex animal production operations has witnessed a correspondingly increased use of antibiotics and antimicrobials. Therefore, targeting the zoonotic diseases caused by the AR bacterial pathogens in animals and the animal production systems could be an effective strategy for improving both human and animal health (Wall *et al.*, 2016; Hu *et al.*, 2017; Adegoke *et al.*, 2016; Singh, 2017).

Early detection of the AR bacteria in environments and animals is important interventions in the One Health framework. Studies on the composition, abundance and diversity of the antibiotic resistomes in environments and clinical settings would lead to identification of the critical control points (CCPs) in the wastewater treatment plants, sewage treatment, biomedical waste management, animal husbandry, and agricultural practices, the food supply chain, pharmaceutical industry effluent management, etc. (Walsh, 2013; Nesme *et al.*, 2014; Vaz-Moreira *et al.* 2014; Pal *et al.*, 2016; Parnanen *et al.*, 2016; Adegoke *et al.*, 2016; Bengtsson-Palme *et al.*, 2017; Ma *et al.*, 2017; Manaia *et al.*, 2018; De, 2019; Li *et al.*, 2022; Kang *et al.*, 2022; Kim & Cha, 2021; Munk *et al.*, 2022; Yin *et al.*, 2022). A full understanding of the resistance mechanisms and the HGT genetic landscape would also allow early identification of the resistance mechanisms to new antibiotics (Hobson *et al.*, 2021).

The Paradigm of Antibiotic Resistomes

The study of ARGs has progressed from the resistance patterns of the isolated pathogens in the axenic cultures during the Golden era of antibiotics to the entire sets of ARGs, called the antibiotic resistomes, in the metagenomic libraries of bacterial communities. The 'resistomes' include all types of ARGs, including the proto-resistance genes and the cryptic or silent resistance genes (Crofts *et al.*, 2017). The present information has been compiled from a collection of hundreds of 'google-searched' high-impact articles.

Tools and Technologies for Studying Antibiotic Resistomes

Traditionally, research on antibiotics and AR has been conducted with aim of treating the infectious diseases of humans and animals in the clinical setting. AR is a genetically encoded selectable phenotype that can be determined by the bacterial growth inhibition assays (broth cultures or disc-diffusion in agar) (Clinical and Laboratory Standards Institute, 2006) or the gene detection techniques such as quantitative PCR (qPCR) or microarrays (Beatson & Walker, 2014; Parnanen *et al.*, 2016). However, the methods for the bacterial axenic cultures are not useful for the non-cultivable bacteria. The minimum inhibitory concentration (MIC) of an antibiotic can be calcu¬lated for each bacterial isolate in a dilution-based assay and the bacterial isolate is scored as susceptible, intermediate, or resistant to that antibiotic. Diag¬nostic laboratories usually analyze the AR phenotypes in clinically important bacteria using standard methods (Clinical and Laboratory Standards Institute, 2006). While the culture-based approaches take 2-3 days to several weeks, the molecular techniques provide results within one day. However, the molecular techniques detect only well-characterized resistance genes.

Standard microbial HGT mechanisms, namely, conjugation, transformation, and transduction have been used for decades of AR research. Demonstration of AR in the commensals in human and animal guts, and its exchange with the pathogens by the HGT mechanisms pointed towards the need for further investigations on its emergence and dissemination in the microbial communities of other natural habitats. The above traditional techniques were inadequate for that purpose. Metagenomics proved to be a powerful tool to detect the composition of any microbial community as well as the abundance and diversity of the ARGs in that community. Presently, two different approaches, viz., the functional metagenomics and the sequence-based metagenomics are employed for antibiotic resistome studies (Schmieder & Edwards, 2012; Mullany, 2014; Bengtsson-Palme *et al.*, 2017; Crofts *et al.*, 2017).

Functional metagenomics involves cloning and expression of the environmental genomic DNA fragments in a heterologous host (often an *E. coli* strain) to construct a metagenomic library, which is then screened against different antibiotics to discover the functions of the genes. This approach has revealed novel AR proteins of previously unknown functions and those not detectable by the sequence alone. Different categories of the ARGs, such as the genes encoding the antibiotics-inactivating proteins, multidrug efflux pumps, and resistance to the folate antagonist have been identified by this approach. Since its first description of the uncultured soil metagenome in 2000 AD, functional metagenomics has led to the discovery of the mcr1 plasmid-mediated colistin resistance determinant in a Chinese pig farm, the *tet* in a human oral microbiome, and 10 novel β-lactamases in the human gut microbiomes (Schmieder & Edwards, 2012; Hu *et al.*, 2017). However, functional metagenomic expression library screening too has limitations: the clone and insert size, differing AR mechanisms, expression and regulatory constraints in the heterologous hosts, false positives, and difficulties in controlling and simulating the conditions for comparison between environments.

On the other hand, sequence-based metagenomics involves extracting and random sequencing of DNA directly from the environmental communities of the cultivable and the non-cultivable bacteria. Typically, the total DNA is extracted from the bacterial community, a random sample is sequenced, and the sequences are then compared to the known (or reference) sequences available in the databanks. This identifies the ARGs, including mutations. Most sequence-based metagenomics studies are performed using the Illumina or Roche/454 pyrosequencing systems. The resistomes can be predicted from the metagenome using reference genes in the databanks. Several thousand different metagenomes have been sequenced from a wide variety of terrestrial and the aquatic environments.

The sequence-based metagenomics too has limitations (Bengtsson-Palme *et al.*, 2017), such as the problems of technical complexity, robustness, accuracy, requirement of the reference genes, cost, etc. The large data volumes require both expertise in bioinformatics and a more advanced informatics infrastructure. The sequence-based identification of an ARG also requires functional confirmation. However, fast refinements in these technologies will bring down the costs and improve the accuracy of prediction about the sources, evolution, and effects of ARGs. Inverse PCR and the long-read sequencing were useful for studying the mobility potential of environmental ARGs, with a potential for developing the AR early warning systems (Parnanen *et al.*, 2016). Metagenomics-based approach can be useful in identifying reservoir resistome signatures for source-attribution of antimicrobial resistance determinants (Duarte, *et al.*, 2021). The resistomes of single clones, culture isolates (Haan & Drown, 2021; Li *et al*, 2022), and multi-species mixed cultures from an ecosystem sample (i.e., culturomics) (Muziasari *et al.*, 2016; Nowrotek *et al.*, 2019) have been studied with various objectives. Alternatively, meta-transcriptomics has the potential to become the main method for detection of the functional resistance genes (Chen *et al.*, 2020). The limitations of these methodologies are being addressed with new and innovative technologies (Apjok G, 2023). Raman spectroscopy-based culture-independent ARG detection in bacterial ecosystems has also been reported (Munck *et al.*, 2015; Rebrosova *et al.*, 2022).

Various ARG databases containing species-specific or pan-species data, and intrinsic and extrinsic resistomes have been created, besides bioinformatics and computational tools, including AI and machine learning algorithms (Gupta *et al*, 2020; Duarte *et al*, 2021; Ma *et al*, 2021; Popa *et al*, 2022; Papp *et al*, 2022). For instance, the Comprehensive Antibiotic Research Database (CARD) has been created to identify putative ARGs in new unannotated genome sequences (Alcock *et al.*, 2020). Resfams is a new curated database of protein families organized by ontology and the associated highly precise and accurate profile hidden Markov models for the AR function (Gibson *et al.*, 2014). The tools for studying the phylogenetic structure and resistomes of the microbial communities have been employed to determine the synteny of the ARGs with the mobile genetic elements (MGEs) (Schmieder & Edwards, 2012). The metadata associated with a given ARG is being generated for modeling the risk of their transmission to the pathogens. WGS-based methods, e.g., the 'Mykrobe' predictor and machine learning approach are being developed and validated for susceptibility/resistance profiling of the bacterial pathogens (Schmieder & Edwards, 2012).

In short, whole sets of the ARGs i.e., the resistomes of any ecosystem can now be determined by employing the above-mentioned next-generation technologies. Although thousands of ARGs have been cataloged, the total number is yet to be determined. Tools and technologies are being further refined and updated. Various potential applications of antibiotic resistomes for AR mitigation are envisaged (Crofts *et al*, 2017; Hu *et al*, 2017; Duarte *et al*, 2021; Ma *et al*, 2021; Kim and Cha, 2021; Iskandar *et al*, 2022).

Antibiotic Resistomes in Various Environments

Thousands of different metagenomes have been sequenced from a wide variety of terrestrial and aquatic environments (Pal *et al*, 2016; Ma *et al*, 2017; Chen *et al*, 2019; Skarzynska *et al*, 2020; Cao *et al*, 2020; Zainab *et al*, 2020; Han *et al*, 2020; Wang *et al*, 2020; Ma *et al*, 2021; Lawther *et al*, 2022; Lee and Yoo, 2022; Li *et al*, 2022; Munk *et al*, 2022; Rhouma *et al*, 2022; Amarasekara, 2023). Bacteria are ubiquitous, generally living in communities of multiple species and inhabiting diverse terrestrial and aquatic environments, including human and animal body niches. ARGs most probably originated in the antibiotic producers as a mechanism of self-defense and were later acquired by the co-inhabitants to defend against the hostile environment, which further evolved and disseminated globally through water, soil, aerosols, migratory animals, etc. It has been recently proposed that the resistance gene flow in nature is 'from the natural environments' (source) 'to the natural environments' (sink) via humans, animals, and plants, as intermediate recipients and disseminators (Hu *et al*., 2017).

Soil microbes have the most diverse pool of ARGs, some of which can be exchanged with the clinical pathogens as suggested by a high level of sequence similarity. For example, the resistance cassettes against five classes of antibiotics (β-lactams, aminoglycosides, amphenicols, sulfonamides, and tetracyclines) in the multidrug-resistant soil bacteria have been found to possess the sequence identity to those from diverse human pathogens (Martínez, 2008; Forsberg *et al*., 2012; Schmieder & Edwards, 2012; Thanner *et al*., 2016). Efflux pumps and genes conferring resistance to vancomycin, tetracycline, or β-lactams used in animal and human healthcare are most commonly found in soil (Canton, 2009; Pal *et al*., 2016). In addition, the ARGs, including the *qnr* and the *blaCTX* genes in bacteria that are phylogenetically related to the non-antibiotic-producing bacteria have also been recently detected (Canton, 2009). The Alaskan soil bacteria with no known exposure to commercial antibiotics carry ARGs to β lactams. ARGs in the soil metagenomes, which have low levels of sequence similarity with those from pathogens, suggest their different roles in natural environments (Schmieder & Edwards, 2012).

Water is among the most important bacterial habitats on the Earth, representing a major way of dissemination of bacteria between different environmental compartments. AR bacteria can be exchanged among the waste, surface, and drinking water sectors of the urban water cycle, and other environments (e.g., soil) and eventually reach humans (Vaz-Moreira *et al.*, 2014). AR bacteria are found widely in aquatic environments, both pristine and those contaminated with antibiotics from agriculture, aquaculture farming, or wastewater treatment plants (Haan & Drown, 2021). Some of the ARGs found in the clinical human pathogens have also been found in bacteria of pristine ecosystems (Vaz-Moreira *et al.*, 2014; Miner *et al.*, 2021). The resistome associated with the fish farms represents the native aquatic ARGs enriched by antibiotic use at the farms (Vaz-Moreira *et al.*, 2014). However, despite an abundance of their functional ARGs in wastewater treatment plants, only a few ARGs are probably transferred to human pathogens (Muziasari *et al.*, 2016). The sludge products of urban and rural wastewater treatment plants are increasingly used as fertilizers for crops, dispersing unknown amounts of ARGs and antibiotics that withstand the standard sewage treatment. The metagenomics approach for the activated sludge identified two novel bleomycin resistance genes (Munck *et al.*, 2015; Su *et al.*, 2017; Manaia *et al.*, 2018). High levels of the ARGs found in bacteria in the river sediments downstream from a wastewater treatment plant warrant further studies (Xiong *et al.*, 2022).

Antibiotics, disinfectants, and metals, even in low concentrations in the wastewater create a selection pressure for the AR (Karkman *et al.*, 2018). The wastewater treatment plants essentially use the microbiological bioremediation to clean up water. The subinhibitory concentrations of antibiotics induce quorum sensing and biofilm formation that allow exchange of the genetic material and acquisition of the AR in aquatic and terrestrial habitats (Martínez, 2008; Larsson, 2014). The deep metagenomic sequencing revealed a stably maintained core set of novel ARGs that conferred resistance to all the antibiotics tested. This unique wastewater resistome has little scope for transfer into the human gut microbiota (Ash, 2015).

A large-scale survey of the ARGs and the bacterial communities from eleven Chinese wastewater treatment plants showed that the treatment process could significantly reduce the abundance and diversity of ARGs, but those conferring resistance to β-lactams and aminoglycosides and three MGEs persisted even after the treatment. Resistomes varied with the wastewater treatment processes, seasons, and regions. The footprint of ARGs during the wastewater treatment process could be tracked and the resistome data can be used for improving the ARG mitigation in the wastewater treatment plants (An *et al.*, 2018).

Spatiotemporal distribution of ARGs and the bacterial communities in the Chinese urban sewage revealed 381 different ARGs across China; seasonal variation in the abundance of ARGs, without geographical clustering was observed. The core resistome accounted for >50% of the total ARGs. This approach provided a baseline for investigating the environmental dissemination of resistance elements and the possibility of using the abundance of ARGs in the sewage as a tool for antibiotic stewardship (Munck *et al.*, 2015). The waste disposal in the peri-urban areas can spread AR from the waste to the soil bacteria. Diverse and abundant ARGs were detected in the peri-urban soils (Xiang *et al.*, 2018).

The incidence of ARGs in drinking water causes potential risks to human health, hence a matter of public concern (Han *et al.*, 2020). A catalog of the antibiotic resistome in the drinking water was established, and the host-tracking of ARGs was conducted in a multinational survey using the metagenomic approach. Sixteen ARG types having 181 subtypes were observed; bacitracin, aminoglycoside, sulfonamide, and β-lactam resistance genes were dominant and hosted by *Acidovorax, Acinetobacter, Aeromonas, Methylobacterium, Methyloversatilis, Mycobacterium, Polaromonasand, Pseudomonas*. This resistome catalog provided a useful reference for future studies on the global surveillance and the risk management of ARGs in drinking water (Ma *et al.*, 2017).

The livestock production effluents, such as wastewater, manure, and dust, increase the density of AR bacteria and ARGs in the environment. The resistome data can be useful for characterizing and quantify the public health risk of livestock effluents (Zhao *et al.*, 2020). AR mechanisms, the majority belonging to the tetracycline resistance in 34 soil, manure, and wastewater samples from the feedlot, the ranch, and the dairy operations were discovered in a study. The soil, manure, and wastewater resistomes differed, and so were dairy operations and the feedlot. In another study, the functional metagenomic of cow dung manure identified 80 different ARGs and a new clade of chloramphenicol acetyltransferases (Wichmann *et al.*, 2014). Antibiotic resistome within the gut of livestock have been reviewed (Ma *et al.*, 2021). The use of antibiotics in agriculture may have resulted in the spread of strains, such as vancomycin-resistant enterococci in both the farm animals exposed to antibiotics and humans in contact with the animals, as well as the maintenance of ARGs in apparently antibiotic-free animals (Schmieder & Edwards, 2012). Human activities can drive the spatial and temporal distribution of the ARGs (Gaze *et al.*, 2013; Xiang *et al.*, 2018). In beef cattle in the United States, environmental pathways of the spread of ARGs may be more risk than the food (meat) supply, because of the food safety system in place (i.e., the treatment of beef at critical control points to kill the pathogens as well as the commensals).

The sequencing, characterization, and analysis of the human microbiomes of the mouth, nasal cavity, skin, gut, and vagina of healthy donors through metagenomics has been undertaken in the Human Microbiome Project (HMP), an initiative of the NIH launched in 2008. Intestinal microbiomes from various populations are also being investigated (Schmieder & Edwards, 2012; Nesme *et al.*, 2014; van Schaik, 2015; Bengtsson-Palme *et al.*, 2017; Crofts, 2017; Munck *et al.*, 2017). Despite the shared core microbiome, the composition of the gut microbiota varies among individuals under the influence of numerous factors. Antibiotics may have long-term consequences on the human microbiota, causing a shift to a different but stable community.

The diverse pool of ARGs in the commensal gut microbiota of healthy individuals could potentially lead to the emergence of new resistant pathogenic strains. Methicillin and fluoroquinolone resistance genes and multidrug efflux pumps were found in the meconium three days after birth, and teicoplanin resis¬tance genes were found on the sixth day in the infant fecal sample. The oral microbiota can also act as a reservoir of the AR microbes, with the opportunity for rapid dissemination. The AR genes resistant to tetracycline and amoxicillin, and a novel tetracycline resistance determinant, tet37, were identified in the metagenomic libraries from the oral microbiota. The human oral and fecal microbiomes differ, both in the composition and the associated resistomes (van Schaik, 2015; Munck *et al.*, 2017).

A clinical resistome has been defined by creating a database of potential ARGs in the 17 most common human bacterial pathogens using >20,000 bacterial genomes. This represented the subset of the environmental resistome that is clinically relevant, and the dataset and the approach provided a baseline for further investigations into the abundance of clinically relevant ARGs across different environments (Munck *et al.*, 2017). In an interesting study, refugees in Germany exhibited ≥5 ARGs, while German residents ≤3 ARGs, irrespective of potential pathogens (Hasler *et al.*, 2018). Climate change, with Monsoon floods, is affecting the spread of ARGs. High rates of AR exist in humans, animals, and environments in India (Laxminarayan & Chaudhury, 2016; Gaur, 2017; Singh *et al.*, 2018).

The gut microbiome of hospitalized patients is one of the most important niches for the exchange of AR genes in hospitals. The conjugative plasmids, especially in the *Enterobacteriaceae* and *Enterococcaceae* pathogens, play a key role in the dissemination of ARGs in the gut of patients (van Schaik, 2015; Millan, 2018). In 252 fecal metagenomes from three countries, the most abundant AR determinants were those for the antibiotics also used in animals and for the antibiotics that have been used for a long (Forslund *et al.*, 2013).

Plastisphere is another example of a global man-made ecosystem investigated to have microbial colonization with antibiotic resistomes (Yang *et al*., 2020). Antibiotic resistomes in bioaerosols may also pose a risk (Lee & Yoo, 2022). Resistomes in microbiomes of the migratory birds are another threat to long-distance migration of ARGs (Cao *et al*., 2020).

Combating of AR in the One Health Frame

The ubiquitous bacteria and the vast number of ARGs cannot be wiped out from the Earth, but the ARG hotspots can certainly be identified, targeted for treatment, and monitored for changes following treatment. Traditional methods of ARG identification and monitoring are far from adequate for the purpose. Metagenomics-based approaches provide information about the diversity, abundance, evolution, and flow of ARGs or resistomes in communities of cultivable and non-cultivable bacteria in various habitats. Strategies to combat AR will require resistome-informed changes to AR surveillance, the stewardship practices, and the antibiotic development pipeline (Petchiappan & Chatterji, 2017).

The current practices to combat AR include the personal and general hygiene, and treatment of the wastewater for irrigation, sludge as organic fertilizer, and other environments. The hygiene practices and bio-remediation of the wastewater and industrial waste disposal add antibiotics, biocides, and toxic metals to the environment, and promote the emergence and exchange of AR in the bacterial communities. The problem of AR bacteria persists where suboptimal treatment methods are practiced. Therefore, the wastewater and the industrial effluent treatment plants need to be re-modeled with modern bio- and chemo-remediation technologies, including membrane filtration, activated carbon, photo-driven nanotechnologies, and ozonation to remove the AR microbes, associated ARGs, residual antibiotics, biocides, and toxic metals (Schmieder & Edwards, 2012; Nolvak *et al*., 2018).

Each wastewater treatment plant is a unique system that would probably need a specific procedure to maximize the removal of the AR bacteria and the ARGs (Manaia *et al*., 2018). The resistome ecology should serve as a guide for the wastewater professionals involved in optimizing wastewater treatment for the removal of AR bacteria and ARGs. The metagenomics-based approach provides better evidence of the effectiveness of the treatment methods for its ability to indicate both the diversity of the bacterial strains and resistomes before and after treatment. In addition, the abundance of ARGs in the sewage system should be incorporated as a tool to monitor antibiotic stewardship. The Metagenomics approach can also improve the risk assessments for AR within agriculture and through the food chain to animals and humans (Schmieder & Edwards, 2012; Thanner *et al.*, 2016; Crofts *et al.*, 2017; Kim & Cha, 2021).

The next-generation technologies need to be employed for surveillance of the potential hotspots of HGT. The environmental resistomes of diverse functional metagenome libraries can also serve as screens for new antibiotic pipeline, assess AR potential of the new/improved antibiotic, and explore alternative strategies for combating the AR, such as inverting the selective advantage of AR, use of the AR enzyme-inhibitors as antibiotic adjuvants (e.g., loperamide to facilitate tetracycline uptake and ticlopidine to inhibit teichoic acid biosynthesis) (Schmieder & Edwards, 2012; Crofts *et al.*, 2017).

Importance of the metagenomics-based ARG surveillance is highlighted in several examples. For instance, early detection of the emergence of the mcr1 gene as a transmissible threat to colistin in Chinese pig farms was made possible by the metagenomics-based AR surveillance program. In other studies, the tet in a human oral microbiome, and 10 novel β-lactamases in the human gut microbiomes were discovered. The resistome-informed innovative methods of wastewater treatment and risk estimation are being developed. The municipal wastewater treatment in the photobioreactors led to the reduced antibiotic resistome proportion, number of the ARG subtypes, and the abundance of individual ARGs in the bacterial community (Nolvak *et al.*, 2018). In another study, epic PCR identified the host distribution of four resistance-associated genes (*tetM*, *int1*, *qacE1*, and *blaOXA*-58) in the influent and the effluent. The bacterial hosts of these ARGs decreased in the wastewater treatment plant effluent. Exhaustive profiling of the ARG bacterial communities in the wastewater treatment plant provided an improved level of precision to the ARG risk estimates (Hultman *et al.*, 2018).

Continued development and updating of technologies for the next-generation surveillance of ARGs is required, e.g., improved computational and bioinformatics tools to create the databases. WGS-based methods can enhance the speed and accuracy of diagnostics. The 'Mykrobe' predictor has been developed to identify the susceptibility profiles for 12 antibiotics from the raw unassembled Illumina platform NGS data of *Staphylococcus aureus* and *Mycobacterium tuberculosis*. A machine learning approach is being developed to accurately predict resistance profiles of multidrug-resistant isolates of *Enterobacteriaceae*. The faster and more accurate diagnostics will decrease the number of empirical and unsuitable antibiotic prescriptions. Discovery of newer antimicrobials can also be guided by antibiotic resistomes (Hobson *et al.*, 2021).

Conclusions and Future Perspectives

AR is a global public health threat and the strategic fight to mitigate it has been jointly initiated by WHO, FAO, and nations worldwide. India has devised the National Action Plan, 2017-2021. The next generation tools and technologies are being developed to improve the strategy to combat AR threats. The entire sets of ARGs, called the resistomes of microbial communities in the terrestrial and the aquatic ecosystems, including clinical settings, and human and animal bodies can now be determined by the next generation technologies and tools. The current 'resistome paradigm' will impact the strategies for combating AR pathogens in the frame of the One Health concept. The resistome will provide more valuable information for AR surveillance and risk analysis, assessment of the hotspots of ARG emergence and exchange, the identification of critical control points in an early warning system, the effectiveness of waste treatment methods, and the stewardship practices in hospitals. Moreover, resistomes would provide screens for the discovery of new antimicrobials and alternative options. The resistomes of different environments in India also need to be studied for above purposes.

References

Adegoke AA. et al. (2016). Antibiotic resistant superbugs: assessment of the interrelationship of occurrence in clinical settings and environmental niches. Molecules. 22:29.

Alcock BP et al. (2020). CARD 2020: antibiotic resistome surveillance with the comprehensive antibiotic resistance database. Nucleic Acids Res. 48 (Database issue):D517–D525.

Amarasekara NR. et al. (2023). Exploring the co-occurrence of antibiotic, metal, and biocide resistance genes in the urban agricultural environment. J. Agric. Food Res. 11:100474.

An X-L. et al. (2018). Tracking antibiotic resistome during wastewater treatment using high throughput quantitative PCR. Environ. Internatl. 117:146-153.

Anon. (2015). Global Action Plan on Antimicrobial Resistance. Publisher: World Health Organization, Geneva, 2015.

Anon. (2016). The FAO Action Plan on Antimicrobial Resistance 2016-2020. Publisher: Food and Agricultural Organization, Rome, Italy, 2016.

Anon. (2017). National Action Plan for Containment of Antimicrobial Resistance, Ministry of Health & Family Welfare, Government of India, New Delhi, India, 2017.

Apjok G. et al. (2023). Characterization of antibiotic resistomes by reprogrammed bacteriophage-enabled functional metagenomics in clinical strains. Nat Microbiol. 8(3):410-423.

Ash C. (2015). Unique wastewater antibiotic resistome. Science. 350(6263):924-925.

Beatson SA. and Walker MJ. (2014). Tracking antibiotic resistance. Science. 345(6203):1454-1455.

Bengtsson-Palme J. et al. (2017). Using metagenomics to investigate human and environmental resistomes. J. Antimicrob. Chemother. 72(10):2690–2703.

Canton R. (2009). Antibiotic resistance genes from the environment: a perspective through newly identified antibiotic resistance mechanisms in the clinical setting. Clin. Microbiol. Infect. 15(Suppl. 1):20-25.

Cao J. et al. (2020). Metagenomic analysis reveals the microbiome and resistome in migratory birds. Microbiome. 8:26.

Chen QL. et al. (2019). Antibiotic resistomes in plant microbiomes. Trends Plant Sci. 24(6):530-541.

Chen YM. et al. (2020). Diverse and abundant resistome in terrestrial and aquatic vertebrates revealed by transcriptional analysis. Sci. Rep. 10:18870.

Clinical and Laboratory Standards Institute. (2006). Methods for Dilution Antimicrobial Susceptibility Tests for Bacteria that Grow Aerobically: Approved Standard, 7th Edition (CLSI Document M7-A7). Clinical and Laboratory Standards Institute, Wayne, USA, 2006.

Crofts TS. et al. (2017). Next-generation approaches to understand and combat the antibiotic resistome. Nat. Rev. Microbiol. 15(7):422-434.

Czatzkowska M. et al. (2022). Impact of anthropogenic activities on the dissemination of ARGs in the environment-A review. Int. J. Environ. Res. Pub. Hlth.19:12853.

De R. (2019). Metagenomics: aid to combat antimicrobial resistance in diarrhea. Gut Pathog. 11:47.

Destoumieux-Garzon D. et al. (2018). The One Health concept: 10 years old and a long road ahead. Front. Vet. Sci. 5:14.

Duarte ASR. et al. (2021). Metagenomics-based approach to source-attribution of antimicrobial resistance determinants- identification of reservoir resistome signatures. Front. Microbiol. 11:601407.

Evans BR. and Leighton FA. (2014). A history of One Health. Rev. sci. tech. Off. int. Epiz.33(2):413-420.

Forsberg KJ. et al. (2012). The shared antibiotic resistome of soil bacteria and human pathogens. Science. 337 (6098):1107-1111.

Forslund K. et al. (2013). Country-specific antibiotic use practices impact the human gut resistome. Genome Res.23:1163-1169.

Gaur RK. (2017). Antibiotic resistance: Alternative approaches. Indian J. Pharmacol. 49:208-210.

Gaze WH. et al. (2013). Influence of humans on evolution and mobilization of environmental antibiotic resistome. Emerg. Infect. Dis. 19(7); http://dx.doi.org/ 10.3201/eid1907.120871.

Gibson MK. et al. (2014). Improved annotation of antibiotic resistance determinants reveals microbial resistomes cluster by ecology. The ISME J. 2014:1-10.

Gupta CL., Tiwari RK. and Cytryn E. (2020). Platforms for elucidating antibiotic resistance in single genomes and complex metagenomes. Environ. Internatl. 138:105667.

Haan TJ. and Drown DM. (2021). Unearthing antibiotic resistance associated with disturbance-induced permafrost thaw in interior alaska. Microorganisms 9:116-127.

Han Z. et al. (2020). Antibiotic resistomes in drinking water sources across a large geographical scale: multiple drivers and co-occurrence with opportunistic bacterial pathogens. Water Res. 183:116088.

Hasler R. et al. (2018). The antibiotic resistome and microbiota landscape of refugees from Syria, Iraq and Afghanistan in Germany. Microbiome 6:37.

Hobson C., Chan AN. and Wright GD. (2021). The Antibiotic Resistome: a guide for the discovery of natural products as antimicrobial agents. Chem. Rev. 121(6):3464-3494.

Hu Y. et al. (2017). The antibiotic resistome: gene flow in environments, animals and human beings. Front. Med. 11(2):161-168.

Hultman J. et al. (2018). Host range of antibiotic resistance genes in wastewater treatment plant influent and effluent. FEMS Microbiol. Ecol. 94:fiy038.

Inda-Díaz JS. et al. (2023). Latent antibiotic resistance genes are abundant, diverse, and mobile in human, animal, and environmental microbiomes. Microbiome 11:44.

Iskandar K. et al. (2022). Antibiotic discovery and resistance: the chase and the race. Antibiotics 11:182.

Kang J. et al. (2022). Shifts of Antibiotic Resistomes in Soil Following Amendments of Antibiotics-Contained Dairy Manure. Int. J. Environ. Res. Pub. Hlth. 19:10804.

Karkman A. et al. (2018). Antibiotic-resistance genes in waste water. Trends Microbiol. 26(3): P220-228.

Khan S. et al. (2017). The use of minimum selectable concentrations (MSCs) for determining the selection of antimicrobial resistant bacteria. Ecotoxicology. 26:283-292.

Kim DW. and Cha CJ. (2021) Antibiotic resistome from the One-Health perspective: understanding and controlling antimicrobial resistance transmission. Exptl. Mol. Med. 53:301-309.

Larsson DGJ. (2014). Antibiotics in the environment. Upsala J. Med. Sci. 119:108-112.

Lawther K. et al. (2022). Resistome analysis of global livestock and soil microbiomes. Front. Microbiol. 13:897905.

Laxminarayan R. and Chaudhury RR. (2016). Antibiotic resistance in India: Drivers and opportunities for action. PLoS Med. 13(3):e1001974.

Lebov J. et al. (2017). A framework for One Health research. One Health. 3:44-50.

Lee G. and Yoo K. (2022). A review of the emergence of antibiotic resistance in bioaerosols and its monitoring methods. Rev. Environ. Sci. Biotechnol. 21:799-827.

Li S. et al. (2022). Antibiotic resistant bacteria and genes in wastewater treatment plants: From occurrence to treatment strategies. Sci. Total Environ. 838(Pt 4):156544.

Ma L. et al. (2017). Catalogue of antibiotic resistome and host tracking in drinking water deciphered by a large-scale survey. Microbiome. 5:154-165.

Ma T., McAllister TA. and Guan LL. (2021). A review of the resistome within the digestive tract of livestock. J. Anim. Sci. Biotechnol. 12:121.

Manaia CM. et al. (2018). Antibiotic resistance in wastewater treatment plants: Tackling the black box. Environ. Internatl.115:312-324.

Martínez JL. (2008). Antibiotics and antibiotic resistance genes in natural environments. Science. 321:265-268.

Martínez JL. and Baquero F. (2014). Emergence and spread of antibiotic resistance: setting a parameter space. Uppsala J. Med. Sci. 119(2):68-77.

Millan AS. (2018). Evolution of plasmid-mediated antibiotic resistance in the clinical context. Trends Microbiol. 26(12):978-985.

Miner KR. et al. (2021). Emergent biogeochemical risks from Arctic permafrost degradation. Nat. Clim. Chang. 11(10):809-819.

Mullany P. (2014). Functional metagenomics for the investigation of antibiotic resistance. Virulence. 5(3):443-447.

Munck C. et al. (2015). Limited dissemination of the wastewater treatment plant core resistome. Nat. Commun. 6:8452.

Munk P. et al. (2022). Genomic analysis of sewage from 101 countries reveals global landscape of antimicrobial resistance. Nat. Commun. 13:7251.

Murray JCL. et al. (2022). Antimicrobial Resistance Collaborators. (2019). Global burden of bacterial antimicrobial resistance in 2019: a systematic analysis. Corrected version. Lancet 399: 629–655.

Muziasari WI. et al. (2016). Aquaculture changes the profile of antibiotic resistance and mobile genetic element associated genes in Baltic Sea sediments. FEMS Microbiol. Ecol. 92:fiw052.

Nesme J. et al. (2014). Large-scale metagenomic-based study of antibiotic resistance in the environment. Curr. Biol. 24:1096-1100.

Nolvak H. et al. (2018). Reduction of antibiotic resistome and integron-integrase genes in laboratory-scale photobioreactors treating municipal wastewater. Water Res.142:363-372.

Nowrotek M. et al. (2019). Culturomics and metagenomics: In understanding of environmental resistome. Front. Environ. Sci. Eng. 13:40.

Ondon BS. et al. (2021). Sources of antibiotic resistant bacteria (ARB) and antibiotic resistance genes (ARGs) in the soil: A review of the spreading mechanism and human health risks. Rev. Environ. Contam. Toxicol. 256:121-153.

Pal C. et al. (2016). The structure and diversity of human, animal and environmental resistomes. Microbiome. 4:54-68.

Palma E., Tilocca B. and Roncada P. (2020). Antimicrobial resistance in veterinary medicine: An Overview. Int. J. Mol. Sci. 21:1914

Papp M. and Solymosi N. (2022). Review and comparison of antimicrobial resistance gene databases. Antibiotics 11:339.

Parnanen K. et al. (2016). Evaluating the mobility potential of antibiotic resistance genes in environmental resistomes without metagenomics. Sci. Rep.6:35790.

Patel S. (2016). Drivers of bacterial genomes plasticity and roles they play in pathogen virulence, persistence and drug resistance. Infect. Genet. Evol. 45:151-164.

Perry J. et al. (2016). The prehistory of antibiotic resistance. Cold Spring Harb. Perspect. Med.; doi: 10.1101.

Petchiappan A. and Chatterji D. (2017). Antibiotic resistance: Current perspectives. ACS Omega 2:7400−9.

Popa SL. et al. (2022). Deep learning and antibiotic resistance. Antibiotics. 11:1674.

Rebrosova K. et al. (2022). Raman Spectroscopy- A novel method for identification and characterization of microbes on a single-cell level in clinical settings. Front. Cell. Infect. Microbiol. 12:866463.

Schmieder R. and Edwards R. (2012). Insights into antibiotic resistance through metagenomic approaches. Future Microbiol.7(1):73-89.

Singh A. (2017). Invited Lead Lecture for XVII Annual Conference of 'Indian Society of Veterinary Pharmacology and Toxicology' and National Symposium on 'Combating Antimicrobial Resistance', Department of Veterinary Pharmacology and Toxicology, COVS, LUVAS, Hisar-125004 (Haryana), Dec. 20-22, 2017.

Singh A. (2020). Response: How COVID-19 is accelerating the threat of antimicrobial resistance. Brit. Med. J. 369:m1983.

Singh AK. et al. (2018). Prevalence of antibiotic resistance in commensal Escherichia coli among the children in rural hill communities of Northeast India. PLoS ONE. 13(6):e0199179.

Su J-Q. et al. (2017). Metagenomics of urban sewage identifies an extensively shared antibiotic resistome in China. Microbiome 5:84.

Thanner S. et al. (2016). Antimicrobial resistance in agriculture. mBio 7(2):e02227-15.

van Schaik W. (2015). The human gut resistome. Phil. Trans. R. Soc. B. 370:20140087.

Vaz-Moreira I. et al. (2014). Bacterial diversity and antibiotic resistance in water habitats: searching the links with the human microbiome. FEMS Microbiol. Rev. 38:761-18.

Wall BA. et al. (2016). Drivers, dynamics and epidemiology of antimicrobial resistance in animal production. Publisher: Food and Agricultural Organization, Rome, Italy, 2016.

Walsh F. (2013). Investigating antibiotic resistance in non-clinical environments. Front. Microbio.4:19-27.

WHO GLASS. (2022). Global antimicrobial resistance and use surveillance system (GLASS) report 2022. World Health Organization, Geneva.

Wichmann F. et al. (2014). Diverse antibiotic resistance genes in dairy cow manure. mBio 5(2):e01017-13.

WOAH. (2022). Strategy on antimicrobial resistance and the prudent use of antimicrobials: preserving the efficacy of antimicrobials. [www.woah.org/]

Xiang Q. et al. (2018). Spatial and temporal distribution of antibiotic resistomes in a peri-urban area is associated significantly with anthropogenic activities. Environ. Pollutn. 235:525-533.

Xie T. et al. (2017). A system dynamics approach to understanding the One Health concept. PLoS ONE. 12(9):e0184430.

Xiong S. et al. (2022). Geographic patterns and determinants of antibiotic resistomes in coastal sediments across complex ecological gradients. Front. Microbiol. 13:922580.

Yang K. et al. (2020). Temporal dynamics of antibiotic resistome in the plastisphere during microbial colonization. Environ. Sci. Technol. 54(18):11322-11332.

Yin X. et al. (2022). An assessment of resistome and mobilome in wastewater treatment plants through temporal and spatial metagenomic analysis. Water Res. 209:117885.

Zampieri M. (2021). The genetic underground of antibiotic resistance. Science 371(6531):783-784.

Zhao Y. et al. (2020). Antibiotic resistome in the livestock and aquaculture industries: Status and solutions, Crit. Rev. Environ. Sci. Technol. DOI: 10.1080/10643389.2020.1777815

Zhu Y-G. et al. (2017). Microbial mass movements. Science. 357(6356):1099-1100.

13

Computational Biology in the Surveillance of Anti-microbial Resistance (AMR) and Rapid Anti-microbial Drug Discovery

Rasanpreet Kaur[1], Mukta Jain[2], Amit Kumar Singh[3], Parul Yadav[1],Ankush[1], Saurabh Gupta[1], Swaroop Kumar Pandey[1], Jagdip Singh Sohal[4*]

[1]Department of Biotechnology, GLA University, Chaumuhan, Mathura Uttar Pradesh, India
[2]P P Savani University, Surat, Gujarat, India
[3]Amity Institute of Microbial Technology, Amity University Rajasthan Delhi-Jaipur Highway, Jaipur, Rajasthan, India
[4]Centre for Vaccines and Diagnostic Research, GLA University Chaumuhan, Mathura, Uttar Pradesh, India

Abstract

The discovery of penicillin by Alexander Fleming in 1924 was one of the greatest milestones in the infections' treatment and management. It was the foundation of the modern era of antibiotic drugs. Antibiotics such as penicillins, cephalosporins, quinolones, tetracycline, macrolides, sulphonamides, aminoglycosides and glycopeptides are the mainstay in managing severe infections. However, the emergence of resistant strains of bacteria hashindered the progress of research in this field. Recently, new approaches to understand the bacteria resistance to antibiotics are being adopted and these involve conjugation of the molecular understanding of bacteria systems and analysis using the Bioinformatics tools. Consequently, many molecules have been developed to limit resistance associated with different bacterial infections. Since AMR is a highly clinically relevant subject hence, there is strong synergy in silico study and in vivo studies to facilitates the discovery of potent antibiotics. In this paper, we seek to give an overview of the in silico approaches to do the surveillance of AMR as well as review the tools needed to discover new anti-microbial agents.

Keywords: Anti-microbial resistance (AMR), Bioinformatics, Computational Biology, *in silico*, drug resistance

Introduction

Until the 20thcentury, bacterial infections were the number one cause of human death. In the 1940s, antibiotics became the lifelines for treating serious infections that saved millions of lives. Despite the advantages derived from the use of antibiotics, resistance to these drugs emerged. Unfortunately, resistance to most antibiotics emerged in time-course even for the most powerful antibiotics developed.Resistance to antibiotics is a challenge to the scientific community in keeping up the pace of antibiotic discovery.World Economic Forum's Global Risks Reporthas listed antibiotic resistance as one of the greatest threats (WEF, 2020).United Nations (UN) has warned that drug-resistant diseases could account for 10 million deaths each year by 2050. By 2030, antimicrobial resistance (AMR) could likelylead up to 24 million people into extreme poverty(IACG,2019). Currently, at least 7,00,000 people die each year due to drug-resistant diseases (IACG,2019). The emergence and widespread of antibiotic-resistant organisms is a global challenge and needs a multi-dimensional approach to address the fundamental issues to minimize drug-resistance.The Antibiotic Resistance Genes Database (ARDB) contains a repository of around 23,000 antibiotic resistance gene or protein sequences conferring resistance against over 240 antibiotics (ARDB). Computational Biology (Bioinformatics) has become one of the important tools in studying antimicrobial resistance. It employs a range of computation techniques to make predictions about the biological phenomenon.

The rapid progression of antibiotic-resistant have led the scientific community to consider different molecules as new anti-microbial agents. Traditional approaches of drug discovery are tedious, time consuming and labor intensive. In this matter Bioinforamtics tools can help screening large panel of molecules (eg. Phytochemicals) in shorter period of time and lead to short-listing of molecles that can be taken up to *in vivo* and *in vitro* studies. In the present paper, we provide the role of the bioinformatics approaches to anti-microbial drug discoveryand its surveillance.

Bioinformatics Strategies to Limit Antibiotic Resistance

Bioinformatics can provide an important platform formodeling a biological living cell and docking proteins to discover effective drug strategies in combating antibiotic resistance. In recent times, various bioinformatics strategies are being used to combat antibiotic resistance.

Whole-genome Bioinformatics Strategies

In recent times, whole-genome sequencing (WGS) of pathogenic organisms has be comean affordable tool for genotyping. Analysis of the whole genomes could provide insights into different related lineages of organisms and can revolutionize disease outbreak analysis. The information generated by Genome sequencing is particularly important in biomolecular modeling and drug design concerning antibiotics resistance. This can also provide insights into disease transmission, virulence, and antimicrobial resistance.

Structural biology and bioinformatics can lead to target identification by screening various bacterial proteins. Computational Biology is also helpful in proposing binding sites for ligand molecules.

In silico Analysis for Antigenic Profiling

Whole-genome sequencing technologies have helped in developing molecular typing tools that have replaced the traditional labor-intensive serovar analysis Serovars prediction can be done *in silico*by analyzing the surface antigen encoding genes. This can help to identify a specific type of marker that can be used for developing cost-effective molecular assays to detect serovars.

Insilico Plasmid Identification

Plasmids are essential mobile genetic elements for the acquisition and spread of antibiotic resistance. Different types of Bioinformatics tools are readily available for use in plasmid extraction and assembling from high throughput sequencing (HTS) data. These tools could be used to access plasmid sequence to explore the nature of plasmid.Assessment of plasmid characteristics and their association with different hosts will provide an understanding of plasmids' contribution in transmitting antibiotics resistant genes.

Metagenomics and Bioinformatics for Antimicrobial Surveillance

AMR surveillance has focused mainly on a few pathogenic species and that can be treated as the tip of the iceberg. Broader species analysis is needed for a better understanding of AMR. It is very much possible that the majority of AMR genes might be found in the commensal bacterial flora of healthy humans and animals or the environment.Metagenomics techniques in conjunction with Bioinformatics can quantify thousands of transmissible resistance genes in a single sample without any predetermined genes. Thus prospects of metagenomics as a tool for AMR surveillance in the future are quite bright because of the advantage over traditional tools. The unique advantage of metagenomics isthe direct application on samples from healthy and clinically ill individuals as well as the potential reservoir. This might result in better surveillance of AMR across host species and all reservoirs.

Comprehensive Antibiotic Resistance Database

The Comprehensive Antibiotic Resistance Database (CARD; https://card.mcmaster.ca) is a rigorously curated resource providing reference gene and protein sequences, detection models, and bioinformatics tools on the molecular basis of bacterial antimicrobial resistance (AMR). CARD is used to focus on providing high-quality reference data and molecular sequences within a controlled vocabulary. CARD has also designed the Antibiotic Resistance Ontology (ARO). CARD can help to identifythe trends in AMR mobility as well as in the identification of previously undescribed and resistance variants.

Bioinformatics Tools for the Targeted Drug Design to Combat AMR

Nowadays bioinformatics techniques such as molecular docking have been used to evaluate ligand-protein interaction and also to estimate binding energy during the docking process. This helps in the*in silico*screening of various molecules with respect to the AMR target and shortlisting of molecules for further *in vitro* and *in vivo* studies. Some commonly used software in bioinformatics include; Swiss-model (online software for homology modelling), AutodockVina 1.1.2 (for ligand-protein docking) (Trott & Olson, 2010), AutoDock Tools 1.5.6 (for preparing ligand and protein in .pdbqt format) (Tools, 2016), Avogadro (for ligand energy minimization) and Chimera 1.8.1 (to prepare and view 3D docked complex), DruLiTo 1.0 (for drug-likeness studies) (Prasanth *et al.*, 2020) and Discovery studio (for visualization of docked sites) (Khan & Htar, 2020).

Protein Sequence Databases

The most significant protein sequence databases include; SWISS-PROT (Swiss Protein) Databank(Chou & Elrod,1999), TrEMBL (translation of DNA sequences in EMBL) (Boeckmann, *et al.*, 2003), UniProt (Universal Protein Resource)(UniProt Consortium, 2014), PIR (Protein Information Resource) (Wu *et al.*, 2003)· and wwPDB (worldwide Protein DataBank). The SWISS-PROT represents one of the comprehensive protein sequence databases. The SWISS-PROT provides information on its entries, which have been generated in both experimental as well computational studies. It also provides links to several other data sources such as GenBank, wwPDB, and various other secondary protein databases namely domains, post-translational modifications, species-specific data collections, etc. The protein information in SWISS-PROT mainly concentrates on model organisms and humans. The TrEMBL by contrast provides information on proteins from all organisms[9].Similarly, the PIR is another comprehensive collection of protein sequences. It provides users several attractive features for example to search for a protein molecule via an '*interactive text search*' and to perform various web-based analyses such as sequence alignment, matching of peptide molecules, and peptide mass calculations (Barker *et al.*, 2003). The UniProt is one of the comprehensive collections of protein sequence resources, which are open to free access. The UniProt database emerged by combining SWISS-PROT, PIR, and TrEMBL collections. It provides all sorts of protein information ranging from sequence to function (UniProt Consortium, 2010). The wwPDB has been exclusively designed to archive every single 3D structure of protein molecules to become freely available to the scientific community. The databank now contains over 83,000 experimentally generated structures. The PDB also constantly develops tools for the users to provide better access to the data (Berman et. al., 2007).

Docking and Molecular Interaction Studies

The best-known docking program is DOCK, which can assign ligand sites on the receptor quite reliably. It also evaluates the quality of the fit. Another program GRID uses a 3D grid to find out protein binding sites for ligands. AUTODOCK is another commonly used suit and is perhaps one of the most cited platforms for the prediction of protein-ligand docking studies (http:// autodock. scripps.edu/). It is run and maintained jointly by The Scripps Research Institute (TSRI) and Olson Laboratory. The High Ambiguity Driven protein-protein Docking (HADDOCK) (http://haddock.science. uu.nl/) is another docking approach for the modeling of bio-molecular complexes (de Vries *et al.*, 2010). The massive generation of data has led to the development of various databases to organize and facilitate studies on molecular interactions. The Biomolecular Interaction Network Database (BIND) is one of the largest available information resources that provide access to pairwise molecular interaction and complexes (Bader *et al.*, 2001). Similarly, The Molecular INTeraction Database (MINT) is another database, which stores information of functional interactions of biological molecules (Licata *et al.* 2012). Chimera can be used for visualising the docked sites of target proteins and ligands, but the detailed visualization and comparison of the docked sites of target proteins and ligands are performed by Discovery Studio and Ligplot.

Drug Likeness Calculations

Many tools are available to predict drug-like properties and ADMET (absorption, distribution, metabolism, excretion, and toxicity). For example, the OSIRIS Property Explorer is a web-based tool, which predicts several

ADMET properties including cLogP, solubility, Toxicity, and Overall Drug-Score(Mehmood *et al.*, 2014). The values are displayed in different colors like green for good, red for bad, and yellow for irrelevant. Although it is a very user-friendly platform, however, independent assessment is needed of its quality. Similarly, ChemSilico is a neural net-based prediction method, which calculates ADMET properties. This tool has been validated and trained using over 35,000 tested compounds. The Pre-ADME is another freely available web-based utility that predicts the ADMET properties of a druggable compound. Similarly PASS Online (Prediction of Activity Spectra for Substances) is a Bayesian-based tool that calculates over 4000 different biological activities including pharmacological effects, mutagenicity, mode of action, toxicity, interaction with metabolic enzymes, and transporters, influence on gene expression, and embryotoxicity. PASS can predict with validation of 85%. It is freely available, but the user has to register first. DREADD (designer receptors exclusively activated by designer drugs) is a recent addition in the toolkit of a computational biologist for the identification of druggable targets for both known and orphan GPCRs (G-protein coupled receptors). It also allows one to study the activities of novel drugs as well. Lipinski's filters using DruLiTo 1.0 software are also applied for examining drug-likeness attributes as including quantity of hydrogen acceptors, the quantity of hydrogen donors, molecular weight, and partition coefficient log P.

Molecular Dynamic Simulations

The MDS techniques aim to provide detailed information on the fluctuations, dynamic processes such as ion transport, and small- and large-scale conformational changes of proteins, nucleic acids, and their complexes occurring in biological systems. They also assist the determination of structures from experimental approaches like XRD and NMR spectroscopy. GROMACS (Groningen Machine for Chemical Simulation) software can be used for simulation studies (Spoel *et al.*, 2005).

Conclusions

Ever since the discovery of penicillin many new molecules have been identified to fight the infections. There is a growing use of these molecules in the treatment of infections and challenges are originating due to the excessive clinical use of antibiotics. And several resistance strains have emerged and threatened the effectiveness of most antibiotics.Molecular understanding of bacterial evolution is the key to preventing bacterial resistance. Lately, bioinformatics has played a vital role in drug discovery and Omics studies. Detailed understanding of the mechanisms of bacterial resistance can be gained using precipitate the

Bioinformatics approach to unravel such resistance mystery and design drugs. Hopefully,*in silico* methods will limit bacteria resistance by doing surveillance and possibly lead to annew drugs for treating infections.

Acknowledgment

We thank Dr. Prasanth Survajhala, Senior scientist- Birla Institute of Scientifc Research and Dr Renuka Survajhala, Manipal University Jaipur.

References

ARDB (Antibiotic Resistance Genes Database). https://ardb.cbcb.umd.edu/

Bader, G. D., Donaldson, I., Wolting, C., Ouellette, B. F., Pawson, T., & Hogue, C. W. (2001). BIND—the biomolecular interaction network database. Nucleic Acids Research, 29(1), 242-245.

Barker, W. C., Garavelli, J. S., Huang, H., McGarvey, P. B., Orcutt, B. C., Srinivasarao, G. Y., ... & Wu, C. (2000). The protein information resource (PIR). Nucleic Acids Research, 28(1), 41-44.

Berman, H., Henrick, K., Nakamura, H., & Markley, J. L. (2007). The worldwide Protein Data Bank (wwPDB): ensuring a single, uniform archive of PDB data. Nucleic Acids Research, 35(suppl_1), D301-D303.

Boeckmann, B., Bairoch, A., Apweiler, R., Blatter, M. C., Estreicher, A., Gasteiger, E., ... & Schneider, M. (2003). The SWISS-PROT protein knowledgebase and its supplement TrEMBL in 2003. Nucleic Acids Research, 31(1), 365-370.

Chou, K. C., & Elrod, D. W. (1999). Protein subcellular location prediction. Protein Engineering, 12(2), 107-118.

de Vries, S. J., Van Dijk, M., &Bonvin, A. M. (2010). The HADDOCK web server for data-driven biomolecular docking. Nature Protocols, 5(5), 883.

Khan, S. U., &Htar, T. T. (2020). Deciphering the binding mechanism of Dexamethasone against SARS-CoV-2 main protease: computational molecular modelling approach. ChemRxivorg, 10.

Licata, L., Briganti, L., Peluso, D., Perfetto, L., Iannuccelli, M., Galeota, E., ... &Cesareni, G. (2012). MINT, the molecular interaction database: 2012 update. Nucleic Acids Research, 40(D1), D857-D861.

Mehmood, M. A., Sehar, U., & Ahmad, N. (2014). Use of bioinformatics tools in different spheres of life sciences. Journal of Data Mining in Genomics & Proteomics, 5(2), 1.

Prasanth, D. S. N. B. K., Murahari, M., Chandramohan, V., Panda, S. P., Atmakuri, L. R., & Guntupalli, C. (2020). In silico identification of potential inhibitors from Cinnamon against main protease and spike glycoprotein of SARS CoV-2. Journal of Biomolecular Structure and Dynamics, 1-15.

Spoel, D., Lindahl, E., Hess, B., Groenhof, G., Mark, A. E., & Berendsen, H. J. (2005). GROMACS: fast, flexible, and free. Journal of computational chemistry, 26(16), 1701-1718.

The Global Risks Report 2020, World Economic Forum. https://www.weforum.org/reports/the-global-risks-report-2020

Tools, A. (2016). 1.5. 6 (ADT)/MGL Tools 1.5. 6, The Scripps Research Institute, CA, USA, 2012.

Trott, O., & Olson, A. J. (2010). AutoDockVina: improving the speed and accuracy of docking with a new scoring function, efficient optimization, and multithreading. Journal of computational chemistry, 31(2), 455-461.

UN Interagency Coordination Group (IACG) on Antimicrobial Resistance Report 2019. https://www.who.int/antimicrobial-resistance/interagency-coordination-group/en/

UniProt Consortium (2010) The Universal Protein Resource (UniProt) in 2010. Nucleic Acids Research, 38: D142-148.

UniProt Consortium (2014), Activities at the Universal Protein Resource (UniProt). Nucleic Acids Research, 42: D191-198.

Wu, C. H., Yeh, L. S. L., Huang, H., Arminski, L., Castro-Alvear, J., Chen, Y., ... & Barker, W. C. (2003). The protein information resource. Nucleic Acids Research, 31(1), 345-347.

14

Genomic Insights into Antimicrobial Resistance: Leveraging Next-Generation Sequencing for Comprehensive Identification and Characterization

Malyaj R Prajapati, Mrinal Srivastava, Aakansha Manav, Surendra Upadhayay, Amit Kumar, Jitender Singh and Ravindra Kumar

College of Biotechnology, Sardar Vallabhbhai Patel University of Agriculture and Technology, Meerut, Uttar Pradesh, India

Abstract

Recent advancements in cost-effective nucleic acid sequencing technologies have revolutionized diagnostic microbiology and microbial surveillance, supported by increased accessibility to bioinformatics software and online resources. Over 40 publicly available bioinformatics tools have been developed for the identification of Antimicrobial Resistance (AMR) determinants in nucleic acid and protein sequences. These tools vary in parameters such as accepted input data types, the presence of search software within AMR determinant databases, and the search approach (mapping or alignment), resulting in distinct advantages and limitations for each method in terms of specificity and sensitivity.The European Nucleotide Archive (ENA) facilitates progress by providing online submission platforms for sequencing and supplementary phenotypic antimicrobial susceptibility data. This enables researchers to analyze, enhance, and test new methods, contributing to the ongoing refinement of AMR identification. Whole Genome Sequencing (WGS) advancements play a crucial role in real-time AMR determinant detection, informing the development of prevention and management strategies against the escalating threat of AMR. Integration of open-source tools and WGS is extending global genomics-based pathogen surveillance and AMR monitoring. However, challenges persist, necessitating the optimization of pipelines and databases, and improvements in phenotypic predictions on datasets. Addressing these issues will enhance the reliability and effectiveness of genomics-driven approaches in the ongoing battle against Antimicrobial Resistance.

Keywords: *AMR; WGS; Bioinformatics tools; NCBI; ENA*

Introduction

The study of infectious diseases, alongside other clinical and natural strengths, is going through fast change introduced on by the approach of reasonable next generation sequencing (NGS) advancements (Koser *et al.*, 2012).These technologies become adopted as routine methods easily, and laboratory techniques are transformed throughout the process. The amount of genomic bacterial data generated is huge. As of this writing, for example, over 200,000 *Salmonella* genomes alone are in the public domain with hundreds being added weekly. A whole genomic DNA sequence characterizes the maximum practicable level of structural detail on the individuating traits of an microbial organism or population. It can therefore be used to provide more accurate microbial genome recognition, evolutionary relations and a detailed catalogue of epidemiologically important characteristics. This has a significant role to play for outbreak research, diagnosis and treatment of infectious diseases, microbiology and epidemiology (Allard *et al.*, 2019). Besides, DNA sequences are also a universal dataset which can theoretically be used to determine any biological function. This means that antimicrobial resistant (AMR) can be detected and to track the development and spread of AMR bacteria in a hospital or the community.

AMR is a worldwide health problem, which causes tens of thousands of deaths annually (O'Neill, 2016). Previously, AMR is detected as a measure of the inhibitory growth effects of a chemotherapeutic agent in a particular laboratory culture population. Despite various additional changes, clinical laboratories have depended on methods of diffusion and dilution to direct clinical care and track AMR over time. The data collected show that the AMR from the genomic sequence for many bacteria can be accurately predicted. The NGS based approach to AMR detection involves robust bioinformatics tools to analyze and visualize the microbial AMR genes and their precursors (Catwright *et al.*, 2013).

In this chapter performed a research literature review and offer open-source tools for antimicrobial resistance (AMR) resources and databases and provide potential perspectives and recommendations.

Sequencing Platform

Ever since the first report of a complete bacterial genome sequence in 1995 (Fleischmann *et al.*, 1995), sequencing technologies have rapidly improved. Second-generation sequencing platforms allow whole bacterial genomes to be sequenced within hours, while third-generation sequencing platforms, that provide longer reads and additional information, such as methylation sites, with even higher speed have been developed (Land *et al.*, 2015). This review assesses the performance of popular sequencing platforms as well as emerging state-of-the art technologies that were available at the time of writing of this review.

Illumina

DNA amplification is by bridge PCR style (Fedurco *et al.*, 2006). This sequencing method works by using the principle of the reversible dye-terminators and polymerases, Clonal amplification of DNA on a surface is involved (Bentley *et al.*, 2002). To form local clonal DNA colonies. DNA fragments and primers are connected to a flow cell and enhanced with a polymerase. The dye is chemically extracted, along with the terminal 3' blocker, facilitating the subsequent cycle. Four kinds of reversible terminator bases (RT-bases) are inserted, and non-incorporated nucleotide sequences are been washed to decide a sequence A digital camera captures pictures of the fluorescent-labeled nucleotides. By inserting each nucleotide one after the other, DNA chains are extended, but then the photo can be captured at a later stage. The limitation of Illumina is not deleting a nucleotide blocker after signal detection, this then hinders the bonding of a fresh nucleotide to the DNA fragment in the next step (Fedurco *et al.*, 2006).The recently released NovaSeq 6000 system can deliver 20 billion reads per run with a maximum paired read length of 150 bp.

SOLiD

Originally released in 2007 by Applied Biosystems, which became Life Technologies after merging with Invitrogen in 2008 and now Thermo Fisher Scientific after its acquisition in 2014), this system utilizes a sequence by ligation method using DNA ligase. Repeated cycles of ligation of fluorescent labeled probes, washing of nonligated probes, and imaging ultimately determines the nucleotide sequence with each base read twice (Rothberg *et al.*, 2011). The technology provides the second highest throughput after Illumina but only accommodates 75 bp as the longest read length (100 bp for paired end read) and without any updated models since the release of 5500xl W instrument in 2013, which is capable of delivering up to 6 billion reads per run.

Ion Torrent

This technology bears similarities to the Roche 454 pyrosequencing platform in that amplification of an adaptor-ligated fragment is performed on a bead using emulsion PCR. In addition, the sequence by synthesis reaction is done on each bead-containing microwell to determine the sequence. Unlike pyrosequencing, base determination is made by measuring pH changes, resulting from the release of hydrogen ions during base incorporation. These pH changes are converted into a voltage signal, the amplitude of which is proportional to the number of bases added sequentially in each cycle. The Ion PGM 314, 316, 318, and S5 instruments can generate 400-bp read length. Currently, the Proton 1, the latest instrument, produces the highest throughput (up to 80 million reads) but still is lower than that output of Illumina and SOLiD systems.

Web server for *in silico* Detection of AMR

The high degree of agreement between both the phenotype as well as genotype correlates with the advancement of new and updated versions of the bioinformatics software. AMR, and the development of well-cured AMR gene databases. In principle, *In silico* AMR detection method based on search algorithm to query input genome sequence data for the existence of a pre-determined group of AMR determinants in the AMR reference databases. (Fig 1).

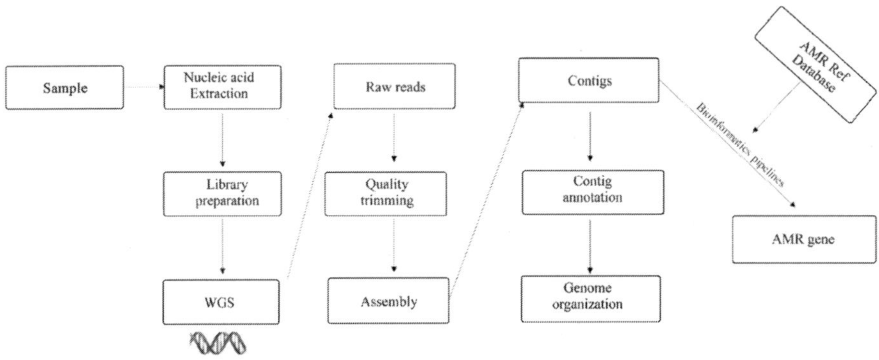

Fig. 1: Workflow for of *in silico* AMR determinant detection

This can be obtained using proprietary programmes provided by private companies or open-access systems comprising different levels of user expertise. Open-access systems are available at public genome data centers such as the Center for Genomic Epidemiology (CGE) http://www.genomicepidemiology.org/online or downloadable for local install from GitHub (https://github.com/), bitbucket(https://bitbucket.org/account/user/genomicepidemiology/projects/DB) and similar.

Several bioinformatics tools can process genome sequence data either as sequencing reads or as assembled sequences (Boolchandani*et al.*, 2019). Generally, the available resources cannot provide quality control of input sequence data, so it is the responsibility of users to ensure the quality of the submitted sequences or assemblies. While using assembly-based approaches, variations between assemblers can compromise the comparability of the result (Alcock *et al.*, 2020). After assembly, most common methods to comparing input data with AMR reference databases dependent on BLAST and Hidden Markov Model searches, among others. BLAST-based methods can provide various outputs based on the default settings for length of gene and percentage sequence identity. This can adversely affect the precision if the settings are too low or too high. In addition, assembly-based approaches are computationally challenging. Despite these limitations, assembly-based approaches could also have additional value in the context of AMR monitoring as they enabled the molecular context of AMR genes to be analyzed, along with their mobilizable potential. Read-based approaches may use various method to align sequencing reads to AMR reference databases, including BWA, Bowtie2, and KMA (Boolchandani*et al.*, 2019). KMA (k-mer alignment) has recently been developed to map raw sequencing readings directly against redundant AMR reference databases (Alcock *et al.*, 2020). The KMA tool was designed specifically for rapid and precise analysis of the bacterial genome as opposed to other mapping approaches, such as BWA, which were established for a large reference genome, such as the human genome, and subsequently applied empirically to microbiology (Clausen *et al.*, 2018). KMA uses the k-mer seeding for speed-up mapping and the Needleman-Wunsch algorithm to precisely align k-mer seed extensions. Multi-mapping readings are overcome using a novel filtering method (ConClave scheme) to ensure correct distribution of templates (Alcock *et al.*, 2020). Read-based approaches allow the identification of AMR genes present in low abundance, which may be skipped if the assemblies are incomplete (Boolchandani*et al.*, 2019).

Independent of the bioinformatics approach preferred, the efficiency of *in silico*AMR is significantly dependent on the availability of reference AMR databases.AMR reference databases may be subdivided into specialized solutions for the identification of resistance to particular antimicrobials and/ or bacterial species or solutions for the detection of virtually every potential AMR determinant in any DNA/amino acid sequence.In addition to their target area, reference AMR databases have significant variations that users need to identify in order to choose the best fit-for-use database.First, the AMR reference databases vary on the requirements for the inclusion of submissions. For example, CARD submissions must have been cited in scientific literature (Alcock *et al.*, 2020). In ResFinder,citation is not a strict necessary (Bortolaia *et al.*, 2020). Genes must have a GenBank accession number and an expert review of NCBI GenBank submissions. Further, the types of submissions vary across databases, with many other databases containing AMR genes and just a few databases, including chromosome gene mutations mediating

AMR. Finally, several available reference AMR databases vary in terms of the format of the submissions (fasta, json, etc.), the ability to download, and the accessibility and frequency of the analysis.

At present, more 50 online tools available in public domain for the prediction *in silico* AMR are documented in the research literature (Zankari *et al.*, 2017). They range from basic reference AMR databases that must be installed in the user's existing bioinformatics pipeline to systems that provide a well-cured database with advanced search tools. These bioinformatics tools provide interfaces of varying complexity that involve different skills in bioinformatics and microbiology to perform sequence analysis and to interpret the results (Table 1). As the characteristics of these tools vary widely, the results obtained from various tools may not be entirely comparable. In addition, using the same method with various input formats of same data (e.g. raw reads vs. assembled sequences, trimmed vs. non-trimmed reads; assemblies generated by different tools, etc.) can different results (McDermott *et al*.,, 2016). A robust genomic approach to the testing of AMR gene content involves precise curated reference databases that should be aligned and harmonized to provide comparable outputs globally. Once it is completed, the bioinformatics analysis approach can undeniably lead to a significant change in the way we perform AMR analysis and compare findings worldwide. Importantly, currently available bioinformatics tools can detect new gene variants, but they are not presently equipped to detect new AMR genes. The identification of novel resistance elements from genomic data is pursued using iterative kmer-based algorithms as well as other machine learning techniques, but these approaches also involve well-characterized reference genomes with phenotypic training dataset (Eyre *et al.*, 2017; Nguyen *et al.*, 2018 & 2019; Myllykangas *et al.*, 2012; Rothberg *et al.*, 2011).

Table 1: Open-source tools for *in silico* antimicrobial resistance detection in bacteria [30].

Resource Name	**Description**	**Link**
CARD (Comprehensive Antibiotic Resistance Database)	A database that provides information on antibiotic resistance genes, their functions, and associated phenotypes.	card.mcmaster.ca
ResFinder	A web-based tool that identifies acquired antimicrobial resistance genes in whole-genome sequencing data.	cge.cbs.dtu.dk/services/ResFinder
ARG-ANNOT	A tool for the annotation of antibiotic resistance genes from sequencing data.	arg-annot.genouest.org
AMR Finder Plus	A tool that detects antimicrobial resistance genes in bacterial genomes using a database of known genes.	ncbi.nlm.nih.gov/pathogens/antimicrobial-resistance/AMRFinder
KmerFinder	A tool that uses k-mer based approaches to identify antimicrobial resistance genes in sequencing data.	cge.cbs.dtu.dk/services/KmerFinder
BacMet	A database that contains information about the genomic determinants of bacterial metal and antibiotic resistance.	bacmet.biomedicine.wisc.edu
GenBank	An extensive database of nucleotide sequences that can be searched for specific antimicrobial resistance genes.	ncbi.nlm.nih.gov/genbank
PATRIC (Pathosystems Resource Integration Center)	A comprehensive resource for bacterial genomes, including tools for analyzing antimicrobial resistance.	patricbrc.org
SRA (Sequence Read Archive)	A repository for raw sequencing data which can be analyzed for antimicrobial resistance.	ncbi.nlm.nih.gov/sra
MentaLiST	A tool that predicts antimicrobial resistance based on sequence data.	mentalist.mpi-inf.mpg.de
AMRscan	A web server for the prediction of antimicrobial resistance based on genomic data.	amrscan.tau.ac.il
EPI-SEQ	A database focused on epidemiological data and antimicrobial resistance gene profiles.	epi-seq.org
CGE (Center for Genomic Epidemiology)	Provides various tools for analyzing genomic data related to antimicrobial resistance and virulence.	cge.cbs.dtu.dk
MyDbFinder	A tool that identifies antimicrobial resistance genes in metagenomic data.	mydbfinder.org
DeepARG	A deep learning-based tool for predicting antibiotic resistance genes from sequences.	deeparg.csail.mit.edu

Resource Name	Description	Link
ABRicate	A command-line tool for running antimicrobial resistance gene searches against various databases.	github.com/tseemann/abricate
Pathogenwatch	A platform for tracking pathogen genomes, including antimicrobial resistance profiles.	pathogenwatch.org
ResistomeDB	A database containing information on resistance genes found in microbial communities.	resistomedb.uw.edu
Bacterial Antimicrobial Resistance Genes Database (BARG)	A database that catalogs known antimicrobial resistance genes in bacteria.	bargdb.org
SnpEff	A tool for annotating and predicting the effects of variants on genes, including resistance genes.	snpeff.sourceforge.net
GlycoPseu	A database for analyzing the glycan composition and related resistance in pseudomonads.	glycopseudomonas.org
AMRdb	A curated database of antimicrobial resistance genes with comprehensive annotations.	amrdb.org
Virulence Factor Database (VFDB)	A database that includes information on virulence factors and their association with antimicrobial resistance.	vfdb.org
Bacterial Genomes Database (BGD)	A resource for accessing and analyzing complete bacterial genome sequences, including resistance genes.	bgd.mun.ca
Antibiotic Resistance Database (ARDB)	A database that catalogs known antibiotic resistance genes and their associated mechanisms.	ardb.tcd.ie
RAPID	A tool for rapid identification of antimicrobial resistance genes from metagenomic data.	rapid-tool.org
KmerDB	A k-mer based database for analyzing sequences and predicting antimicrobial resistance.	kmerdb.org
UniProt	A comprehensive protein sequence database that includes annotations for antimicrobial resistance proteins.	uniprot.org
Pathogen Genome Database (PGD)	A database dedicated to pathogenic microbes, providing insights into resistance mechanisms.	pgd.mpi-bremen.de
TAXONOMY	NCBI Taxonomy database that can be used to explore microbial taxonomy and resistance profiles.	ncbi.nlm.nih.gov/taxonomy

Resource Name	Description	Link
RAPID-AR	A web server for rapid identification of antibiotic resistance genes using high-throughput sequencing data.	rapid-ar.com
Genome Detective	A tool for analyzing microbial genomes, including identifying resistance genes.	genomedetective.com
Bacterial Antimicrobial Resistance Gene Database (BARDB)	A comprehensive resource for known antimicrobial resistance genes in bacteria.	bardb.com
ResFinder 4.0	An updated version of ResFinder with enhanced features for identifying resistance genes.	cge.cbs.dtu.dk/services/ResFinder
BacGene	A resource for exploring bacterial genomes and their associated resistance mechanisms.	bacgene.org
MRSA Finder	A web tool for identifying methicillin-resistant Staphylococcus aureus and its resistance genes.	cge.cbs.dtu.dk/services/MRSAfinder
AMR Gene Finder	A tool for identifying antimicrobial resistance genes based on sequence alignment.	amrgene.org
NCBI Pathogen Detection	A platform for detecting pathogens and their resistance genes from sequencing data.	ncbi.nlm.nih.gov/pathogens
MetaSub	A project focused on characterizing the microbiome of urban environments, including antimicrobial resistance.	metasub.org
Resistome Analysis	A tool for analyzing and comparing resistomes across different environments or bacterial strains.	resistome.org
MetaARG	A metagenomic database specifically for antimicrobial resistance genes.	metaarg.org
ARGs-OAP	A web-based tool for identifying and analyzing antimicrobial resistance genes in metagenomic datasets.	args-oap.org
ABRicate Web	A web version of the ABRicate tool for finding antimicrobial resistance genes in genomic data.	abricate.web
MycoRes	A resource for identifying antimicrobial resistance in mycobacteria, particularly in clinical isolates.	mycores.org
TIGER (Tool for Identifying Genes in E. coli)	A tool designed for identifying resistance genes in E. coli genomes.	tiger.org
Panres	A database that catalogs pan-genomic resistance genes across different bacterial species.	panres.org

Resource Name	Description	Link
PATRIC Resistance Analysis	Part of PATRIC, this tool focuses specifically on analyzing resistance genes in bacterial genomes.	patricbrc.org
ARFinder	A tool that predicts antimicrobial resistance genes based on nucleotide sequences.	arfinder.org
PathoScope	A tool for metagenomic data analysis, including detection of antimicrobial resistance genes.	pathoscope.org
Microbial Genomics	A resource for genomic data, providing tools for resistance gene detection in microbial genomes.	microbialgenomics.org

Future Perspectives

The significant advantage of employing NGS technologies for detecting and monitoring AMR lies in its potential to align with the One Health Surveillance System, facilitating accurate comparisons across various reservoirs. This extension is not limited to the phenotypic antimicrobial class but extends to the precise genetic mechanisms, offering a more comprehensive understanding of AMR dynamics. The realization of One Health objectives has historically faced challenges due to the high costs associated with evaluating animal and environmental samples using classical methods that focus on metabolic and biochemical characterization. However, as NGS technology becomes more accessible, it is anticipated that metagenomics will gain popularity, enabling the exploration of different microbial communities and their potential roles in resistance ecology.

This shift suggests a transformation of One Health Monitoring into a nucleotide surveillance of microbial communities. With the ability to generate and publish data promptly, the vision of creating a "weather map" for bacterial infections and resistance becomes conceivable. This dynamic approach holds promise for providing real-time insights into the dynamics of AMR, paving the way for more informed and timely intervention strategies across human, animal, and environmental health domains.

Conclusion

The progress in NGSand the utilization of online tools for real-time identification of AMR determinants are pivotal for the development of effective prevention and management strategies against the escalating threat of AMR. The availability of various open-resource tools plays a crucial role in expanding the prediction of AMR determinants, contributing to global pathogen surveillance and genomic-level AMR monitoring.While these advancements showcase promising potential, certain prerequisites for a successful transition must be addressed. This includes the establishment of curated AMR databases to ensure a high degree of concordance between phenotypes and genotypes, the implementation of benchmarking designs, proficiency testing schemes, and the facilitation of options sharing among researchers. Despite these strides, a critical need for standardization in pipelines and databases persists. Additionally, there is a pressing demand for refining phenotypic predictions based on genomic data, which would enhance the reliability and accuracy of AMR identification. By addressing these challenges, the field can further solidify its foundation and contribute substantially to the global efforts aimed at mitigating the consequences of Antimicrobial Resistance.

References

Alcock, B. P., Raphenya, A. R., Lau, T. T., Tsang, K. K., Bouchard, M., Edalatmand, A., ... & McArthur, A. G. (2020). CARD 2020: antibiotic resistome surveillance with the comprehensive antibiotic resistance database. Nucleic acids research, 48(D1), D517-D525.

Allard, M. W., Stevens, E. L., & Brown, E. W. (2019). All for one and one for all: the true potential of whole-genome sequencing. The Lancet. Infectious diseases.

Arango-Argoty, G., Garner, E., Pruden, A., Heath, L. S., Vikesland, P., & Zhang, L. (2018). DeepARG: a deep learning approach for predicting antibiotic resistance genes from metagenomic data. Microbiome, 6(1), 1-15.

Bentley, S. D., Chater, K. F., Cerdeno-Tarraga, A. M., Challis, G. L., Thomson, N. R., James, K. D., ... & Oliver, K. (2002). O= Neil. S., Rabbinowitsch, E., Rajandream, MA, Rutherford, K., Rutter, S., Seeger, K., Saunders, D., Sharp, S., Squares, R., Squares, S., Taylor, K., Warren, T., Wietzorrek, A., Woodward, J., Barrell, BG, Parkhill, J., and Hopwood, DA, 141-147.

Boolchandani, M., D'Souza, A. W., &Dantas, G. (2019). Sequencing-based methods and resources to study antimicrobial resistance. Nature Reviews Genetics, 20(6), 356-370.

Bortolaia, V., Kaas, R. S., Ruppe, E., Roberts, M. C., Schwarz, S., Cattoir, V., ... &Aarestrup, F. M. (2020). ResFinder 4.0 for predictions of phenotypes from genotypes. Journal of Antimicrobial Chemotherapy, 75(12), 3491-3500.

Cartwright, E. J., Patel, M. K., Mbopi-Keou, F. X., Ayers, T., Haenke, B., Wagenaar, B. H., & Quick, R. (2013). Recurrent epidemic cholera with high mortality in Cameroon: persistent challenges 40 years into the seventh pandemic. Epidemiology & Infection, 141(10), 2083-2093.

Clausen, P. T., Aarestrup, F. M., & Lund, O. (2018). Rapid and precise alignment of raw reads against redundant databases with KMA. BMC bioinformatics, 19(1), 1-8.

Clausen, P. T., Zankari, E., Aarestrup, F. M., & Lund, O. (2016). Benchmarking of methods for identification of antimicrobial resistance genes in bacterial whole genome data. Journal of Antimicrobial Chemotherapy, 71(9), 2484-2488.

Clausen, P. T., Zankari, E., Aarestrup, F. M., & Lund, O. (2016). Benchmarking of methods for identification of antimicrobial resistance genes in bacterial whole genome data. Journal of Antimicrobial Chemotherapy, 71(9), 2484-2488.

de Man, T. J., &Limbago, B. M. (2016). SSTAR, a stand-alone easy-to-use antimicrobial resistance gene predictor. MSphere, 1(1).

Eyre, D. W., De Silva, D., Cole, K., Peters, J., Cole, M. J., Grad, Y. H., ... & Paul, J. (2017). WGS to predict antibiotic MICs for Neisseria gonorrhoeae. Journal of Antimicrobial Chemotherapy, 72(7), 1937-1947.

Fedurco, M., Romieu, A., Williams, S., Lawrence, I., &Turcatti, G. (2006). BTA, a novel reagent for DNA attachment on glass and efficient generation of solid-phase amplified DNA colonies. Nucleic acids research, 34(3), e22-e22.

Fleischmann, R. D., Adams, M. D., White, O., Clayton, R. A., Kirkness, E. F., Kerlavage, A. R., & Merrick, J. M. (1995). Whole-genome random sequencing and assembly of Haemophilus influenzae Rd. Science, 269(5223), 496-512.

Gupta, S. K., Padmanabhan, B. R., Diene, S. M., Lopez-Rojas, R., Kempf, M., Landraud, L., &Rolain, J. M. (2014). ARG-ANNOT, a new bioinformatic tool to discover antibiotic resistance genes in bacterial genomes. Antimicrobial agents and chemotherapy, 58(1), 212-220.

Hasman, H., Clausen, P. T., Kaya, H., Hansen, F., Knudsen, J. D., Wang, M., ... &Hammerum, A. M. (2019). LRE-Finder, a Web tool for detection of the 23S rRNA mutations and the optrA, cfr, cfr (B) and poxtA genes encoding linezolid resistance in enterococci from whole-genome sequences. Journal of Antimicrobial Chemotherapy, 74(6), 1473-1476.

Hendriksen, R. S., Bortolaia, V., Tate, H., Tyson, G. H., Aarestrup, F. M., & McDermott, P. F. (2019). Using genomics to track global antimicrobial resistance. Frontiers in public health, 7, 242.

Hunt, M., Mather, A. E., Sánchez-Busó, L., Page, A. J., Parkhill, J., Keane, J. A., & Harris, S. R. (2017). ARIBA: rapid antimicrobial resistance genotyping directly from sequencing reads. Microbial genomics, 3(10).

Inouye, M., Dashnow, H., Raven, L. A., Schultz, M. B., Pope, B. J., Tomita, T., & Holt, K. E. (2014). SRST2: rapid genomic surveillance for public health and hospital microbiology labs. Genome medicine, 6(11), 1-16.

Jia, B., Raphenya, A. R., Alcock, B., Waglechner, N., Guo, P., Tsang, K. K., & McArthur, A. G. (2016). CARD 2017: expansion and model-centric curation of the comprehensive antibiotic resistance database. Nucleic acids research, gkw1004.

Kaya, H., Hasman, H., Larsen, J., Stegger, M., Johannesen, T. B., Allesøe, R. L., & Larsen, A. R. (2018). SCCmecFinder, a web-based tool for typing of staphylococcal cassette chromosome mec in Staphylococcus aureus using whole-genome sequence data. Msphere, 3(1).

Köser, C. U., Holden, M. T., Ellington, M. J., Cartwright, E. J., Brown, N. M., Ogilvy-Stuart, A. L.,& Croucher, N. J. other authors (2012). Rapid whole-genome sequencing for investigation of a neonatal MRSA outbreak N Engl J Med, 366, 2267-227510.

Lakin, S. M., Dean, C., Noyes, N. R., Dettenwanger, A., Ross, A. S., Doster, E., & Boucher, C. (2017). MEGARes: an antimicrobial resistance database for high throughput sequencing. Nucleic acids research, 45(D1), D574-D580.

Land, M., Hauser, L., Jun, S. R., Nookaew, I., Leuze, M. R., Ahn, T. H., ... & Ussery, D. W. (2015). Insights from 20 years of bacterial genome sequencing. Functional & integrative genomics, 15(2), 141-161.

Lanza, V. F., Baquero, F., Martínez, J. L., Ramos-Ruíz, R., González-Zorn, B., Andremont, A.,&Coque, T. M. (2018). In-depth resistome analysis by targeted metagenomics. Microbiome, 6(1), 1-14.

Liu, B., & Pop, M. (2009). ARDB—antibiotic resistance genes database. Nucleic acids research, 37(suppl_1), D443-D447.

McDermott, P. F., Tyson, G. H., Kabera, C., Chen, Y., Li, C., Folster, J. P., & Zhao, S. (2016). Whole-genome sequencing for detecting antimicrobial resistance in nontyphoidal Salmonella. Antimicrobial agents and chemotherapy, 60(9), 5515-5520.

Moura, A., Soares, M., Pereira, C., Leitão, N., Henriques, I., & Correia, A. (2009). INTEGRALL: a database and search engine for integrons, integrases and gene cassettes. Bioinformatics, 25(8), 1096-1098.

Myllykangas, S., Buenrostro, J., & Ji, H. P. (2012). Overview of sequencing technology platforms. In Bioinformatics for high throughput sequencing (pp. 11-25). Springer, New York, NY.

Naas, T., Oueslati, S., Bonnin, R. A., Dabos, M. L., Zavala, A., Dortet, L., &Iorga, B. I. (2017). Beta-lactamase database (BLDB)–structure and function. Journal of enzyme inhibition and medicinal chemistry, 32(1), 917-919.

Nguyen, M., Brettin, T., Long, S. W., Musser, J. M., Olsen, R. J., Olson, R., & Davis, J. J. (2018). Developing an in silico minimum inhibitory concentration panel test for Klebsiella pneumoniae. Scientific reports, 8(1), 1-11.

Nguyen, M., Long, S. W., McDermott, P. F., Olsen, R. J., Olson, R., Stevens, R. L., & Davis, J. J. (2019). Using machine learning to predict antimicrobial MICs and associated genomic features for nontyphoidal Salmonella. Journal of Clinical Microbiology, 57(2).

O'Neill, J. (2016). Tackling drug-resistant infections globally: final report and recommendations.

Pal, C., Bengtsson-Palme, J., Rensing, C., Kristiansson, E., & Larsson, D. J. (2014). BacMet: antibacterial biocide and metal resistance genes database. Nucleic acids research, 42(D1), D737-D743.

Rothberg, J. M., Hinz, W., Rearick, T. M., Schultz, J., Mileski, W., Davey, M., & Bustillo, J. (2011). An integrated semiconductor device enabling non-optical genome sequencing. Nature, 475(7356), 348-352.

Saha, S. B., Uttam, V., & Verma, V. (2015). u-CARE: user-friendly Comprehensive Antibiotic resistance Repository of Escherichia coli. Journal of clinical pathology, 68(8), 648-651.

Van Goethem, M. W., Pierneef, R., Bezuidt, O. K., Van De Peer, Y., Cowan, D. A., &Makhalanyane, T. P. (2018). A reservoir of 'historical'antibiotic resistance genes in remote pristine Antarctic soils. Microbiome, 6(1), 1-12.

Wattam, A. R., Davis, J. J., Assaf, R., Boisvert, S., Brettin, T., Bun, C., & Stevens, R. L. (2017). Improvements to PATRIC, the all-bacterial bioinformatics database and analysis resource center. Nucleic acids research, 45(D1), D535-D542.

Xavier, Basil Britto, Anupam J. Das, Guy Cochrane, Sandra De Ganck, Samir Kumar-Singh, Frank MøllerAarestrup, Herman Goossens, and Surbhi Malhotra-Kumar. "Consolidating and exploring antibiotic resistance gene data resources." Journal of clinical microbiology 54, no. 4 (2016): 851-859.

Yin, X., Jiang, X. T., Chai, B., Li, L., Yang, Y., Cole, J. R., ... & Zhang, T. (2018). ARGs-OAP v2. 0 with an expanded SARG database and Hidden Markov Models for enhancement characterization and quantification of antibiotic resistance genes in environmental metagenomes. Bioinformatics, 34(13), 2263-2270.

Zankari, E., Allesøe, R., Joensen, K. G., Cavaco, L. M., Lund, O., &Aarestrup, F. M. (2017). PointFinder: a novel web tool for WGS-based detection of antimicrobial resistance associated with chromosomal point mutations in bacterial pathogens. Journal of Antimicrobial Chemotherapy, 72(10), 2764-2768.

Zhou, C. E., Smith, J., Lam, M., Zemla, A., Dyer, M. D., & Slezak, T. (2007). MvirDB—a microbial database of protein toxins, virulence factors and antibiotic resistance genes for bio-defence applications. Nucleic acids research, 35(suppl_1), D391-D394.

15

Pharmacological Plausibilities to Overcome Antimicrobial Resistance

***Anu Rahal*[1] *and Amit Kumar*[2]**

[1]*Division of Animal Health, ICAR-Central Institute for Research on Goats (CIRG), Makhdoom, Farah, Mathura, Uttar Pradesh, India*
[2]*Division of Animal Biotechnology, College of Biotechnology, Sardar Vallabhbhai Patel University of Agriculture and Technology (SVPUAT) Meerut, Uttar Pradesh, India*

Abstract

Antimicrobial resistance (AMR) is a one of the major public health crisis recognised globally. Microbial infections find a frequent occurrence in animals and humans, leading to reduced growth rates and fertility, diminished production of meat and milk, occasionally leading to head loss, and are therefore, labelled as a major concern for animal welfare. In the dearth of alternative prophylactic measures, antibiotics remain the principal tool for their management. Once an antibiotic is used rampantly in a host population, resistance against it is inevidently seen in the analogous parasitic population and the hunt for a new antibiotic molecule becomes imperative. Discovery and development of a new antimicrobial drug is a time and cost expensive procedure with limited assurance of success. As a result, the past few decades have witnessed only a very few new classes of antibiotics. If the AMR can be restricted or reverted, the success rate of antimicrobial therapy will be boosted and lot of public health issues be avoided.

Introduction

The epidemiological risk and hazards to global health security posed by AMR has been reiterating in several World Health Assembly (WHA) declarations and has been prioritized under the Global Health Security Agenda (GHSA). The Indian Ministry of Health & Family Welfare (MoHFW) has also identified AMR as one of the top priorities for collaborative work with WHO and the first National Action Plan on AMR has been implemented (2017-2022). India ranked fifth in antibiotic consumption in food producing animals (ruminants, pigs, and poultry) in 2010. Even though there has been a gradual reduction of 3.6% in antibiotic consumption during 2011-2019 (Koya *et al.*, 2022), with mounting incomes and shifting in dietary patterns in favour of the consumption of animal protein, especially for poultry, the veterinary antibiotic utilization is projected to further rise by 312%, elevating India to the fourth rank by 2030 (Van Boeckel *et al.*, 2015). FAO has already reported some of the peak resistance rates among common commensal and environmental bacteria against antibiotics like penicillin, cephalosporins, erythromycin and co-trimazoles in India (INFAAR). Resistance to the broad-spectrum fluoroquinolones and third generation cephalosporin antibiotics is already more than 70% in *Escherichia coli*, *Klebsiella pneumoniae*, and, *Acinetobacter baumannii* and more than 50% in *Pseudomonas aeruginosa*. Even the microbial resistance to carbapenems, the last-resort antibiotics, is extremely high among gram-negative microorganisms (Sumanth *et al.*, 2016). To overcome these incidences, it is impulsive to understand the microbe and drug interaction in host system.

The main cause of AMR is the misuse and overexposure of antibiotics, which often reduces the efficacy of newly discovered antibiotics and their derivatives. The development of AMR is principally based upon the alterations in pharmacokinetic and pharmacodynamic mechanism as regard to the interaction of drug in the microbe. While the pharmacokinetic mechanisms include enzymatic inactivation, changing cell permeability through porin loss or increase in expression of efflux pumps and mechanical protection provided by biofilm formation, the pharmacodynamic means mainly refer to a modification of drug targets. AMR is inevitable and relentless, but the process has been accelerated by the misuse of antibiotics in both humans and animals.

Pharmacokinetic Consideration

All the drug molecules enter the site of action through passive diffusion usually through porins but, being a xenobiotic, they are actively extruded by the cellular defense procedures. For therapeutic success, a minimal therapeutic level of drug needs to be maintained for certain duration of time. By hypothesis, the drug therapy can be made effective if the activity of efflux pumps is reduced or their expression is masked, or else the drugs are redesigned, so that they are no longer suitable substrates for the efflux systems, and thus their clinical efficacy is restored (Kourtesi *et al.*, 2013). Out of the three rational approaches in the direction of confronting drug resistance, reducing the efflux of clinically relevant antibiotics, probably through a potent efflux pump inhibitors or a modulator seems to carry a great prospective.

Efflux pump modulation: All the major efflux pump families- MFS, ABC, SMR, and MATE are widely distributed in Gram-positive and Gram-negative bacteria, while the RND super family is specific to Gram-negative microorganisms. In Gram-positive bacteria, the MFS family is the most relevant efflux pump group, the best studied members of this family being NorA from *Staph. aureus* and PmrA from *Streptococcus pneumoniae* (Lorca *et al.*, 2007; Gill *et al.*, 1999; Ubukata *et al.*, 1989). Efflux pump activity modulators have been clinically proven to either decrease the intrinsic bacterial resistance to antibiotics or quash the resistance acquired in resistant strains, even with multiple target mutations, and also diminish the frequency of emergence of new resistant (mutant) strains (Lomovskaya, 1999). Over expression of efflux pumps in clinically resistant strains has already been observed (DeMarco, 2007). The over expression of efflux pumps can be induced by the antibiotics itself during the course of treatment or by host-produced endogenous molecules (Piddock, 2006a), accounting for the slow development of refractoriness in the course of chronic treatment. The problem gets even more perplexed when the overexpression is induced by unrelated drug molecules and even domestic antimicrobials like disinfectants and household chemicals. In this regard, the interconnectedness of ecosystems, particularly water bodies like rivers and ponds holding high levels of antibiotic-resistant microbial population and their resistance genes also play an overwhelming role in the spread of AMR. *Staphylococcus aureus* exposed to increasing concentrations of ethidium bromide developed higher levels of resistance to fluoroquinolones and biocides compared to the parent strain, and this increase in resistance was related to a several-fold increase in the expression of norA efflux gene, which in turn was due to a deletion in its promoter region (70bp). Omeprazole, a proton pump inhibitor agent used to treat gastroesophageal reflux disease, and its newly synthesized derivative analogues can inhibit norfloxacin transport by NorA (Vidaillac *et al.*, 2007). Interestingly, a single modulator can affect the activity of multiple efflux pumps. Paroxetine, a serotonin reuptake inhibitor, inhibits drug efflux by NorA as well as other non-MFS drug efflux pumps, such as those of the MATE family (Kuroda and Tsuchiya, 2009; Kaatz *et al.*, 2003).

Efflux pump Inhibitors: Several known drug molecules /compounds are substrates and serve as inducer or inhibitor of efflux pumps alongwith new natural and synthetic products being reported (Wright and Sutherland, 2007). Celecoxib alone is not bactericidal but in combination at lower concentrations increases the sensitivity of the bacteria to the antibiotics. These effects of celecoxib are probably due to the inhibition of efflux transporters that are involved in extruding antibiotics out of bacterial cells (Kalle and Rizvi, 2011). Although several drug combinations carry such potential but only a few have been proved and none of these are still clinically available, their use may be useful for increasing the susceptibility of different bacterial species to antibiotics.

Natural efflux pump Inhibitors: Several natural molecules eg. plant alkaloid reserpine, kaempferol rhamnoside, and capsaicin inhibit activity of efflux pump NorA of *Staph aureus* (Kalia *et al.*, 2012; Holler *et al.*, 2012). While reserpine, kaempferol and rhamnoside directly bind to the efflux pump and competitively inhibits its activity during drug/H+antiport (Holler *et al.*, 2012), the capsaicin-mediated inhibition mechanism is unclear. Another MFS multidrug efflux pump, *bmr* is closely related to NorA from *S. aureus* (Neyfakh, 1992). Ethidium bromide efflux through *bmr* was completely abolished by reserpine (Neyfakh *et al.*, 1991). Reserpine is also reported to modulate the activities of two dissimilar MFS-associated chloramphenicol efflux pumps, CmlR1 and CmlR2, from Gram-positive *Streptomyces coelicolor* (Vecchione *et al.*, 2009). Reserpine could also inhibit the drug efflux pump, Lde, which confers resistance to the fluoroquinolones ciprofloxacin and norfloxacin present in Gram-positive pathogen *Listeria monocytogenes* (Godreuil *et al.*, 2003).

Role of P-glycoprotein (P-gp) in drug resistance mechanism: P-gp, one of the key members of the superfamily of the ATP-binding cassette (ABC) efflux proteins, recognizes many antibiotics as its substrate (Van Bambeke *et al.*, 2000, 2003), and could therefore effectively modulate their intracellular concentration and hence their activity. P-gp-mediated efflux of azithromycin partially reduced its cellular accumulation and hence, diminished the antimicrobial activity towards phagocytized *Staphylococcus aureus* (Seral *et al.*, 2003a, b). In humans also, P-gp-mediated export of drugs causes reduced intracellular concentration, resulting in suboptimal dosing. The direct binding of drugs to P-gp has also been demonstrated, although the precise mechanism of transport is still debated. The transport of several anthelmintics (ivermectin, benzimidazoles and imidazothiazole derivatives) by human P-gp has been reported (Nare, B. *et al.*, 1994; Naito *et al.*, 1998; Brayden and Griffin, 2008), suggesting drug efflux to be a key factor in development of resistance in helminths that contain functionally related transport proteins. Chloroquine resistance is attributed to a verapamil-sensitive efflux pump (Peel, 2001), similar to ABC transporter P-glycoproteins of multidrug-resistant human cancer cells. A recent study supports an energy-driven extrusion as the major basis of chloroquine resistance in *P. falciparum*.

Mechanism to intervene drug resistance determinants: Different options exist for inhibiting the activity of AMR determinants, like inhibition of the energy supply required for the activity of efflux pumps: alteration in the membrane potential and inhibition of ATP generation. However, these potential inhibitors may be lethal to the host cells and are consequently of no clinical use (Olivares *et al.*, 2013). The search for bacteria-specific elements which fasten to the energized state of the inner plasma membrane and hence modulate the efflux pump activity as TonB in *P. Aeruginosa,* may be helpful (Zhao *et al.*, 1998).

One of the straight forward approach to inhibit efflux pumps is to prevent their activation by protons, such as in the case of drug/H + antiporters. Since these efflux pumps require protons for potentiation, proton scavenging molecules can effectively block the activity of these efflux pumps.

RND efflux system has a proven role in invasion, adherence and colonization of the host cell. Therefore, the inhibition of RND pumps viz. BRA1080 (a dipeptide in *Brucella suis*), BMEI1742 (a mitochondrial transporter in *Brucella mellitnesis*), and BRA0749-BRA0750 (oligopeptide importer) can both increase the susceptibility to antibiotics and reduce the virulence of bacterial pathogens (Halling *et al.*, 2005). A major obstacle, however, may arise from the fact that multiple efflux manipulation may cause unexpected toxicities due to the variety of their physiological roles.

Conclusion

In regards to AMR, the pharmacokinetic/pharmacodynamic index of antibiotics is a rather hot topic, as wrong therapeutic regimens not only do not allow the desired clinical result but it also promotes the development of resistance, because what fails to kill bacteria fortifies AMR. To overcome AMR, understanding the mechanisms of efflux pump regulation, specifically during disease pathophysiology and drug treatment is inevitable. If the pathogen efflux pumps are selectively inhibited, it will lead to greater intracellular concentrations of the drug in the pathogen and better killing and will overcome the rising problem of drug resistance due to extrusion of therapeutic drugs from their site of action i.e. the pathogen. If the efflux pump of host can be selectively activated, it will reduce the chances of drug accumulation and toxicity in the host. This will also increase the safety of the drug. This understanding will also be helpful for monitoring the scope and extend of resistance and allow development of ideal antimicrobial combinations or synergists with no common mechanisms of resistance, and even, revert the genetic changes involved in resistance to specifically target drug resistant parasites. This arduous work is very challenging to implement, and a huge help can be provided by drug delivery systems that allow delivering antibiotics at the right concentrations, for the right period of time, and also at the right place, as in the case of drug targeting.

References

Brayden, D.J. and Griffin, J. (2008) Avermectin transepithelial transport in MDR1- and MRP-transfected canine kidney monolayers.Vet. Res. Commun.32, 93–106.

DeMarco C.E., Cushing L. A., Frempong-Manso E. et al. (2007). Efflux-related resistance to norfloxacin, dyes, and biocides in bloodstream isolates of Staphylococcus aureus. Antimicrobial Agents and Chemotherapy. 51(9): 3235–3239.

Gill, M.J., Brenwald, N.P. and Wise, R. (1999). Identification of an efflux pump gene, pmrA, associated with fluoroquinolone resistance in Streptococcus pneumoniae. Antimicrob. Agents Chemother. 43: 187–189.

Godreuil, S., Galimand, M., Gerbaud, G., Jacquet, C. and Courvalin, P. (2003). Efflux pump lde is associated with fluoroquinolone resistance in Listeria monocytogenes. Antimicrobial Agents and Chemotherapy. 47(2): 704–708.

Halling, S. M., Peterson-Burch, B. D., Bricker, B. J. et al., (2005). Completion of the genome sequence of Brucella abortus and comparison to the highly similar genomes of Brucella melitensis and Brucella suis. J. Bacteriology. 187 (8): 2715–2726.

Holler, J.G., Christensen, S.B., Slotved, H.C., Rasmussen, H.B., Guzman, A., Olsen, C.E., Petersen, B. and Molgaard, P. (2012). Novel inhibitory activity of the Staphylococcus aureus NorA efflux pump by a kaempferol rhamnoside isolated from Persea lingue Nees. J. Antimicrob. Chemother. 67:1138–1144.

Kaatz, G. W., Moudgal, V. V., Seo S. M. et al. (2003). Phenylpiperidine selective serotonin reuptake inhibitors interfere with multidrug efflux pump activity in Staphylococcus aureus. International Journal of Antimicrobial Agents, 22(3):254–261.

Kalle A. M. and Rizvi. A. (2011). Inhibition of bacterial multidrug resistance by Celecoxib, a Cyclooxygenase-2 Inhibitor. Antimicrobial Agents and Chemotherapy, 55(1):439–442.

Kourtesi, A. Ball, R., Huang, Y. Y. et al. (2013). Microbial efflux systems and inhibitors: approaches to drug discovery and the challenge of clinical implementation. The Open Microbiology Journal,.7:34–52.

Koya, S.F., Ganesh, S., Selvaraj, S., Wirtz, V.J., Galea, S., Rockers, P.C. (2022). Antibiotic consumption in India: Geographical variations and temporal changes between 2011 and 2019. JAC-Antimicrobial Resistance, 4(5):dlac112

Kuroda, T. and Tsuchiya, T. (2009). Multidrug efflux transporters in the MATE family. Biochimica et Biophysica Acta, 1794 (5):763–768.

Lomovskaya, O., Lee, A., Hoshino, K. et al. (1999). Use of a genetic approach to evaluate the consequences of inhibition of efflux pumps in Pseudomonas aeruginosa. Antimicrobial Agents and Chemotherapy. 43: 1340–1346.

Lorca, G.L., Barabote, R.D., Zlotopolski, V., Tran, C., Winnen, B., Hvorup, R.N., Stonestrom, A.J., Nguyen, E., Huang, L.W., Kim, D.S., et al. (2007). Transport capabilities of eleven Gram-positive bacteria: Comparative genomic analyses. Biochim. Biophys. Acta. 1768:1342–1366.

Naito, S. et al. (1998). Development of novel reversal agents, imidazothiazole derivatives, targeting MDR1- and MRP-mediated multidrug resistance. Oncol. Res.10:123–132.

Nare, B. et al. (1994). Benzimidazoles, potent anti-mitotic drugs: substrates for the P-glycoprotein transporter in multidrug-resistant cells. Biochem. Pharmacol.48: 2215–2222.

Neyfakh, A. (1992). The multidrug efflux transporter of Bacillus subtilisis a structural and functional homolog of the Staphylococcus NorA protein. Antimicrobial Agents and Chemotherapy. 36(2): 484–485.

Neyfakh, A.A., Bidnenko, V.E. and LanBoChen, L.B.C. (1991). Efflux-mediated multidrug resistance in Bacillus subtilis: similarities and dissimilarities with the mammalian system. Proceedings of the National Academy of Sciences of the United States of America. 88(11): 4781–4785.

Olivares, J., Bernardini, A., Garcia-Leon, G., Corona, F. and Martinez, J.L. (2013).The intrinsic resistome of bacterial pathogens. Front. Microbiol. 2013:4.

Peel, S.A. (2001). The ABC transporter genes of Plasmodium falciparum and drug resistance. Drug Res. Updates. 4: 66–74.

Piddock, L. (2006). Clinically relevant chromosomally encoded multidrug resistance efflux pumps in bacteria. Clinical Microbiology Review, 19:382–402.

Seral, C., Carryn, S., Tulkens, P. M. and Bambeke, F. V. (2003). Influence of P-glycoprotein and MRP efflux pump inhibitors on the intracellular activity of azithromycin and ciprofloxacin in macrophages infected by Listeria monocytogenes or Staphylococcus aureus. J. Antimicrob. Chemother. 51:1167– 1173.

Seral, C., Michot, J. M., Chanteux, H., Mingeot-Leclercq, M. P., Tulkens, P. M. and Bambeke, F. V. (2003). Influence of P-glycoprotein inhibitors on accumulation of macrolides in J774 murine macrophages. Antimicrob. Agents Chemother.47:1047–1051.

Sumanth, G. et al. (2016). Trends in antibiotic resistance among major bacterial pathogens isolated from blood cultures tested at a large private laboratory network in India, 2008–2014. International Journal of Infectious Diseases. 50 (2016): 75-82.

Ubukata, K., Itoh-Yamashita, N. and Konno, M. (1989). Cloning and expression of the norA gene for fluoroquinolone resistance in Staphylococcus aureus. Antimicrob. Agents Chemother. 33: 1535–1539.

Van Bambeke, F., E. Balzi, and P. M. Tulkens. (2000). Antibiotic efflux pumps. Biochem. Pharmacol.60:457–470.

Van Bambeke, F., J. M. Michot, and P. M. Tulkens. (2003). Antibiotic efflux pumps in eukaryotic cells: occurrence and impact on antibiotic cellular pharmacokinetics, pharmacodynamics and toxicodynamics. J. Antimicrob. Chemother.51:1067–1077.

Van Boeckel, Thomas P., et al. (2015). Global trends in antimicrobial use in food animals. Proceedings of the National Academy of Sciences. 112.18 (2015): 5649-5654.

Vecchione, J. J., Alexander Jr., B. and Sello, J. K. (2009). Two distinct major facilitator superfamily drug efflux pumps mediate chloramphenicol resistance in Streptomyces coelicolor. Antimicrobial Agents and Chemotherapy. 53(11): 4673–4677.

Vidaillac C., Guillon J., Arpin C., et al. (2007). Synthesis of omeprazole analogues and evaluation of these as potential inhibitors of the multidrug efflux pump NorA of Staphylococcus aureus. Antimicrobial Agents and Chemotherapy, 51(3):831–838.

Wright G. D. and Sutherland A. D. (2007). New strategies for combating multidrug-resistant bacteria. Trends in Molecular Medicine, 13(6):260–267.

Zhao, Q.; Li, X.Z.; Mistry, A.; Srikumar, R.; Zhang, L.; Lomovskaya, O.; Poole, K. (1998). Influence of the TonB energy-coupling protein on efflux-mediated multidrug resistance in Pseudomonas aeruginosa. Antimicrob. Agents Chemother. 42:2225–2231.

Zhou, X., Jia, F., Liu, X., Wang, Y. (2012). Total Alkaloids of Sophorea alopecuroides-induced down-regulation of AcrAB-ToLC efflux pump reverses susceptibility to ciprofloxacin in clinical multidrug resistant Escherichia coli isolates. Phytother. Res. 26: 1637–1643.

Index